Respiratory Medicine

Series Editors

Sharon I. S. Rounds
Brown University
Providence, RI, USA

Anne Dixon
University of Vermont, Larner College of Medicine
Burlington, VT, USA

Lynn M. Schnapp
University of Wisconsin - Madison
Madison, WI, USA

More information about this series at http://www.springer.com/series/7665

J. Francis Turner, Jr. • Prasoon Jain
Kazuhiro Yasufuku • Atul C. Mehta

Editors

From Thoracic Surgery to Interventional Pulmonology

A Clinical Guide

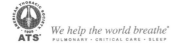

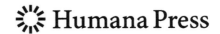

Editors
J. Francis Turner, Jr.
Director of Interventional Pulmonology
Director of Pulmonary Rehabilitation
Pulmonary & Critical Care Medicine
Wyoming Medical Center
Casper, Wyoming
USA

Kazuhiro Yasufuku
Division of Thoracic Surgery
University of Toronto
Toronto, ON
Canada

Prasoon Jain
Pulmonary and Critical Care
Louis A Johnson VA Medical Center
Clarksburg, WV
USA

Atul C. Mehta
Buoncore Family Endowed Chair in Lung
Transplantation, Respiratory Institute
Cleveland Clinic
Cleveland, OH
USA

ISSN 2197-7372   ISSN 2197-7380   (electronic)
Respiratory Medicine
ISBN 978-3-030-80297-4   ISBN 978-3-030-80298-1   (eBook)
https://doi.org/10.1007/978-3-030-80298-1

This Humana imprint is published by the registered company Springer Nature Switzerland AG
The registered company address is: Gewerbestrasse 11, 6330 Cham, Switzerland

We humbly dedicate this book to Professor Dr. Ko-Pen Wang. A pioneer in the art and science of Bronchoscopy and Interventional Pulmonology and an inspiration to us all.

Preface

We are privileged to introduce this new collaborative work in the field of interventional pulmonology.

From Thoracic Surgery to Interventional Pulmonology: A Paradigm Shift is an exciting alliance between thoracic surgery and interventional pulmonology experts that seeks to outline and discuss options available to practitioners surrounding 15 difficult topics which regularly confront interventional pulmonologists and thoracic surgeons.

As minimally invasive techniques and devices have rapidly advanced owing to technological improvements, the options for treatment of difficult airway, pleural disease, as well as staging and diagnosis of cancer have leapfrogged forward at an amazing pace.

With this advancement, we must ever serve our patients to offer the most efficacious options for their individual needs.

As such, this book offers reviews of specific questions with each chapter written with the collaboration of both an interventional pulmonologist and thoracic surgeon.

With this timely subject matter tailored to some of the most difficult questions in pulmonary medicine and thoracic surgery, we hope the readers will gain insight into the powerful collaboration available between our disciplines for the improved care of our patients.

Casper, Wyoming, USA   J. Francis Turner, Jr.
Clarksburg, WV, USA   Prasoon Jain
Toronto, ON, Canada   Kazuhiro Yasufuku
Cleveland, OH, USA   Atul C. Mehta

Contents

Contributors

Ghulam Abbas, MD, MHCM, FACS Chief, Division of Thoracic & Esophageal Surgery Professor, Dept of Cardiovascular & Thoracic Surgery Medicine, WVU Medicine, Morgantown, WV, USA

Ritesh Agarwal, MD, DM Department of Pulmonary Medicine, Postgraduate Institute of Medical Education and Research (PGIMER), Chandigarh, India

Sameer K. Avasarala, MD Division of Allergy, Pulmonary, and Critical Care, Vanderbilt University Medical Center, Nashville, TN, USA

Jamie L. Bessich, MD Interventional Pulmonology Program, Division of Pulmonary, Sleep and Critical Care Medicine, New York University Grossman School of Medicine, New York, NY, USA

Martina Bonifazi, MD Department of Biomedical Sciences and Public Health, Università Politecnica delle Marche, Ancona, Italy

Pulmonary Diseases Unit, Azienda Ospedali Riuniti, Ancona, Italy

Robert F. Browning Jr., MD, FACP, FCCP, DAABIP Interventional Pulmonology, Pulmonary and Critical Care Medicine Service, Walter Reed National Military Medical Center, Bethesda, MD, USA

Normand R. Caron, MD, PhD Thoracic Surgery, Harry S. Truman Memorial Veterans Hospital, Columbia, MO, USA

Kasia Czarnecka-Kujawa, MD, FRCPC, MPH Division of Respirology, Toronto General Hospital, University Health Network, University of Toronto, Toronto, ON, Canada

Division of Thoracic Surgery, Toronto General Hospital, University Health Network, University of Toronto, Toronto, ON, Canada

Himanshu Deshwal, MD Division of Pulmonary, Sleep and Critical Care Medicine, New York University Grossman School of Medicine, New York, NY, USA

Sahajal Dhooria, MD, DM Department of Pulmonary Medicine, Postgraduate Institute of Medical Education and Research (PGIMER), Chandigarh, India

Rajeev Dhupar, MD, MBA, FACS University of Pittsburgh School of Medicine, Pittsburgh, PA, USA

VAPHS, Pittsburgh, PA, USA

Erik E. Folch, MD, MSc Massachusetts General Hospital, Harvard Medical School, Boston, MA, USA

J. Francis Turner, Jr., MD, FACP, FCCP, FCCM, ATSF Director of Interventional Pulmonology, Director of Pulmonary Rehabilitation, Pulmonary & Critical Care Medicine, Wyoming Medical Center, Casper, Wyoming, USA

Stefano Gasparini, MD Department of Biomedical Sciences and Public Health, Università Politecnica delle Marche, Ancona, Italy

Pulmonary Diseases Unit, Azienda Ospedali Riuniti, Ancona, Italy

Erin A. Gillaspie, MD, MPH Department of Thoracic Surgery, Vanderbilt University Medical Center, Nashville, TN, USA

Rajiv Goyal, MD, MRCP Department of Pulmonary Medicine, Jaipur Golden Hospital, New Delhi and Rajiv Gandhi Cancer Institute, New Delhi, India

David Griffin, MD, FACS Intermountain Medical Center, Murray, UT, USA

Sarah Hadique, MD, FCCP Department of Pulmonary and Critical Care, West Virginia University, Morgantown, WV, USA

Associate Professor, Department of Pulmonary and Critical Care, West Virginia University, Morgantown, WV, USA

Bethany Hampole, MD Department of Thoracic and Cardiovascular Surgery, Loyola University Health System, Maywood, IL, USA

Prasoon Jain, MD, FCCP Pulmonary and Critical Care, Louis A Johnson VA Medical Center, Clarksburg, WV, USA

Jeremy C. Johnson, DO Pulmonary and Critical Care Medicine, Harry S. Truman Memorial Veterans Hospital and University of Missouri, Columbia, MO, USA

Satish Kalanjeri, MD, FCCP, MRCP Pulmonary and Critical Care Medicine, Harry S. Truman Memorial Veterans Hospital and University of Missouri, Columbia, MO, USA

Samuel V. Kemp, MD(Res), MBBS, MRCP National Heart & Lung Institute, Imperial College, London, UK

Nottingham City Hospital, Nottingham, UK

Amie J. Kent, MD Department of Cardiothoracic Surgery, New York University Grossman School of Medicine, New York, NY, USA

Sandeep Khandhar, MD, FACS Virginia Cancer Specialists USON, Inova Fairfax, University of Virginia, Fairfax, VA, USA

Danai Khemasuwan, MD, MBA, FCCP Virginia Commonwealth University Medical Center, Richmond, VA, USA

Hyun S. Kim, MD Massachusetts General Hospital, Harvard Medical School, Boston, MA, USA

Pyng Lee, MD, FCCP, FRCP, PhD Division of Respiratory and Critical Care Medicine, Department of Medicine, National University Hospital, Singapore

Yong Loo Lin Medical School, National University of Singapore, Singapore

Amit K. Mahajan, MD, FCCP, DAABIP Department of Surgery, Inova Schar Cancer Institute, Inova Fairfax Hospital, Falls Church, VA, USA

Fabien Maldonado, MD, FCCP Division of Allergy, Pulmonary, and Critical Care, Vanderbilt University Medical Center, Nashville, TN, USA

Sean McKay, MD, FACP, FCCP, DAABIP Interventional Pulmonology, Pulmonary and Critical Care Medicine Service, Walter Reed National Military Medical Center, Bethesda, MD, USA

Atul C. Mehta, MD, FACP, FCCP Buoncore Family Endowed Chair in Lung Transplantation, Respiratory Institute, Cleveland Clinic, Cleveland, OH, USA

Matthew Middendorf, MD Interventional Pulmonology, Pulmonary and Critical Care Medicine Service, Walter Reed National Military Medical Center, Bethesda, MD, USA

Philip Mullenix, MD, FACS, FCCP Department of Cardiothoracic Surgery, Walter Reed National Military Medical Center, Bethesda, MD, USA

Catherine L. Oberg, MD David Geffen School of Medicine at the University of California in Los Angeles, Los Angeles, CA, USA

Priya P. Patel, MD Department of Surgery, Inova Schar Cancer Institute, Inova Fairfax Hospital, Falls Church, VA, USA

Samaan Rafeq, MD Interventional Pulmonology Program, Division of Pulmonary, Sleep and Critical Care Medicine, New York University Grossman School of Medicine, New York, NY, USA

Armando Sabbatini Thoracic Surgery Unit, Azienda Ospedali Riuniti, Ancona, Italy

Inderpaul Singh Sehgal, MD, DM Department of Pulmonary Medicine, Postgraduate Institute of Medical Education and Research (PGIMER), Chandigarh, India

Pallav L. Shah, MD, MBBS, FRCP Royal Brompton Hospital, London, UK

National Heart & Lung Institute, Imperial College, London, UK

Chelsea and Westminster Hospital NHS Foundation Trust, London, UK

Ankur Sinha, MD Division of Pulmonary and Critical Care Medicine, Maimonides Medical Center, Brooklyn, NY, USA

Maher Tabba, MD, MS, FCCP, FACP Division of Pulmonary and Critical Care and Sleep Medicine, Tufts Medical Center, Boston, MA, USA

Wickii T. Vigneswaran, MD, MBA, FACS Department of Thoracic and Cardiovascular Surgery, Loyola University Health System, Maywood, IL, USA

Tatiana Weinstein, MD Division of Pulmonary, Sleep and Critical Care Medicine, New York University Grossman School of Medicine, New York, NY, USA

Kazuhiro Yasufuku, MD, PhD, FRCSC Division of Thoracic Surgery, Toronto General Hospital, University Health Network, University of Toronto, Toronto, ON, Canada

Chapter 1
Rigid Versus Flexible Bronchoscopy

Sameer K. Avasarala, Erin A. Gillaspie, and Fabien Maldonado

History

Rigid Bronchoscope

Professor Gustav Killian at the Poliklinik of Freiburg University (Germany) is credited with performing the first therapeutic rigid bronchoscopy on March 30, 1897 [1]. An animal bone was extracted from the right bronchus of a 63-year-old farmer [2]. A Mikulicz-Rosenheim rigid esophagoscope with rigid forceps was used for the procedure [1]. It was not the first rigid bronchoscopy Professor Killian had performed, but it was the first with a therapeutic intent [3, 4]. Chevalier Jackson was the first to perform rigid bronchoscopy in the United States [2]. He is widely regarded as an innovator in the field of otorhinolaryngology. It is reported that his clinical practice leads to a decline in the mortality rate of airway foreign body from 98% to 2% [5].

The advent of the flexible bronchoscope (FB) in the 1960s leads to a profound decline in the use of the rigid bronchoscope (RB). The development of the FB is regarded as disruptive technology; the ongoing utility of the RB came into question [6]. However, due to technological advances, the use of the RB saw a resurgence in the late twentieth century. Edwin Boyles is credited with developing the optical telescope with forward and angle viewing. Other key landmarks in the history of rigid bronchoscopy include the use of the carbon dioxide laser by Laforet (1976), the application of neodymium-doped yttrium aluminum garnet

S. K. Avasarala (✉) · F. Maldonado
Division of Allergy, Pulmonary, and Critical Care, Vanderbilt University Medical Center, Nashville, TN, USA

E. A. Gillaspie
Department of Thoracic Surgery, Vanderbilt University Medical Center, Nashville, TN, USA

© The Author(s), under exclusive license to Springer Nature
Switzerland AG 2021
J. F. Turner, Jr. et al. (eds.), *From Thoracic Surgery to Interventional
Pulmonology*, Respiratory Medicine,
https://doi.org/10.1007/978-3-030-80298-1_1

(Nd:YAG) laser by Toty (1981), and endobronchial electrosurgery being performed by Hooper Jackson (1985) [6, 7]. The initial report by Toty et al. described the use of Nd:YAG to treat 164 patients with benign or malignant central airway obstruction [7]. The refinement of the laser photo resection is credited to Jean-François Dumon, who is widely considered the father of interventional pulmonology [8]. In 1990, Jean-François Dumon published his landmark case series (188 prosthesis, 66 patients) which reported the use of the dedicated, silicone tracheobronchial stent [9].

Flexible Bronchoscope

The prototype device now known as the FB was developed in 1964; its creation is credited to Shigeto Ikeda [1]. The initial iteration of a usable instrument contained over 15,000 glass fibers. Later, the Machida bronchoscope incorporated a working channel; it was used to obtain bronchoscopic biopsies using a flexible forceps [10]. The FB continued to undergo refinement, evolving into the ubiquitous device that we currently use across specialties. Over the last three decades, there have been significant technological advances with the design of the FB. Improvements in lighting, image processing, and compatibility with accessories and devices allow the FB to remain an important tool for physicians and surgeons who manipulate the airways. Advancement in stent manufacturing and design has also led to a wider selection of stents that can be placed via a FB [11].

Design

The design of the RB varies significantly from the FB. In general, the FB is a more fragile, technologically advanced piece of equipment. The latest generation provides excellent visualization of the tracheobronchial tree via the use of charge-coupled device (CCD) chips.

Rigid Bronchoscope

Although a RB can be used in a variety of complex procedures, its design is unassuming. In simplicity, it is a straight metallic conduit to the airway. This tube allows airway visualization and provides a channel to pass and manipulate a variety of tools. Rigid bronchoscopes have three main components: barrel, multifunctional head, and an optic with a light source [1]. At present, a handful of companies manufacture rigid bronchoscopes and related equipment: Lymol Medical (Woburn, Massachusetts, USA), KARL STORZ Endoscopy-America (El Segundo, California,

USA), Novatech (La Ciotat, France), and Richard Wolf Medical Instruments (Vernon Hills, Illinois, USA). Although made by different manufacturers, the general structure of the bronchoscope is similar.

Barrel

The barrel of a rigid bronchoscope is a hollow metal tube, with a beveled distal tip. They come in a variety of lengths and color-coded diameters. The outer diameter of rigid barrels ranges from 3 mm to 18 mm. The length of the rigid barrels ranges from 33 to 43 cm. The tracheal barrels are shorter and bronchial barrels have side ventilation ports. When the rigid barrel is engaged in a mainstem, the side ventilation ports allow for contralateral ventilation. The proximal end of the barrel connects to the multifunctional head.

Selecting the appropriate diameter of a barrel is an important consideration. It is predicated on several variables, including the indication and the patient's anatomy. Diameters that are too large may be difficult to pass through the glottis or stenotic airway. Barrels that are too narrow create challenges for adequate ventilation, constrain the use of instruments, or are not useful in dilating an airway. Smaller diameter barrels can be more easily introduced into the mainstem bronchi and bronchus intermedius. However, limitations in the internal diameter may hinder the ability to use multiple tools simultaneously.

Multifunctional Head

The multifunctional head (also referred to as a universal barrel) is an interface which allows rotation and attachment of the barrel to a variety of accessories and the ventilation system. A ventilation circuit is attached via the ventilation port; a closed or open ventilation strategy may be used. Depending on the type of RB that is used, the multifunctional head can be an independent piece which attaches to the barrel or be a unified extension of the barrel itself. There are a variety of instruments that can be introduced through the axial or lateral ports of the RB. These include grasping forceps, large biopsy forceps, suction catheters, laser fibers, or a microdebrider. Additionally, a FB can be passed through the RB to access airways that are beyond the reach of the rigid bronchoscope.

Optics and Light Source

There are several optics and light sources that can be used to illuminate a RB. Like other RB-related equipment, lighting equipment is produced by several manufacturers. The visualization system is comprised of two pieces, an optic (also referred to as a telescope) and a light source. The optic is made from a thin glass rod, which is connected to a proximal light source via fiber-optic cable.

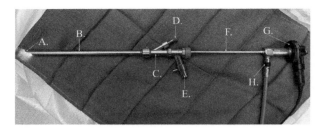

Fig. 1.1 Assembled rigid bronchoscope. Most models of rigid bronchoscopes must be fully assembled for use. A fully assembled rigid bronchoscopy is comprised of several interchangeable pieces: barrel (B) with beveled tip (A), multifunctional head (C), lateral port of multifunctional head (D), adapter for jet ventilation (E), telescope (F), light source (H), and camera (G)

An illuminated optic is typically paired with a camera to allow the endoscopic image to be projected on a display. The traditional way of direct visualization via the eyepiece of the optic is rarely used nowadays. Depending on the video processor unit available at a given institution, there are a variety of adapters that can be used to attach the optic and light source to the monitor.

The assembly of the barrel, multifunctional head, and optic (with light source) allows for the formation of a robust tool that is essential in the armamentarium of airway specialists (Fig. 1.1).

Flexible Bronchoscope

Flexible bronchoscopes have undergone tremendous evolution over the last four decades. Most practitioners currently use a true video bronchoscope, which did not become available until 1987 [1]. It was at that time that a CCD chip was able to be miniaturized and used within an endoscope. Older models used optical fibers as a conduit for image transmission through the insertion tube and handle, to an eyepiece or display [12].

The latest generation of bronchoscopes allows options for magnification, insertion tube rotation, use of narrow band imaging, and up to 210-degree tip angulation [13]. Although specifications vary considerably among manufacturers, the FB is comprised of several key components: cable for light source and imaging processing, control level, suction channel, catheter insertion channel, and the insertion tube. The insertion tube contains important parts that allow the FB to visualize, illuminate, and maneuver (Fig. 1.2). Flexible bronchoscopes with fiber-optic bundles are still used but mostly in the context of hybrid bronchoscopes [1]. In these models, the insertion tube contains the fiber-optic bundle, which transmits images to the CCD chip that is housed in the control head.

The size of the working channel is an important variable in the selection of a FB for a given procedure. Flexible bronchoscopes with a large working channel (2.8 mm) allow for more meaningful suctioning and easier passage of instruments

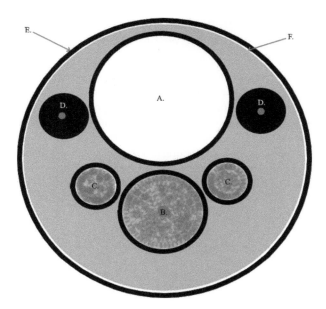

Fig. 1.2 Cross-sectional schematic of the insertion tube of a flexible bronchoscope. The insertion tube of flexible bronchoscope houses several key fragile components. The instrument channel (A) allows for suctioning or passage of tools. The image guide fiber bundle (B) allows for visualization. The light guide fiber bundles (C) allow for illumination. Angulation wires (D) allow for anteflexion and retroflexion of the distal end of the flexible bronchoscope. These components are wrapped in a metal mesh (F), which is surrounded by the external covering of the insertion tube (E)

via the working channel. Although there are tools that can be passed through a 2.0 mm working channel, the applications remain limited. For example, a 1.9 mm cryoprobe can be passed through a 2.0 mm working channel, but the significant amount of friction between the probe and inner walls of the working channel may make it challenging to use.

Contemporary Applications

Rigid bronchoscopy is a procedure that is performed by trained interventional pulmonologists, thoracic surgeons, and otorhinolaryngologists. It has a wide array of applications in the management of both benign and malignant airway diseases. The structure of the barrel provides a large working field within the major airways such as the trachea, mainstem bronchi, and bronchus intermedius. The complementary use of the FB and RB within a single procedure allows access and the ability to intervene on many areas of the tracheobronchial tree. For interventional pulmonologists and thoracic surgeons, both bronchoscopes are invaluable tools in a variety of clinical scenarios: central airway obstruction, tracheobronchial stent management, massive hemoptysis, and airway foreign bodies [14].

Central Airway Obstruction

Historically, 20–30% of patients with primary lung cancer developed central airway obstruction [15]. More contemporary data suggest an incidence around 13% [16]. In addition to malignancy, there are a variety of benign disorders that can compromise central airways: post-tracheostomy tracheal stenosis, post-intubation tracheal stenosis, idiopathic subglottic stenosis, complications of lung transplantation, or complications of inflammatory disorders [17, 18]. The most common cause of benign central airway stenosis is post-intubation traumatic stricture [19]. Anatomically, central airway obstruction can be classified by its extent and type. Extent is determined by the length of involvement; the type may be categorized as extrinsic, intrinsic, or mixed.

It is estimated that management of central airway obstruction accounts for 70% of all rigid bronchoscopies performed [20]. The RB has a variety of advantages in the management of central airway obstruction. The large barrel can be used to secure, core, and dilate the airway. It also acts a passageway for the FB and other endoscopic tools. More recently, the RB has been used as a conduit for application of spray cryotherapy in the management of central airway tumors [21]. The barrel provides a large egress channel for nitrogen to escape, which mitigates the risk of the development of pneumothorax (Fig. 1.3). This risk is present since the gas expands by a factor of several hundred once released from the catheter [22].

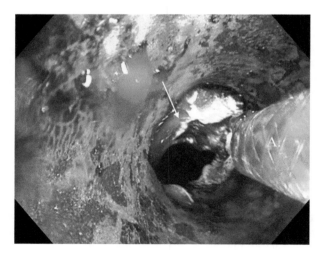

Fig. 1.3 Rigid bronchoscopy with spray cryotherapy. The barrel of the rigid bronchoscope allows for the procurement of a relatively large, secure working field within the airway. This is advantageous in a variety of scenarios. When performing spray cryotherapy, the rigid bronchoscope provides for a large egress channel. This is essential since the liquid nitrogen that exits the distal tip of the cryotherapy catheter (A) expands several hundred-fold while freezing the target (frost highlighted by the white arrow). Without adequate egress, this rapid expansion poses a risk for pneumothorax development secondary to barotrauma

The RB has advantages when performing ablative therapy. It allows the concurrent use of multiple instruments, including a rigid suction catheter. In this scenario, an ablative therapy such as ND:YAG laser can be used to devitalize a tumor while the large bore suction catheter is in place to quickly control any bleeding. Timely use of the RB has important implications for patients with central airway obstruction. In a retrospective study that evaluated 32 patients with central airway obstruction (malignant or benign) requiring an admission to the intensive care unit, emergent rigid bronchoscopy with dilation, laser debulking, or silicone stent insertion led to improvements in clinical status. Twenty (62.5%) patients were able to be immediately transferred to a lower level of care after intervention [23].

Flexible bronchoscopy also has applications in central airway obstruction. When inserted through an endotracheal tube or laryngeal mask airway, it can serve as a useful tool in selected patients with central airway obstruction. Generally, a FB is more readily available than a RB. Of the 1115 therapeutic procedures captured in the AQuIRE Registry, 382 (34%) were performed with a FB [24]. Flexible bronchoscopy has the advantage of being able to be performed under moderate sedation [25]. Most endoscopic ablative tools (electrocautery, argon plasma coagulation, certain lasers, cryoprobe, and spray cryotherapy) can be used through the working channel of a FB. Mechanical debulking using flexible forceps is possible, although it is not as effective as using the dedicated RB debulking forceps [25].

Stent Management

Rigid bronchoscopy is an extremely useful tool in airway stent management. A RB can be used to place, revise, or remove stents [26]. Traditional management of silicone stents requires the use of a RB. Case reports of silicone stents being placed without the use of a RB have been published, but this is not generally recommended [27].

To deploy a silicone stent, a stent of an appropriate size, shape, and length is selected. This stent is folded, lubricated, and loaded into a stent delivery device. The delivery device passed through the barrel of the RB; the handles of the delivery apparatus are manipulated to deploy the stent at its intended site. Large grasping forceps are used to change the stent's position post-deployment (Fig. 1.4). The same forceps can be used to remove a silicone or other type of stent [28].

Self-expanding metallic stents can be deployed via the use of a FB or RB. Depending on the size of the stent, some may even be deployed under direct visualization through the working channel [29–31]. Due to increased maneuverability of the FB, lobar stenting may be achieved [32–34]. Most stents placed via a FB are done via guidewire and the use of fluoroscopy. Stent deployment with the exclusive use of the RB is limited to the trachea, mainstem bronchi, or bronchus intermedius.

The RB is a powerful tool that can be used for the removal of stents [35]. This is particularly important in the management of uncovered metallic stents that have been in the airway for some time, as there is often granulation tissue and scarring

Fig. 1.4 Silicone stent placement. The rigid bronchoscope is an essential tool in the management of silicone tracheobronchial stents. The internal diameter of the barrel provides a conduit for stent delivery, repositioning, or removal. Grasping forceps (A) can be used to manipulate the silicone stent to achieve optimal placement

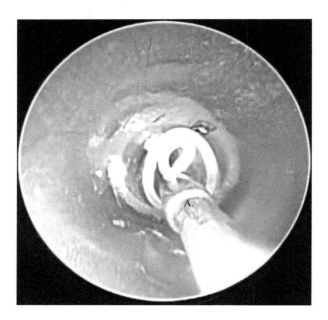

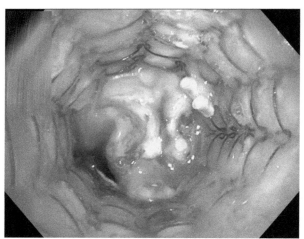

Fig. 1.5 Metallic stent complications. Stent-related complications occur commonly, and they require prompt intervention. Granulation tissue formation is a well-known complication. This endoscopic view showcases a near-complete tracheal obstruction due to an admixture of in-stent granulation tissue and mediastinal tissue. This patient had a metallic tracheal stent in situ for several months, with radiographic evidence of airway dehiscence

[36]. These stents can get completely embedded into the airway [37]. In scenarios such as airway compromise due to granulation tissue overgrowth, hemoptysis due to stent-related complications, or stent-related infections, these stents must be removed (Fig. 1.5). Removal of these stents can be very challenging and can lead to complications as severe as loss of the airway and death. In July of 2005, the US Food and

Drug Administration issued a warning pertaining to the use of covered and uncovered metallic tracheal stents in patients with benign airway disorders [38]. The use of a RB in these situations allows for the securement of a larger, secure working field. Even with the use of the RB, manipulation of these stents and surrounding tissue can cause significant bleeding or the formation of a defect in the airway.

Follow-up surveillance bronchoscopies for post-stent placement monitoring can be easily performed via FB. However, there is no clear data to suggest these bronchoscopies are needed. One study suggest that follow-up surveillance bronchoscopy within 4–6 weeks of stent placement may be useful. It is important to know that only half of the follow-up bronchoscopies in this study were performed exclusively with the use of a FB, the rest were with a RB or a FB in combination with a RB [39]. Another study suggests that routine surveillance bronchoscopy after stent insertion is not an effective practice [40]. Stent-related complications were detected in only nine asymptomatic patients, less than half of which needed a therapeutic intervention.

Massive Hemoptysis

Massive hemoptysis is a medical emergency. It is a life-threatening condition that can lead to severe hypoxia, hemodynamic stability, and death. There is no clear consensus of what volume of blood is considered massive hemoptysis. Common causes include lung cancer, bronchiectasis, and certain pulmonary infections [41]. In clinical practice, a multimodality approach is needed to diagnose and manage massive hemoptysis [42]. The use of chest computed tomography and the FB can help with localization of bleeding and guide intervention [41].

Rigid bronchoscopy can be a useful therapeutic tool in massive hemoptysis. It allows for the securement of the airway with a large working channel in which multiple therapeutic tools can be used simultaneously. In scenarios of unilateral bleeding, the side ventilation ports of the barrel can be used to provide adequate ventilation to non-bleeding lung, while the distal end of the barrel is engaged in and isolating the bleeding lung. In addition to identifying and treating bleeding, techniques via rigid bronchoscopy can be useful to clear the airway after bleeding has ceased. Tools such as the rigid suction catheter and cryoprobe are effective in removing large clots from the major airways.

Both the FB and RB can be used independently or in tandem for managing hemoptysis. Flexible bronchoscopy can identify the source in a majority of cases presenting with massive hemoptysis; however, its diagnostic yield is lower in identifying a source for mild or moderate cases [43]. While the FB is useful for airway examination and localization of bleeding, its interventional scope is limited. Perhaps one of the best uses is in blocking the site of bleeding with a balloon occlusion device [44].

In combination with bronchoscopy, it is essential to identify the underlying cause of bleeding and arrange for concurrent intervention such as radiation therapy or bronchial artery embolism embolization [45, 46].

Foreign Body Removal

Typically, foreign body aspiration occurs in children, the elderly, or adults with neurological or neuromuscular disease [47]. The collection of foreign bodies removed by Chevalier Jackson is on display at the Mütter Museum in Philadelphia, Pennsylvania. This display includes over 2000 objects that were removed during Dr. Jackson's career [8].

Several points of controversy exist when deciding using either a RB or FB for the removal of foreign bodies within the adult airway. A similar debate exists in the gastroenterology literature [48]. In pediatric medicine, many consider foreign body removal via rigid bronchoscopy as the standard of care [49]. This is because the airways of a child are narrower, and there is a higher risk of complete airway obstruction. The RB barrel allows for a secure ventilation route, with a lower chance of complete airway obstruction. In contrast, there is data to support a FB centered approach for the removal of foreign bodies in pediatric airways [50].

When used appropriately, a FB has a high success rate in the removal of inhaled foreign bodies. In most instances, flexible bronchoscopy can be considered an appropriate initial approach for the extraction in adults. Rigid bronchoscopy may be the preferred approach in scenarios presenting with respiratory distress, when extraction is expected to be challenging, or flexible bronchoscopy has already failed [47]. Rigid bronchoscopy is most useful for removal of foreign bodies from the major or proximal airways (trachea, left or right mainstem bronchus, or bronchus intermedius). It has limited application in more distal airways, which is an area in which flexible bronchoscopy can be useful.

Data has shown that foreign body removal with a FB has a high success rate. A retrospective bronchoscopy database has shown that over 90% of foreign bodies were successfully removed with no major complications, using a FB [51]. In general, the use of FB allows for a more thorough examination of the airways. It is also very useful in the clinical scenarios in which the neck cannot be manipulated, which would prevent intubation via a RB [47].

Foreign bodies that could damage the airway (thumbtacks, nails, glass, etc.) need to be removed with extreme caution, often necessitating the use of the protective stainless steel RB barrel or an endotracheal tube [50]. Larger foreign bodies may not be able to be removed using a FB endotracheal tube. These must be removal via the barrel or the RB or be engaged at the distal end of the barrel and removed en bloc with the RB [50].

Contraindications

There is significant overlap in the list of contraindications for flexible and rigid bronchoscopy. A majority of which are relative, and they are summarized in Table 1.1. Severe respiratory failure may preclude safe performance of therapeutic bronchoscopy. In some instances, extracorporeal life support may be used to help facilitate bronchoscopy. At present, related data is limited to case reports [52–54].

Table 1.1 Contraindications for flexible and rigid bronchoscopy

	Flexible bronchoscopy	Rigid bronchoscopy
Absolute	Refractory hypoxemia, hemodynamic instability, lack of informed consent, inexperience of operator, life-threatening arrhythmias	Limited mouth opening, unstable midline facial fractures, obstructions at the larynx, and limitation in cervical spine hyperextension or rotation (caution in patients with rheumatoid arthritis and atlantoaxial subluxation and instability), absolute contraindications for flexible bronchoscopy
Relative	Severe hypoxemia, recent myocardial infarction, coagulopathy, pulmonary hypertension, elevated increased intracranial pressure, pregnancy	High oxygenation requirements with high PEEP needs, relative contraindications for flexible bronchoscopy

Abbreviations
FB Flexible bronchoscope, *RB* Rigid bronchoscope, *Nd:YAG* Neodymium-doped yttrium aluminum garnet, *CCD* Charge-coupled device

There often concerns surrounding the performance of therapeutic bronchoscopy (flexible or rigid) in patients with space-occupying brain lesions. This is not a rare scenario since bronchoscopy is often performed in patients with metastatic cancer. In a study by Grosu et al., 12 patients with space-occupying lesions underwent rigid bronchoscopy with general anesthesia, without complication. Due to a small sample size, the results cannot be generalized. Larger studies are needed to assess the safety of bronchoscopy under general anesthesia in this specific patient population.

Complications

Overall, therapeutic bronchoscopy is a safe procedure. Whether performed with a FB or a RB, the most concerning complication is the development of malignant cardiac arrhythmias secondary to severe hypoxia. Local complications with flexible bronchoscopy are usually related to use of concurrent therapeutic tools: airway tear with balloon dilation, hemorrhage with cryotherapy, or airway fire with hot ablation modalities [55, 56].

With the use of a RB, traumatic complications such as tracheal or bronchial wall rupture may also occur. Less severe complications such as injury to the teeth, gums, or the larynx can often be avoided with a careful intubation technique.

The AQuIRE Registry captured 1115 therapeutic bronchoscopy procedures performed over 15 centers within the United States [24]. Only 44 complications were reported, 24 of which resulted in an adverse event. Six complications resulted in death. Most patients in this registry had primary lung cancer. It is important to note there was significant variation in use of rigid bronchoscopy among the contributing centers. Outcomes related to each modality of bronchoscopy are detailed below.

When performed by appropriately trained individuals, rigid bronchoscopy is a safe procedure. In a prospective study that analyzed 3449 procedures using a RB [57], major complications occurred in 48 procedures; hypoxemic respiratory failure was the most serious complication. Data from the AQuIRE Registry also showed low complication rates among therapeutic procedures performed with a RB ($n = 733$) [24]. The overall complication rate was 3.4% (25 patients); 0.5% (four patients) had a complication that resulted in death. Most patient underwent rigid bronchoscopy as their first therapeutic bronchoscopy ($n = 542$). Of this group, 17.5% (95) died within 30 days. In a retrospective study that analyzed 775 rigid bronchoscopies between 1992 and 1999 at a tertiary care hospital, 103 patients had complications (13.4%), but most were mild [58]. Three deaths occurred; two were due to severe hemorrhage and one due to respiratory failure. An overall procedure-related mortality rate was reported to be 0.4%. Most of the patients in this study had advanced lung cancer. On analysis, risk factors associated with severe complications included patients with underlying respiratory, cardiac, or hematologic disorders and patients with tumors or foreign bodies in their airway. Patients with neoplastic carinal involvement were at the highest risk of developing complications.

In a single-center retrospective study that evaluated 79 therapeutic rigid bronchoscopy procedures, major bleeding occurred in 3.8% of patients and postoperative respiratory failure occurred in 5.1% of patients [59]. The overall 30-day mortality rate was 7.6%. Ninety percent of patients in this study had malignant disease.

The AQuIRE Registry also captured data for therapeutic bronchoscopy performed with a FB ($n = 382$) [24]. A 5% overall complication rate was reported in this group. Less than half of these lead to an adverse event. Complication rate leading to death was also low (0.5%). In summary, a large body of medical literature attests to the safety of therapeutic airway interventions being performed using the RB or FB.

Training and Future

Appropriate training is essential to attaining procedural competency. Bronchoscopy is commonly performed by a variety of specialties (critical care medicine, pulmonology, anesthesiology, general surgery, otorhinolaryngology, and thoracic surgery); flexible bronchoscopy training is highly variable. Metrics used to assess competency and minimum procedural requirement vary by professional organization. The Accreditation Council for Graduate Medical Education Program Requirements for graduate medical education in Pulmonary Disease and Critical Care Medicine states that fellows must perform at least 100 flexible bronchoscopy procedures during their training [60].

The joint American Association of Bronchology and Interventional Pulmonology, Association of Interventional Pulmonary Program Directors, American College of Chest Physicians, American Thoracic Society, and Association of Pulmonary and Critical Care Medicine Program Directors summary addresses the minimum number of therapeutic procedures that must be performed at a given institution for accreditation of an interventional pulmonology fellowship [61]. A recommendation of an annual institutional case volume of 50 rigid bronchoscopies was made.

However, readiness for independent practice is determined by the program director of the interventional pulmonology fellowship. Australia, some European nations, and China have their own forms of formal training or certification [62].

Simulation-based training appears to be beneficial in learning flexible bronchoscopy skills [63–65]. A study by Mallow et al. showed that bronchoscopists with former video game playing experience may have lower airway collision rates [66]. A systemic review and meta-analysis concluded that simulation-based bronchoscopy training is effective [67]. Overall, simulation training was found to be beneficial when compared to no intervention. The differences between training and clinical instruction were not significant [67].

There are no validated metrics to assess therapeutic flexible bronchoscopy skills. There is some literature that speaks to training with a RB. A study among anesthesiologists suggested that the technical skill of rigid bronchoscopy can be acquired within ten repetitions on a manikin [68]. The scoring system RIGID-TASC has been studied to assess the skills of basic rigid bronchoscopy. It is a checklist-based tool that assesses key steps in rigid bronchoscopy, from bronchoscope assembly to bronchoscope guidance and time to procedure completion. Scores can distinguish rigid bronchoscopy skills among novice, intermediate, and expert operators [69].

Although the design of the FB has been undergoing significant evolution, RB design has remained relatively stagnant. Novel robotic rigid bronchoscopy platforms are being evaluated. A study on ex vivo animal models and cadavers has shown that a robotic rigid bronchoscopy platform was able to successfully reduce central airway obstruction and force applied to a patient's head and neck [70].

Conclusions

In summary, the FB and RB work in tandem to successfully manage a variety of airway diseases. The ability to be facile with both tools is an essential skill of any physician who manages complex airway diseases. Both instruments have evolved over the course of the past few decades. The list of accessory equipment that can be paired with either of these bronchoscopes continues to grow. There is significant overlap in their indications; complementary use in the appropriate clinical scenarios can lead to positive outcomes with low complication rates.

References

1. Ernst A, Herth FJF. Principles and practice of interventional pulmonology. 1st ed. New York: Springer New York. Imprint: Springer.; 2013. https://doi.org/10.1007/978-1-4614-4292-9.
2. Alraiyes AH, Machuzak MS. Rigid bronchoscopy. Semin Respir Crit Care Med. 2014;35(6):671–80. https://doi.org/10.1055/s-0034-1395500.
3. Becker HD, Marsh BR. History of the rigid bronchoscope. Basel: Karger, Prog Respir Res; 2000. p. 2–15.
4. Bolliger CT, Mathur PN. Interventional bronchoscopy. Basel/New York: Karger; 2000.

5. Giddings CE, Rimmer J, Weir N. Chevalier Jackson: pioneer and protector of children. J Laryngol Otol. 2013;127(7):638–42. https://doi.org/10.1017/S0022215113001084.
6. Tellis GJ. Disruptive technology or visionary leadership? J Prod Innov Manag. 2006;23(1):34–8.
7. Toty L, Personne C, Colchen A, Vourc'H G. Bronchoscopic management of tracheal lesions using the neodymium yttrium aluminium garnet laser. Thorax. 1981;36(3):175–8. https://doi.org/10.1136/thx.36.3.175.
8. Panchabhai TS, Mehta AC. Historical perspectives of bronchoscopy. Connecting the dots. Ann Am Thorac Soc. 2015;12(5):631–41. https://doi.org/10.1513/annalsats.201502-089ps.
9. Dumon J-F. A dedicated tracheobronchial stent. Chest. 1990;97(2):328–32. https://doi.org/10.1378/chest.97.2.328.
10. Levin DC, Wicks AB, Ellis JH Jr. Transbronchial lung biopsy via the fiberoptic bronchoscope. Am Rev Respir Dis. 1974;110(1):4–12.
11. Avasarala SK, Freitag L, Mehta AC. Metallic endobronchial stents: a contemporary resurrection. Chest. 2019;155(6):1246–59. https://doi.org/10.1016/j.chest.2018.12.001.
12. Hsia DW, Tanner NT, Shamblin C, Mehta HJ, Silvestri GA, Musani AI. The latest generation in flexible bronchoscopes: a description and evaluation. J Bronchol Interv Pulmonol. 2013;20(4):357–62.
13. America O: diagnostic bronchoscope (BF-H190). 2020. https://medical.olympusamerica.com/products/bronchoscope/diagnostic-bronchoscope-bf-h190. Accessed 10/19/2020.
14. Batra H, Yarmus L. Indications and complications of rigid bronchoscopy. Expert Rev Respir Med. 2018;12(6):509–20. https://doi.org/10.1080/17476348.2018.1473037.
15. Ginsberg RJ, Vokes E, Ruben A. In: DeVita VT, Hellman S, Rosenberg SA, editors. Cancer: principles and practice of oncology. 5th ed. Philadelphia: Lippincott-Raven; 1997.
16. Daneshvar C, Falconer WE, Ahmed M, Sibly A, Hindle M, Nicholson TW, et al. Prevalence and outcome of central airway obstruction in patients with lung cancer. BMJ Open Respir Res. 2019;6(1):e000429. https://doi.org/10.1136/bmjresp-2019-000429.
17. Murgu SD, Egressy K, Laxmanan B, Doblare G, Ortiz-Comino R, Hogarth DK. Central airway obstruction: benign strictures, tracheobronchomalacia, and malignancy-related obstruction. Chest. 2016;150(2):426–41. https://doi.org/10.1016/j.chest.2016.02.001.
18. Oberg CL, Holden VK, Channick CL. Benign central airway obstruction. Semin Respir Crit Care Med. 2018;39(6):731–46. https://doi.org/10.1055/s-0038-1676574.
19. Casas DB, Fernández-Bussy S, Folch E, Aldeyturriaga JF, Majid A. Non-malignant central airway obstruction. Arch Bronconeumol (English Edition). 2014;50(8):345–54.
20. Petrella F, Borri A, Casiraghi M, Cavaliere S, Donghi S, Galetta D, et al. Operative rigid bronchoscopy: indications, basic techniques and results. Multimed Man Cardiothorac Surg. 2014;2014:1–6.
21. DiBardino DM, Lanfranco AR, Haas AR. Bronchoscopic cryotherapy. Clinical applications of the cryoprobe, cryospray, and cryoadhesion. Ann Am Thorac Soc. 2016;13(8):1405–15. https://doi.org/10.1513/AnnalsATS.201601-062FR.
22. Browning R, Turner JF Jr, Parrish S. Spray cryotherapy (SCT): institutional evolution of techniques and clinical practice from early experience in the treatment of malignant airway disease. J Thorac Dis. 2015;7:S405–S14.
23. Colt HG, Harrell JH. Therapeutic rigid bronchoscopy allows level of care changes in patients with acute respiratory failure from central airways obstruction. Chest. 1997;112(1):202–6. https://doi.org/10.1378/chest.112.1.202.
24. Ost DE, Ernst A, Grosu HB, Lei X, Diaz-Mendoza J, Slade M, et al. Complications following therapeutic bronchoscopy for malignant central airway obstruction: results of the AQuIRE registry. Chest. 2015;148(2):450–71. https://doi.org/10.1378/chest.14-1530.
25. Shepherd RW, Radchenko C. Bronchoscopic ablation techniques in the management of lung cancer. Ann Transl Med. 2019;7(15):362. https://doi.org/10.21037/atm.2019.04.47.
26. Chin CS, Litle V, Yun J, Weiser T, Swanson SJ. Airway stents. Ann Thorac Surg. 2008;85(2):S792–S6.
27. Gesthalter YB, Seeley EJ. Flexible bronchoscopic deployment of a silicone bronchial stent. J Bronchology Interv Pulmonol. 2020;27(1):e10–e2. https://doi.org/10.1097/LBR.0000000000000635.

28. Corporation© B: Bryan-Dumon™ Series II rigid bronchoscope and stent placement kit user manual. 2008. http://www.lymolmedical.com/images/UserManualBronchSmall8-13.pdf. Accessed 09/17/2020.
29. Thoracent: BONASTENT tracheal/bronchial stent. 2017. https://thoracent.com/tracheal-bronchial-stents. Accessed 09/15/2018.
30. Systems MM. AERO® fully covered tracheobronchial stent. 2018. http://endotek.merit.com/files/docs/401871001_D_Aero_Brochure.pdf. Accessed 09/18/2018.
31. Atrium: atrium iCAST™ balloon expandable covered stent. http://www.atriummed.com/en/interventional/icast.asp. Accessed 09/18/2018.
32. Sethi S, Gildea TR, Almeida FA, Cicenia JC, Machuzak MS. Clinical success stenting distal bronchi for "lobar salvage" in bronchial stenosis. J Bronchol Interv Pulmonol. 2018;25(1):9–16. https://doi.org/10.1097/lbr.0000000000000422.
33. Majid A, Kheir F, Chung J, Alape D, Husta B, Oh S, et al. Covered balloon-expanding stents in airway stenosis. J Bronchology Interv Pulmonol. 2017;24(2):174–7. https://doi.org/10.1097/lbr.0000000000000364.
34. Folch E, Keyes C. Airway stents. Ann Cardiothorac Surg. 2018;7(2):273–83. https://doi.org/10.21037/acs.2018.03.08.
35. Lunn W, Feller-Kopman D, Wahidi M, Ashiku S, Thurer R, Ernst A. Endoscopic removal of metallic airway stents. Chest. 2005;127(6):2106–12.
36. Murthy SC, Gildea TR, Mehta AC. Removal of self-expandable metallic stents: is it possible? Seminars in respiratory and critical care medicine: Copyright© 2004 by Thieme Medical Publishers, Inc., 333 Seventh Avenue, New York, NY 10001; 2004. p. 381–5.
37. Khemasuwan D, Gildea TR, Machuzak MS. Complex metallic stent removal: decade after deployment. J Bronchol Interv Pulmonol. 2014;21(4):358–60. https://doi.org/10.1097/lbr.0000000000000101.
38. Lund ME, Force S. Airway stenting for patients with benign airway disease and the Food and Drug Administration advisory: a call for restraint. Chest. 2007;132(4):1107–8. https://doi.org/10.1378/chest.07-0242.
39. Lee HJ, Labaki W, Yu DH, Salwen B, Gilbert C, Schneider ALC, et al. Airway stent complications: the role of follow-up bronchoscopy as a surveillance method. J Thorac Dis. 2017;9(11):4651–9. https://doi.org/10.21037/jtd.2017.09.139.
40. Matsuo T, Colt HG. Evidence against routine scheduling of surveillance bronchoscopy after stent insertion. Chest. 2000;118(5):1455–9. https://doi.org/10.1378/chest.118.5.1455.
41. Hirshberg B, Biran I, Glazer M, Kramer MR. Hemoptysis: etiology, evaluation, and outcome in a tertiary referral hospital. Chest. 1997;112(2):440–4.
42. Davidson K, Shojaee S. Managing massive hemoptysis. Chest. 2020;157(1):77–88. https://doi.org/10.1016/j.chest.2019.07.012.
43. Sakr L, Dutau H. Massive hemoptysis: an update on the role of bronchoscopy in diagnosis and management. Respiration. 2010;80(1):38–58.
44. Radchenko C, Alraiyes AH, Shojaee S. A systematic approach to the management of massive hemoptysis. J Thorac Dis. 2017;9(Suppl 10):S1069–s86. https://doi.org/10.21037/jtd.2017.06.41.
45. Sopko DR, Smith TP. Bronchial artery embolization for hemoptysis. Semin Intervent Radiol. Thieme Medical Publishers;. 2011;28:48.
46. Langendijk JA, ten Velde GPM, Aaronson NK, de Jong JMA, Muller MJ, Wouters EFM. Quality of life after palliative radiotherapy in non-small cell lung cancer: a prospective study. Int J Radiat Oncol Biol Phys. 2000;47(1):149–55. https://doi.org/10.1016/S0360-3016(99)00540-4.
47. Hewlett JC, Rickman OB, Lentz RJ, Prakash UB, Maldonado F. Foreign body aspiration in adult airways: therapeutic approach. J Thorac Dis. 2017;9(9):3398–409. https://doi.org/10.21037/jtd.2017.06.137.
48. Tseng CC, Hsiao TY, Hsu WC. Comparison of rigid and flexible endoscopy for removing esophageal foreign bodies in an emergency. J Formos Med Assoc/Taiwan yi zhi. 2016;115(8):639–44. https://doi.org/10.1016/j.jfma.2015.05.016.

49. Dikensoy O, Usalan C, Filiz A. Foreign body aspiration: clinical utility of flexible bronchoscopy. Postgrad Med J. 2002;78(921):399–403.
50. Swanson KL. Airway foreign bodies: what's new? Seminars in respiratory and critical care medicine. New York: Thieme Medical Publishers, c1994;; 2004. p. 405–11.
51. Sehgal IS, Dhooria S, Ram B, Singh N, Aggarwal AN, Gupta D, et al. Foreign body inhalation in the adult population: experience of 25,998 bronchoscopies and systematic review of the literature. Respir Care. 2015;60(10):1438–48. https://doi.org/10.4187/respcare.03976.
52. Doyle DJ, Hantzakos AG. Anesthetic management of the narrowed airway. Otolaryngol Clin North Am. 2019;52(6):1127–39. https://doi.org/10.1016/j.otc.2019.08.010.
53. Chacon-Alves S, Perez-Vela JL, Grau-Carmona T, Dominguez-Aguado H, Marin-Mateos H, Renes-Carreno E. Veno-arterial ECMO for rescue of severe airway hemorrhage with rigid bronchoscopy after pulmonary artery thromboendarterectomy. Int J Artif Organs. 2016;39(5):242–4. https://doi.org/10.5301/ijao.5000493.
54. Park AH, Tunkel DE, Park E, Barnhart D, Liu E, Lee J, et al. Management of complicated airway foreign body aspiration using extracorporeal membrane oxygenation (ECMO). Int J Pediatr Otorhinolaryngol. 2014;78(12):2319–21. https://doi.org/10.1016/j.ijporl.2014.10.021.
55. Kim JH, Shin JH, Shim TS, Oh YM, Song HY. Deep tracheal laceration after balloon dilation for benign tracheobronchial stenosis: case reports of two patients. Br J Radiol. 2006;79(942):529–35. https://doi.org/10.1259/bjr/17839516.
56. Salaria ON, Suthar R, Abdelfattah S, Hoyos J. Perioperative management of an airway fire: a case report. A A Pract. 2018;10(1):5–9. https://doi.org/10.1213/xaa.0000000000000620.
57. Lukomsky GI, Ovchinnikov AA, Bilal A. Complications of bronchoscopy: comparison of rigid bronchoscopy under general anesthesia and flexible fiberoptic bronchoscopy under topical anesthesia. Chest. 1981;79(3):316–21. https://doi.org/10.1378/chest.79.3.316.
58. Drummond M, Magalhães A, Hespanhol V, Marques A. Rigid bronchoscopy: complications in a University Hospital. Journal of Bronchology & Interventional Pulmonology. 2003;10(3):177–82.
59. Murgu S, Laxmanan B, Stoy S, Egressy K, Chaddha U, Farooqui F, et al. Evaluation of safety and short-term outcomes of therapeutic rigid bronchoscopy using total intravenous anesthesia and spontaneous assisted ventilation. Respiration. 2020;99(3):239–47. https://doi.org/10.1159/000504679.
60. ACGME: ACGME program requirements for graduate medical education in pulmonary disease and critical care medicine (internal medicine). https://www.upstate.edu/pulmcc/pdf/Pulm.pdf. Accessed 09/19/2020.
61. Mullon JJ, Burkart KM, Silvestri G, Hogarth DK, Almeida F, Berkowitz D, et al. Interventional pulmonology fellowship accreditation standards: executive summary of the Multisociety Interventional Pulmonology Fellowship Accreditation Committee. Chest. 2017;151(5):1114–21. https://doi.org/10.1016/j.chest.2017.01.024.
62. Aslam W, Lee HJ, Lamb CR. Standardizing education in interventional pulmonology in the midst of technological change. J Thorac Dis. 2020;12(6):3331–40. https://doi.org/10.21037/jtd.2020.03.104.
63. Cold KM, Konge L, Clementsen PF, Nayahangan LJ. Simulation-based mastery learning of flexible bronchoscopy: deciding factors for completion. Respiration. 2019;97(2):160–7. https://doi.org/10.1159/000493431.
64. Kennedy CC, Maldonado F, Cook DA. Simulation-based bronchoscopy training: systematic review and meta-analysis. Chest. 2013;144(1):183–92. https://doi.org/10.1378/chest.12-1786.
65. Blum MG, Powers TW, Sundaresan S. Bronchoscopy simulator effectively prepares junior residents to competently perform basic clinical bronchoscopy. Ann Thorac Surg. 2004;78(1):287–91.
66. Mallow C, Shafiq M, Thiboutot J, Yu DH, Batra H, Lunz D, et al. Impact of video game cross-training on learning bronchoscopy. a pilot randomized controlled trial. ATS Scholar. 2020:atsscholar. 2019-0015OC.

67. Kennedy CC, Maldonado F, Cook DA. Simulation-based bronchoscopy training. Chest. 2013;144(1):183–92. https://doi.org/10.1378/chest.12-1786.
68. Royds J, Buckley MA, Campbell MD, Donnelly GM, James MFM, Mhuircheartaigh RN, et al. Achieving proficiency in rigid bronchoscopy-a study in manikins. Ir J Med Sci. 2019;188(3):979–86. https://doi.org/10.1007/s11845-018-1944-5.
69. Mahmood K, Wahidi MM, Osann KE, Coles K, Shofer SL, Volker EE, et al. Development of a tool to assess basic competency in the performance of rigid bronchoscopy. Ann Am Thorac Soc. 2016;13(4):502–11. https://doi.org/10.1513/AnnalsATS.201509-593OC.
70. Gafford JB, Webster S, Dillon N, Blum E, Hendrick R, Maldonado F, et al. A concentric tube robot system for rigid bronchoscopy: a feasibility study on central airway obstruction removal. Ann Biomed Eng. 2020;48(1):181–91. https://doi.org/10.1007/s10439-019-02325-x.

Chapter 2
Biopsy for Diffuse Lung Diseases: Surgical Vs Cryobiopsy

Stefano Gasparini, Martina Bonifazi, and Armando Sabbatini

Introduction

The term "diffuse parenchymal lung diseases (DPLDs)" includes a wide spectrum of heterogeneous entities with different etiologies, prognosis, as well as treatment options. Due to the recent progresses in therapeutic landscape of DPLPs, the distinction between idiopathic pulmonary fibrosis (IPF), the most prevalent and severe form, and other diseases has become essential for a proper management [1]. However, an accurate diagnosis of IPF is a challenging process, as, according to the ATS/ERS guidelines [2], it requires an integrated multidisciplinary approach involving pulmonologists, radiologists, and, in more complex cases, also pathologists. The diagnostic work-up of DPLDs, indeed, includes a thorough clinical history, mainly focused on familial background, environmental/occupational exposure and drug intake, a careful physical examination, lung function tests, high-resolution computed tomography (HRCT), bronchoalveolar lavage, and, in case of still inconclusive results, a lung tissue sample. In this context, the role of conventional transbronchial lung biopsy is limited to the exclusion of specific disorders (i.e., sarcoidosis, carcinomatous lymphangitis, organizing pneumonia), since the small sample size, the rate of crush artifacts, and the high likelihood to sample mostly centrilobular areas do not allow to properly identify more complex and spatially heterogeneous morphological patterns [3].

S. Gasparini (✉) · M. Bonifazi
Department of Biomedical Sciences and Public Health, Università Politecnica delle Marche, Ancona, Italy

Pulmonary Diseases Unit, Azienda Ospedali Riuniti, Ancona, Italy
e-mail: s.gasparini@univpm.it

A. Sabbatini
Thoracic Surgery Unit, Azienda Ospedali Riuniti, Ancona, Italy

© The Author(s), under exclusive license to Springer Nature
Switzerland AG 2021
J. F. Turner, Jr. et al. (eds.), *From Thoracic Surgery to Interventional Pulmonology*, Respiratory Medicine,
https://doi.org/10.1007/978-3-030-80298-1_2

19

Surgical lung biopsy (SLB) is currently considered as the gold standard when lung tissue is required [2], but it is characterized by appreciable costs and risks, with a mortality rate of 2–4% within 90 days [4], even higher in patients with an underlying histological pattern of usual interstitial pneumonia (UIP) [5]. Moreover, many subjects are not eligible because of a combination of advanced stage, aging, and comorbidities.

More recently, a valuable, less invasive, sampling technique for morphologic assessment of DPLDs has been proposed to support clinicians in facing the dilemma between the need of a complete clinical picture and the risks to obtain it: the transbronchial lung cryobiopsy (TBLC) [3]. For instance, recent advances in comprehension of DPLDs pathogenesis have coupled with exciting evolutions in technologies related to tissue sampling, no longer an exclusive domain of thoracic surgeons. The growing amount of data supporting risk-benefit profile of TBLC in this context has led to its routine adoption as alternative tool to obtain lung tissue in selected interventional pulmonology centers worldwide [6].

However, the role of TBLC in the diagnostic work-up of DPLDs has yet to be fully established, as evidence-based data on a direct comparison between SLB and TBLC are still lacking. As a result, nowadays, the choice between the two procedures is mainly based on operator's experience and local resources, rather than on a standardized cost-effective algorithm.

In the present chapter, current evidence on diagnostic impact of these techniques in the multidisciplinary approach to DPLDs will be discussed, mainly focusing on the risk-benefit profile of each procedure separately and when combined in a sequential algorithm.

Surgical Lung Biopsy

SLB, whether it be performed via open thoracotomy (open lung biopsy, OLB) or video-assisted thoracoscopy (VATS), is currently recommended by scientific societies as the gold standard to obtain an exhaustive morphological picture in the context of DPLDs [2]. Independent of the surgical method exploited, the diagnostic yield of the procedure is overall excellent, exceeding 90% in most of studies [4, 7]. In particular, a recent systematic review and meta-analysis of literature, including more than 2000 patients from 23 investigations, documented a median diagnostic yield of 95% (range, 42%–100%), and subgroup analyses did not detect any significant difference according to biopsy site, biopsy number, and the surgical lung biopsy method [4]. Although concerns have been risen on whether or not to sample the lingula and middle lobe, most of studies suggested the use of HRTC as guidance to choose the optimal target, avoiding areas of end-stage fibrotic lung [4, 7].

However, data on safety profile was not entirely reassuring, as the 30- and 90-day mortality rates from the 16 studies included in the pooled analysis were respectively 2.2% (95% confidence interval [CI], 1.0–4.0) and 3.4% (95% CI, 1.8–5.5). The composite postoperative mortality was 3.6% (95% CI, 2.1–5.5), but a significant heterogeneity among individual studies was observed ($I2$, 65.4%; chi-square, 43.35; $P < 0.0001$). To explore potential sources of heterogeneity, a number of subgroup analyses were performed on the basis of eligibility criteria in individual studies, and data suggested that strong predictors of a higher mortality risk included age > 70 years, immunocompromised status, mechanical ventilation dependence, and a severe respiratory impairment (diffusing capacity of the lung for carbon monoxide <35% or forced vital capacity <55% predicted) [4]. Further factors of a worse outcome from literature were male sex and the presence of comorbidities, expressed as a Charlson score ≥3 [8]. Evidence on role of surgical method (OLB vs VATS) appeared more controversial, as studies reported heterogenic results [4, 8]. Overall, a safer profile, in terms of morbidity, mortality, and hospital length of stay, has been suggested with VATS compared to OLB, although the majority of data were derived from observational studies [4, 7, 8]. Of note, in a recent large retrospective record-linkage analysis between national healthcare datasets in England, data on inhospital, 30-day, and 90-day mortality rate in 2820 patients who underwent SLB for the diagnosis of DPLDs over 10 years (1997 to 2008) documented a threefold significant higher risk of death with open surgery compared to VATS (adjusted odds ratio 2.94 [95% CI, 1.41–6.11]). Moreover, based on this retrospective analysis, the mortality risk in patient aged <65 years with no comorbidities was 1.6%, while in older, less healthy subjects, it increased to 4.7% [8].

Interestingly, patients with an underlying usual interstitial pneumonia (UIP) pattern at histology, especially in the context of a final diagnosis of IPF, experienced a higher short-term mortality rate, mainly caused by the onset of acute exacerbation, characterized by diffuse alveolar damage superimposed on chronic background of fibrosing features [5]. For instance, although IPF clinical course is usually characterized by an inexorable chronic progression, some patients may develop, at a certain point, a critical, acute worsening of the disease, known as acute exacerbation (AE), leading to respiratory failure and death in more than half of cases [2]. Multivariate analyses showed that male sex and advanced stage are significantly associated with the risk of AE. SLB has been also identified a trigger of AE onset, occurring usually within 30 days after the procedure, and potential causative factors include an inflammatory response to the invasive approach, stretch injury during single lung ventilation, exposure to high oxygen concentrations, and ischemia-reperfusion [9–12].

To minimize risks related to general anesthesia and one-lung ventilation, awake VATS biopsy has been recently proposed as a safer, alternative method for lung sampling [12, 13]. Awake thoracic surgery has been increasingly adopted in different settings, including the management of pneumothorax, wedge resection, lobectomy, and lung volume reduction procedures, with satisfactory results. Recent data on technical feasibility, safety, and diagnostic yield of awake VATS for the diagnosis of DPLDs, although derived from limited case series, showed an excellent risk-benefit profile, independent of the method exploited for regional anesthesia, either by thoracic epidural anesthesia or intercostal block [12, 13]. In particular, no postoperative mortality nor major morbidity occurred, and the median length of hospital stay, as well as procedure-related costs, was overall lower than those of standard technique [12, 13]. However, due to the lack of direct comparisons, the role of awake VATS, although promising, has yet to be validated in larger cohorts.

SLB may also result in postoperative nonlethal complications, including infections, prolonged air leakage, respiratory failure, and continuing pain complaint at 7–12 months at the biopsy site [9].

Therefore, due to the non-negligible mortality and morbidity burden carried by SLB, risks and benefits of this diagnostic approach should be carefully balanced case-by-case, taking into account factors associated with poorer outcomes and the impact of an accurate diagnosis on management of disease. Moreover, a detailed discussion with the patient is highly recommended. Once the decision of performing SLB has been collectively taken, the choice between surgical methods should be based on surgical expertise, sources, and individual patient characteristics. However, referring patients to the closest center with experience on less invasive uniportal videothoracoscopic approach should be preferred.

Transbronchial Lung Cryobiopsy (TBLC)

The first use of cryotechnology for bronchoscopic procedures dates back to 1977, as therapeutic tool in the context of airway occlusions. The ingenious novelty lies in using a flexible cryoprobe through a flexible bronchoscope to obtain parenchymal lung tissue, as recently proposed in a number of studies worldwide reporting their successful experiences in various populations, including patients with DPLDs, focal opacities, and transplant recipients.

Technical Aspects

Cryotechnology is composed of console, cryogen, and cryoprobe (Figs. 2.1 and 2.2). It operates by the Joule-Thomson effect, according to which a compressed gas released at high flow rapidly expands and creates very low temperature at the tip of the probe, leading to the adjacent adhesion of the tissue. Although nitric oxide may achieve lower temperatures (minus 80°–89°), carbon dioxide is nowadays the most common cooling agent used, as in the majority of countries, a regulatory rule hampers the use of the first one in endoscopic suites. The cryoprobe (Fig. 2.2), available in two different diameters (1.9 mm and 2.4 mm), is inserted through the operating channel of the flexible bronchoscope under fluoroscopic guidance into the periphery of the lung. The procedure may be performed either under deep sedation in spontaneous breathing or jet ventilation in "intubated" patients (endotracheal tube or rigid tracheoscope), or under conscious sedation without airways control. Once the probe has been positioned at 10–20 mm from the pleura, perpendicular to the thoracic wall under fluoroscopy guidance, it is cooled for 3 to 6 seconds (Fig. 2.3). Then, the cryoprobe with the frozen lung tissue attached to the tip is withdrawn together with

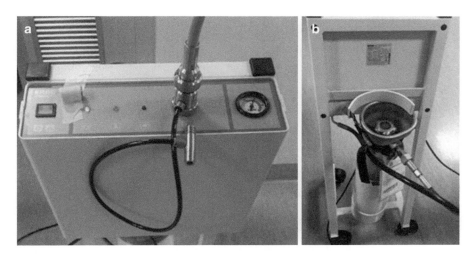

Fig. 2.1 (**a** and **b**) Console (**a**) and gas cylinder (**b**)

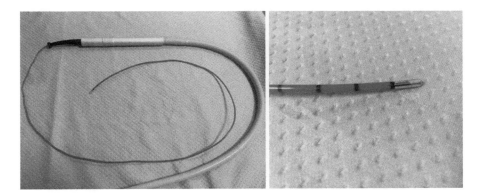

Fig. 2.2 The cryoprobe

the bronchoscope, and samples are thawed in saline and put into formalin. In some centers, a bronchial blocker, such as Fogarty balloon, is prophylactically placed at the entrance of the selected lobar bronchus to minimize potential post-procedural bleedings and inflated immediately after each sampling (Fig. 2.4). The number of biopsies ranges from two to six, and their mean size varies from 11 mm^2 to 157 mm^2, with a mean diameter of around 5–6 mm (Figs. 2.5 and 2.6). From the data published so far, a higher size of probe, a longer activation time, and carrying out the procedure under deep sedation with airways control positively correlate with a larger sample size. The utility of sampling different segments or even different lobes is currently under investigation.

A chest radiograph is performed after the procedure routinely in some centers or only in case of suspected pneumothorax.

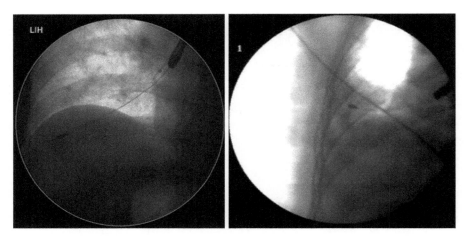

Fig. 2.3 Images obtained under fluoroscopy guidance, showing the probe positioned at 10–20 mm from the pleura, perpendicular to the thoracic wall

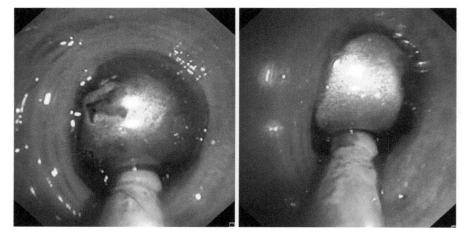

Fig. 2.4 Endoscopic image showing the Fogarty balloon inflated immediately after the sampling to manage post-procedural bleedings

Diagnostic Yield and Safety Profile

The summary estimate of TBLC diagnostic yield (DY) from meta-analyses of studies was overall around 80% [14–17], regardless of the criteria used for defining diagnostic samples (that were either the identification of a specified histological pattern or the final multidisciplinary diagnosis). In detail, the pooled estimates by diagnostic definitions were 0.83 (CI 0.64–0.97, I^2 90.20%, $p < 0.001$) from studies considering multidisciplinary discussion as the final diagnosis (3 studies including

Fig. 2.5 Image showing
the size of cryobiopsy
samples

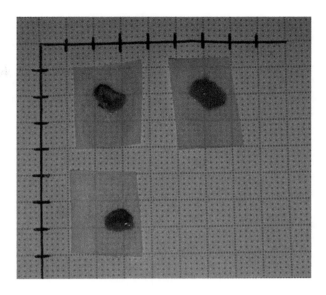

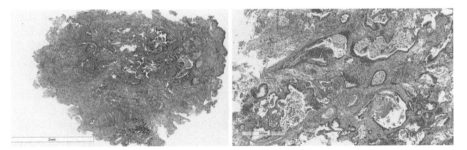

Fig. 2.6 Tissue sections from cryobiopsy showing chronic fibrosis and microhoneycombing

312 patients), 0.80 (0.72–0.87, I^2 68.10%, $p < 0.001$) from studies referring to the detection of specific histological patterns (8 studies including 564 patients), and 0.90 (0.76–0.99, I^2 95.40%, $p < 0.001$) from the two studies that did not specify the diagnostic criteria. The pooled DY by procedural aspects, in terms of type of sedation and airways control, were 0.81 (CI 0.76–0.86) from studies with patients undergoing the procedure intubated under deep sedation (11 studies including 625 patients) and 0.83 (CI 0.64–0.97) from studies with patients not intubated under conscious sedation (3 studies including 142 patients) [14].

Overall, the safety profile was characterized by a mortality rate at the very least negligible (<0.5%) [14–17]. Pneumothorax and mild-to-moderate bleeding were the main adverse events. Pneumothorax rate was highly variable among studies, ranging from 0 to 20%, with pooled estimates around 10%, and chest tube drainage was required in more than half of cases. The heterogeneity among results likely reflects the proportion of baseline clinical risk factors for its onset, such as underlying UIP, pattern, the fibrosis severity at HRCT, the distance from the pleura, and the operator skills.

Data on bleeding rates were even more difficult to be summarized, as definitions on its severity were hugely different among studies. Overall, severe life-threatening bleeding were nearly anecdotal, while mild-to-moderate bleeding were commonly observed [14–17]. Anyhow, it is worth noting that in one of the largest cohort in which a bronchial blocker, such as Fogarty balloon, was prophylactically used, no moderate bleeding occurred [14].

This underlies that the routine use of preventive bronchial blockers and an effective airways control under deep sedation are highly recommended to reduce and manage such complication, suggesting also that the procedure should be performed in centers with experience in the field of interventional pulmonology.

Data on comparison between TBLC and forceps transbronchial biopsy in diagnostic work-up of DPLDs and lung tumors, derived from eight studies, showed that specimen area and DY were significantly superior in the cryobiopsy group, without substantial differences in safety profile [17].

Although data on DY and safety profile of TBLC were overall satisfying, its role in diagnostic work-up of DPLDs has been questioned, due to the lack of studies on a direct comparison with SLB. However, in a retrospective analysis of a prospective clinical protocol, Ravaglia et al. reported a comparison between TBLC and SLB in a large cohort of patients from clinical practice. In detail, data on DY and safety were retrospectively retrieved from 150 patients in VATS group and 297 in TBLC group. As expected, the DY of SLB (98,7%) was higher than that of TBLC (82,8%), but the latter procedure offered significant advantages in terms of safety. Mortality due to adverse event after SLB was observed in four patients (2.7% of total), caused by acute exacerbation of IPF in all cases. In the TBLC group, only one patient died after 7 days (0.3% of total) with acute exacerbation of IPF (coexistence of diffuse alveolar damage and UIP pattern at autopsy) following massive pneumothorax (treated with drainage and high-flow oxygen) and prolonged air leak. Pneumothorax was the most common complication after cryobiopsy, occurring in 60 patients (20.2%), 46 cases (15.5% of total) requiring drainage. No patients needed intervention to control bleeding and there were no cases with persistent fever or pneumonia/empyema. Other complications were transient respiratory failure (two patients, 0.7%) and neurologic manifestations (seizures in two patients, 0.7%). Regarding the length of hospitalization, the median time was 6,1 days after SLB and 2,6 days after TBLC ($p < 0,0001$), with elderly patients being at higher risk of prolonged hospital stay.

A further confirmation of valuable role of TBLC in this context came from a study addressing the impact of this technique on increasing diagnostic confidence in the multidisciplinary process leading to the final diagnosis in comparison to SLB [18]. Tomassetti et al., indeed, in their cross-sectional study, involving 117 patients, documented a major increase in diagnostic confidence after the addition of TBLC, which was not significantly different from that of SLB, with similar interobserver agreement in IPF diagnosis. However, a methodologic limitation of this study is that it was focused on diagnostic agreement among experts, rather than on diagnostic accuracy, although the first has been widely accepted of a reliable surrogate [18].

Cryobiopsy and/or Surgical Lung Biopsy

Diagnosis of DPLDs is a dynamic multidisciplinary process, requiring close communication between clinicians, radiologists, and pathologists. According to current thinking and international guidelines, SLB should be the procedure of choice when a pathological assessment is needed for diagnostic confirmation, due to its excellent accuracy [2]. However, SLB requires endotracheal intubation, general anesthesia, chest tube placement, and typically hospitalization for several days. Mortality rate, overall estimated around 2–6% at 90 days, may increase to 18.8% in patients ultimately diagnosed with IPF [14]. These data suggest that the benefits of diagnostic confirmation must be weighed against the potential risks of life-threatening complications, especially when IPF is suspected, and, thus, in clinical practice, only 10–20% of patients with fibrotic DPLDs actually undergo a SLB, as many subjects are not eligible because of a combination of advanced stage, age, comorbidities, respiratory failure, and pulmonary hypertension. Furthermore, once the surgical biopsy has been obtained, the interobserver concordance between expert pathologists is not always as high as expected, suggesting that the bigger is not necessarily the better, as some histological patterns may not be clearly classified regardless of the dimension of the samples provided [3].

TBLC has been recently advocated as a suitable substitute in this context, as it is characterized by a better safety profile compared to SLB with a satisfying diagnostic yield, even if lower than the gold standard. However, considering the acceptable risks related to TBLC, this procedure and SLB should not be necessarily intended as real competitors in clinical practice, as one patient could undergo TBLC and then subsequently VATS if the first approach is nondiagnostic [14]. Taking into account estimates from meta-analyses on mortality of SLB (3.6%, CI 95% 2.1–5.5) and on diagnostic yield of TBLC (81%, 95% CI 75–87), a diagnostic algorithm including TBLC as the first option and SLB as the subsequent step has been recently proposed by Ravaglia et al. In detail, two possible scenarios could occur: (1) in the worst scenario, 25% of patients undergo surgical lung biopsy because of a nondiagnostic previous cryobiopsy and surgical lung biopsy has the highest mortality (5,5%) and (2) in the best scenario, only 13% of patients undergo surgical lung biopsy because of a nondiagnostic previous cryobiopsy and surgical biopsy has the lowest mortality (2,1%) (Fig. 2.7) [14]. The "final" risk of mortality will range between 0,3 and 1,4%. In other words, even in the worst scenario, the mortality rate related to this diagnostic approach would be significantly lower than the overall mortality of VATS alone [14].

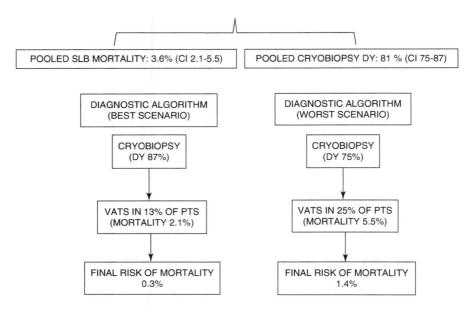

Fig. 2.7 Adapted from Ravaglia et al. [14]. The final risk of mortality of a diagnostic algorithm including TBLC as the first option and SLB as the subsequent step in case of inconclusive results

Conclusion

In conclusion, current data suggest that TBLC plays a remarkable role in the diagnostic work-up of DPLDs, as it offers significant advantages in terms of safety compared to SLB, guaranteeing an excellent diagnostic profile. However, the absence of clinical trials directly comparing the two procedures, due to ethical reasons, makes it difficult to completely elucidate the relative risks and benefits. In this context, TBLC and SLB should not be considered as competitors, as they could be integrated in complementary diagnostic pathways, with TBLC as the first diagnostic approach, reserving the more invasive surgical procedure in case of not adequate or inconclusive results.

Fifty years have been just passed from the first transbronchial lung biopsy performed by Andersen in 1965. Since then, interventional pulmonology has experienced an outstanding evolution, and TBLC, this exciting renewal of an old technique, represents a further step in such process. However, further prospective studies are needed to better define relevant technical aspects of TBLC, such as the optimal number of biopsies to obtain and the utility to sample different segments or even different lobes, in order to standardize the procedure as much as possible

References

1. Wells AU, Kokosi M, Karagiannis K. Treatment strategies for idiopathic interstitial pneumonias. Curr Opin Pulm Med. 2014;20:442–8.
2. Raghu G, Collard HR, Egan JJ, Martinez FJ, Behr J, Brown KK, Colby TV, Cordier JF, Flaherty KR, Lasky JA, Lynch DA, Ryu JH, Swigris JJ, Wells AU, Ancochea J, Bouros D, Carvalho C, Costabel U, Ebina M, Hansell DM, Johkoh T, Kim DS, King TE Jr, Kondoh Y, Myers J, Muller NL, Nicholson AG, Richeldi L, Selman M, Dudden RF, Griss BS, Protzko SL, Schunemann HJ, Fibrosis AEJACoIP. An official ATS/ERS/JRS/ALAT statement: idiopathic pulmonary fibrosis: evidence-based guidelines for diagnosis and management. Am J Respir Crit Care Med. 2011;183:788–824.
3. Poletti V, Benzaquen S. Transbronchial cryobiopsy in diffuse parenchymal lung disease. A new star in the horizon. Sarcoidosis Vasc Diffuse Lung Dis. 2014;31:178–81.
4. Han Q, Luo Q, Xie JX, Wu LL, Liao LY, Zhang XX, Chen RC. Diagnostic yield and postoperative mortality associated with surgical lung biopsy for evaluation of interstitial lung diseases: a systematic review and meta-analysis. J Thorac Cardiovasc Surg. 2015;149:1394–401. e1391
5. Knipscheer BJ, van Moorsel CH, Grutters JC. Non-specific and usual interstitial pneumonia, short-term survival after surgical biopsy. Lung. 2015;193:449–50.
6. Poletti V, Casoni GL, Gurioli C, Ryu JH, Tomassetti S. Lung cryobiopsies: a paradigm shift in diagnostic bronchoscopy? Respirology. 2014;19:645–54.
7. Nguyen W, Meyer KC. Surgical lung biopsy for the diagnosis of interstitial lung disease: a review of the literature and recommendations for optimizing safety and efficacy. Sarcoidosis Vasc Diffuse Lung Dis. 2013;30:3–16.
8. Hutchinson JP, McKeever TM, Fogarty AW, Navaratnam V, Hubbard RB. Surgical lung biopsy for the diagnosis of interstitial lung disease in England: 1997-2008. Eur Respir J. 2016;48:1453–61.
9. Kaarteenaho R. The current position of surgical lung biopsy in the diagnosis of idiopathic pulmonary fibrosis. Respir Res. 2013;14:43.
10. Maldonado F, Moua T, Skalski J. Parenchymal cryobiopsies for interstitial lung diseases: a step forward in disease management. Respirology. 2014;19:773–4.
11. Pompeo E, Cristino B, Rogliani P, Dauri M, Awake Thoracic Surgery Research G. Urgent awake thoracoscopic treatment of retained haemothorax associated with respiratory failure. Ann Transl Med. 2015;3:112.
12. Ambrogi V, Mineo TC. VATS biopsy for undetermined interstitial lung disease under non-general anesthesia: comparison between uniportal approach under intercostal block vs. three-ports in epidural anesthesia. J Thorac Dis. 2014;6:888–95.
13. Pompeo E, Rogliani P, Cristino B, Schillaci O, Novelli G, Saltini C. Awake thoracoscopic biopsy of interstitial lung disease. Ann Thorac Surg. 2013;95:445–52.
14. Ravaglia C, Bonifazi M, Wells AU, Tomassetti S, Gurioli C, Piciucchi S, Dubini A, Tantalocco P, Sanna S, Negri E, Tramacere I, Ventura VA, Cavazza A, Rossi A, Chilosi M, La Vecchia C, Gasparini S, Poletti V. Safety and diagnostic yield of transbronchial lung cryobiopsy in diffuse parenchymal lung diseases: a comparative study versus video-assisted thoracoscopic lung biopsy and a systematic review of the literature. Respiration. 2016;91:215–27.
15. Sharp C, McCabe M, Adamali H, Medford AR. Use of transbronchial cryobiopsy in the diagnosis of interstitial lung disease-a systematic review and cost analysis. QJM. 2016.
16. Johannson KA, Marcoux VS, Ronksley PE, Ryerson CJ. Diagnostic yield and complications of transbronchial lung cryobiopsy for interstitial lung disease. A systematic review and meta-analysis. Ann Am Thorac Soc. 2016;13:1828–38.
17. Ganganah O, Guo SL, Chiniah M, Li YS. Efficacy and safety of cryobiopsy versus forceps biopsy for interstitial lung diseases and lung tumours: a systematic review and meta-analysis. Respirology. 2016;21:834–41.
18. Tomassetti S, Wells AU, Costabel U, Cavazza A, Colby TV, Rossi G, Sverzellati N, Carloni A, Carretta E, Buccioli M, Tantalocco P, Ravaglia C, Gurioli C, Dubini A, Piciucchi S, Ryu JH, Poletti V. Bronchoscopic lung cryobiopsy increases diagnostic confidence in the multidisciplinary diagnosis of idiopathic pulmonary fibrosis. Am J Respir Crit Care Med. 2016;193:745–52.

Chapter 3
Management of Lung Nodules: A Paradigm Shift

Prasoon Jain, Sarah Hadique, Ghulam Abbas, and Atul C. Mehta

Introduction

Lung cancer is the leading cause of cancer-related mortality in the United States accounting for nearly 154,000 deaths annually. Early lung cancers do not cause many symptoms. Historically, in the absence of any effective screening tests, less than one-third of the patients with lung cancer presented with early-stage disease. An overwhelming majority of lung cancers in the past were detected in advanced stages for which surgical cure was no longer an option. The growing acceptance of the low-dose computed tomography (LDCT) for lung cancer screening is changing the paradigm with the expectation that two-thirds of all lung cancers in the screening population will be detected in the early stage, hence will be surgically resectable. The major breakthrough in this area came with publication of National Lung Screening Trial (NLST). In this multicenter randomized prospective study, screening with low-dose computed tomography (LDCT) led to a 20% relative reduction in lung cancer mortality among high-risk individuals [1]. However, LDCT is far from

P. Jain (✉)
Pulmonary and Critical Care, Louis A Johnson VA Medical Center, Clarksburg, WV, USA

S. Hadique
Associate Professor, Department of Pulmonary and Critical Care, West Virginia University, Morgantown, WV, USA

G. Abbas
Chief, Division of Thoracic & Esophageal Surgery Professor, Dept of Cardiovascular & Thoracic Surgery Medicine, WVU Medicine, Morgantown, WV, USA

A. C. Mehta
Buoncore Family Endowed Chair in Lung Transplantation, Respiratory Institute, Cleveland Clinic, Cleveland, OH, USA

© The Author(s), under exclusive license to Springer Nature
Switzerland AG 2021
J. F. Turner, Jr. et al. (eds.), *From Thoracic Surgery to Interventional Pulmonology*, Respiratory Medicine,
https://doi.org/10.1007/978-3-030-80298-1_3

a perfect screening test. In NLST, 27% of subjects had noncalcified nodules on LDCT. More than 90% of those who had lung nodules on CT underwent further diagnostic tests. The majority of the lung nodules were nonmalignant with positive predictive value of 3.8% [2]. In keeping with results from NLST, a more population-based study from the Netherlands (Nelson trial) showed a 26% reduction in lung cancer-related deaths with 69% of all cancer detected via screening being still stage I tumors [3].

Commonly, lung nodule is also discovered as an incidental finding when a chest CT is performed for an unrelated indication. This is not a trivial problem given that more than 80 million annual CT studies are performed in the United States alone [4]. Appropriate management of incidental nodules also requires careful further assessment of risk of malignancy and need for further workup.

Lung nodules detected on CT screening are often small and not readily accessible for biopsy. Many elderly patients with numerous comorbidities are found to have lung nodules with CT imaging. Identifying underlying pathology is critical for appropriate management, and the key challenge is to accomplish this task with minimum risk to the patients. Any procedure-related complication can be viewed as a net harm from CT screening in a patient who does not have underlying malignancy. Need for a higher diagnostic yield and lower complications are the two main catalysts for recent technological advances in the field of bronchoscopy. The same needs have also brought interventional pulmonologists and thoracic surgeons to work more closely than ever before.

The management of incidentally found nodule remains controversial. For those with ≥8–10 mm nodules, positron emission tomography (PET) scan is often helpful in further risk stratification [5] (Fig. 3.1). Although the gold standard for diagnosis of small lung nodules is surgical biopsy [6], in many instances, tissue diagnosis is not warranted, and a video-assisted thoracic surgery (VATS) or robotic pulmonary segmentectomy with curative intention without tissue diagnosis is the most

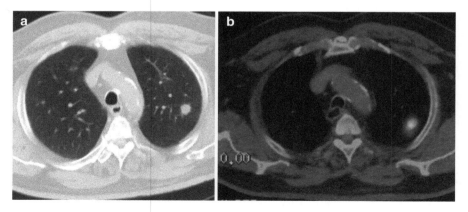

Fig. 3.1 Suspicious left upper nodule in a smoker, highly suspicious for lung cancer (**a**). FDG PET scan showed increased uptake (**b**) without any additional findings. Patient underwent left upper lobe resection that revealed adenocarcinoma

preferred approach. In our experience at West Virginia University, 93% of all patients who underwent robotic segmentectomy or lobectomy without preoperative tissue diagnosis for suspicious lung nodules were found to have malignant lesions (personal communication). Similarly, other institutional reports have shown accuracy rates of 85% and 95% for suspicious nodules resected without tissue diagnosis [7, 8]. In this regard, we agree with National Comprehensive Cancer Network (NCCN) Guidelines that do not require preoperative tissue diagnosis for highly suspicious clinical stage I and II non-small cell lung cancer [9].

However, this still leaves a large number of indeterminate lung nodules that require tissue diagnosis before an appropriate treatment can be offered. Also included in this category are high-risk patients who cannot undergo surgical resection due to medical reasons or refuse surgery due to personal preference. Appropriate management of these patients is a daunting task. Traditional bronchoscopy has little to offer in this situation.

In this chapter, we discuss the current role of advanced bronchoscopic techniques in overall management of pulmonary nodules. First, we discuss the role and limitations of various techniques used for obtaining tissue biopsy from peripheral nodules. We further discuss how interventional pulmonologists are moving beyond the diagnostic role and assisting thoracic surgeons and radiation oncologists in management of lung nodules. We also discuss the potential future role of bronchoscopic treatments for peripheral lung nodules. Finally, we briefly discuss the emerging role of hybrid theaters in which thoracic surgeons, interventional pulmonologist, and others work together to provide advanced care and research on pulmonary nodules.

Biopsy Techniques

Obtaining tissue diagnosis for peripheral lesions <3 cm is not easy. In recent years, several techniques have become available with their associated advantages and limitations [10, 11]. Choosing an appropriate technique requires a comprehensive clinical assessment. Cost and availability of local expertise must be taken into account. No predetermined clinical pathway can meet every individual need. Practicing clinicians must never be enticed to choose the most modern or expensive procedure. They should not hesitate to refer patients to regional centers of excellence if a need for an advanced procedure is determined but cannot be offered locally due to non-availability of expertise or equipment.

Transthoracic Needle Aspiration

Transthoracic needle aspiration (TTNA) under computed tomography guidance is commonly used for obtaining biopsy specimen from solitary lung nodules and masses. The procedure is technically simple and has a sensitivity of more than 90%

and specificity of 100% for malignant lung nodules [12]. Sensitivity is lower for nodules smaller than 2 cm in some but not in all studies; pooled sensitivity is still greater than 90% for such lesions [13, 14]. CT-guided TTNA is also suitable for predominantly ground glass opacities [15]. The main problem with CT-guided TTNA is 20–40% risk of pneumothorax [12]. Chest tube is needed in 5–10% of patients [16]. High incidence of procedure-related pneumothorax is of concern because many of the patients undergoing this procedure have significant underlying lung disease such as chronic obstructive pulmonary disease. Risk of major bleeding is another concern observed in up to 3% of patients. Risk of air embolism and death is exceedingly low.

Lesions close to pleural surface are most suitable for CT-guided TTNA. Bronchoscopy is more useful for centrally located lesions. High risk of pneumothorax also precludes CT-guided TTNA for lesion surrounded by emphysematous bullae.

Conventional Bronchoscopy

The main advantage of bronchoscopy over CT-guided TTNA is its unparallel safety record with <2–3% risk of major bleeding or pneumothorax. Still, conventional bronchoscopy has a limited role in obtaining tissue specimen from lung nodules <3 cm in size. The pooled sensitivity of conventional bronchoscopy is 34% for lesions <2 cm and 63% for lesions >2 cm [17]. Yield is exceedingly low for lesions <1 cm, and for lesions not visible on fluoroscopy. Conventional bronchoscopy is not indicated for these lesions. A higher yield can be expected for a lesion with a positive bronchus sign [18–20] (Fig. 3.2). It is important to look for more easy targets of

Fig. 3.2 A solitary lung nodule with positive bronchus sign. Bronchoscopy is more likely to provide diagnostic specimen from such nodules

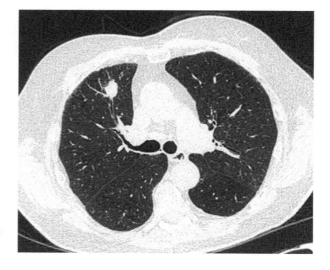

Fig. 3.3 Chest CT showing a right upper lobe nodule with enlarged right paratracheal lymph node. FDG-PET showed high uptake in nodule and paratracheal lymph node. Convex probe endobronchial ultrasound from lymph node revealed adenocarcinoma. No biopsy was deemed necessary from lung nodule

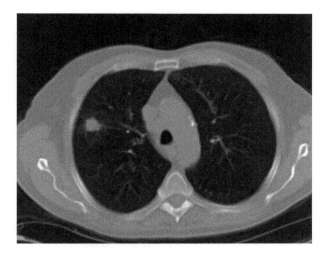

biopsy if the lung nodule is not easily accessible. For example, sampling of enlarged mediastinal lymph nodes with convex probe endobronchial ultrasound may not only provide diagnosis but also provide essential staging information for most appropriate therapy (Fig. 3.3). Diagnostic yield is increased when multiple sampling procedures including peripheral transbronchial needle aspiration (P-TBNA) are performed during bronchoscopy [21]. Unfortunately, P-TBNA continues to be underutilized during bronchoscopy. Data from AQuIRE registry reveals that P-TBNA is used in <20% of patients undergoing bronchoscopy for confirming diagnosis of peripheral lung cancer [22].

Lesions <1–1.5 cm are often invisible on fluoroscopy. The same can be said about predominantly ground glass opacities. A substantial proportion of lung nodules detected on low-dose CT screening have these characteristics. It is intuitive to understand why conventional bronchoscopy has such low yield for these lesions. Several other factors limit successful acquisition of diagnostic tissue with conventional bronchoscopy in peripheral lung nodules. The top three reasons are (1) inability to identify the correct bronchoscopic pathway to the lesion, (2) inability to maneuver biopsy instrument to the lesion, and (3) inability to be certain that biopsy instrument has reached its correct intended destination. Several new bronchoscopic techniques developed over the past decade to increase diagnostic yield for lung nodules have revolved around tackling these three basic issues. The new bronchoscopic techniques include virtual bronchoscopy navigation (VBN), development of ultrathin bronchoscope, electromagnetic navigation bronchoscopy (ENB), radial probe endobronchial ultrasound (RP-EBUS), and robotic bronchoscopy. Application of these techniques has served to offset some of the problems associated with conventional bronchoscopy.

Virtual Bronchoscopy Navigation

In this technique, thin CT images are used to construct virtual bronchoscopy images. The system allows the operator to select the target ahead of the actual procedure and determine the bronchoscopic route to the target (Fig. 3.4). According to a review, the diagnostic yield of VBN was 73.8% overall, and 67.4% for lesions smaller than 2 cm in diameter [23]. Virtual bronchoscopy navigation can be used with conventional bronchoscopy, but its full potential is realized when used with thin bronchoscopes in combination with radial probe endobronchial ultrasound. Ishida and associates performed a randomized study to investigate usefulness of VBN-assisted bronchoscopy with radial probe EBUS in 199 patients with ≤3 cm peripheral pulmonary lesion [24]. Median size of the lesion was 1.8 cm. A thin videobronchoscope

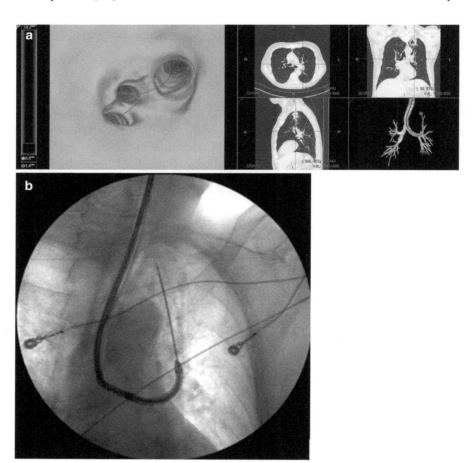

Fig. 3.4 Cavitary mass in apical segment of left upper lobe in a smoker. Virtual bronchoscopy navigation using Lung Point™ directed the bronchoscopist to approach the nodule through apical segment of left upper lobe (**a**). Biopsy using standard forceps revealed adenocarcinoma (**b**)

of 4 mm outer diameter was used in all patients. The diagnostic yield was significantly higher in VBN-guided procedures (80.4% vs. 67%, $p = 0.032$). Bronchoscopy time was also shortened in VBN group. Virtual bronchoscopy images constructed on the basis of chest CT agreed with actual bronchoscopic images 98% of the time.

In recent years, many bronchoscopes have become available that have a small outer diameter but a working channel that can accommodate some biopsy instruments (Fig. 3.5). Use of ultrathin bronchoscopes allows operators to navigate deeper into the lung. A large study has confirmed the added value of using ultrathin bronchoscope with VBN and radial probe EBUS. The diagnostic yield was 74% for <3 cm lesions when biopsy was performed using ultrathin bronchoscope (3 mm outer diameter with 1.7 mm working channel) along with virtual bronchoscopy navigation and radial probe EBUS [25]. In comparison, diagnostic yield was 59% when bronchoscopy was performed using 4 mm bronchoscope using radial probe EBUS and guide sheath method. The ability to navigate to fifth-generation airways with ultrathin 3 mm bronchoscope compared to fourth-generation airways with 4 mm bronchoscope was thought to be the major reason for the difference in the diagnostic yield in two groups.

There are two main issues that limit the usefulness of VBN and ultrathin bronchoscopes for biopsy of small peripheral nodules. First, even though VBN can direct the operator to follow a correct path to the lesion, it does not help with maneuverability which becomes increasingly difficult as the operator navigates to most distal airways. Second, and perhaps more importantly, the small working channel of ultrathin bronchoscopes does not always allow use of standard biopsy forceps or peripheral TBNA procedure. This is the most likely reason for failure of VBN-assisted ultrathin bronchoscopy to significantly improve diagnostic yield compared to non-VBN-assisted bronchoscopy in a study involving 350 patients with <3 cm peripheral pulmonary lesions [26].

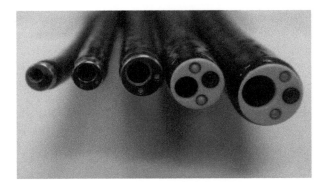

Fig. 3.5 Flexible bronchoscopes of different sizes: from left to right, 2.8 mm bronchoscope with 1.2 mm working channel, 3.0 mm bronchoscope with 1.7 cm working channel, 4.0 mm bronchoscope with 2.0 mm working channel, 4.8 mm bronchoscope with 2.0 mm working channel, and 5.9 mm bronchoscope with 3.0 mm working channel. (Reproduced with permission from Fielding [99])

Electromagnetic Navigation Bronchoscopy (ENB)

Electromagnetic navigation bronchoscopy (ENB) is a revolutionary technique that goes a step beyond VBN. In addition to VBN, ENB involves placement of patient in a magnetic field during bronchoscopy, use of micro-sensor tip called locatable guide (LG) to obtain its exact position in the thorax, and integrating this information with the CT data obtained before the procedure. Evolutionary history and the technical details of ENB are subjects of several recent reviews [27–28]. The first large clinical study using this technique was reported from the Cleveland Clinic Foundation in 2006 [29]. In this study, ENB was used to obtain biopsy from 54 peripheral lung lesions, more than 50% of which were <2 cm in diameter. The diagnostic yield was 74% and pneumothorax rate was 3.5%. The diagnostic yield in subsequent studies has varied from 33% to 97% [27]. A meta-analysis in 2014 showed a diagnostic sensitivity of 71%, and negative predictive value of 52% [30]. The NAVIGATE study provides the most definitive data on diagnostic yield of electromagnetic navigation bronchoscopy. In this multicenter study, the sensitivity and negative predictive value of EMB were 69% and 56%, respectively, in 1157 patients with a mean nodule size of 20 mm [31]. The procedure is safe. The interim results from initial 1000 patients from the same study showed a pneumothorax rate of 4.9%. Procedure-related bleeding was reported in 2.3% of patients and respiratory failure in 0.6% of subjects [32]. Many operators perform ENB under general anesthesia. However, GA for this purpose is not needed. Similar diagnostic yield can be achieved when the procedure is performed under intravenous sedation in experienced hands [33].

Several limitations of ENB in biopsy are readily apparent. Not all studies have reported a high diagnostic yield. For example, the AQuIRE registry has reported a diagnostic yield of 38.5% with the use of ENB for peripheral nodules [22]. This is proposed to be due to selection of more difficult cases for biopsy. However, it may be argued that these are types of cases in which advanced technologies such as ENB need to show a clear superiority over more conventional techniques. An important problem with ENB is that it does not provide real-time confirmation of accurate navigation to the target. Due to this reason, radial probe endobronchial ultrasound (RP-EBUS) is commonly used during ENB procedure for location and verification of the target. Combination of RP-EBUS and ENB has a higher diagnostic yield compared to diagnostic yield of either individual procedure. For example, in a prospective randomized study, the diagnostic yield of combination of ENB and RP-EBUS was 88%, compared to diagnostic yield of 69% with RP-EBUS and 59% with ENB alone [34]. In addition, ENB technology has been hampered by navigation error or CT-body divergence, which is thought to be a major barrier to improving diagnostic yield with this technique. Recently, superDimension ENB system (Medtronic, Minneapolis, Minnesota, USA) has secured FDA approval for fluoroscopic navigation system which allows better visualization of fluoroscopically invisible lesions and allows re-registration once LG reaches close to the target using standard ENB technique. The re-registration of nodule using real-time fluoroscopic data is thought to reduce CT to body divergence and may help improve diagnostic yield. These platforms are discussed later in this chapter. Another approach to correct this problem is real-time confirmation of target location with cone-beam CT. Encouraging early results have been reported with combination of ENB and cone-beam CT [35].

Radial Probe Endobronchial Ultrasound

Radial probe endobronchial ultrasound (RP-EBUS) uses a miniature 20 MHz ultrasound probe housed within a flexible catheter that can be introduced through the working channel to localize the peripheral pulmonary lesion [36] (Fig. 3.6). The ultrasound probe rotates within the bronchus producing radial 360-degree images

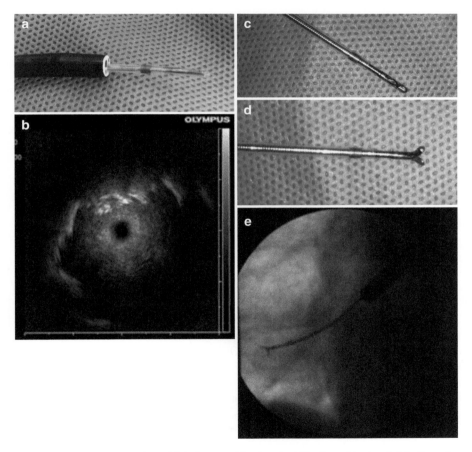

Fig. 3.6 Radial probe endobronchial ultrasound is placed within the guide sheath (**a**). Once the lesion is localized (**b**), ultrasound probe is removed leaving guide sheath in place. Biopsy instruments are introduced through the guide sheath (**c**, **d**). Biopsies are obtained under fluoroscopy (**e**). ((**b**, **e**) were reproduced with permission from Eberhardt [100])

of the surrounding lung parenchyma. Normal lung gives a snowstorm appearance. A tumor surrounding the bronchus with RP-EBUS appears hypo-echoic with a clear hyper-echoic line separating it from surrounding lung. The ultrasound probe can be introduced directly through the working channel of a thin bronchoscope. More commonly, the ultrasound mini probe covered with a disposable catheter called guide sheath is introduced into the bronchus through the working channel [37] (Fig. 3.6a–e). In this method, the ultrasound probe is removed once the lesion is located leaving the guide sheath within the working channel. Biopsy instruments can be introduced through the guide sheath to obtain tissue specimens. The diagnostic yields are reported to be similar with direct bronchoscopic and guide sheath methods in one randomized study [38].

RP-EBUS provides a real-time confirmation of target localization prior to biopsy (Fig. 3.7). In a study involving 467 patients, the overall diagnostic yield was 67% [39]. The diagnostic yield was 58% for 1–2 cm lesions, 72% for 2.1–3 cm lesions, 77% for 3.1–4 cm lesions, and 87% for >4 cm lesions. The yield was highly dependent on location of ultrasound probe in relation to the lesion. The diagnostic yield was 84% when the probe could be placed within the lesion and the tumor surrounded the probe from all sides. However, the diagnostic yield decreased to 48% when the probe was located adjacent to the lesion.

In a meta-analysis from 16 earlier studies involving 1420 patients, the pooled diagnostic sensitivity of RP-EBUS was 73% [40]. A similar diagnostic yield was reported in another meta-analysis involving 3052 subjects [41].

In a more recent meta-analysis that included 7872 subjects from 57 studies, the overall diagnostic yield of RP-EBUS was 70.6% [42]. Factors associated with higher diagnostic yield in these meta-analyses are lesion size, prevalence of malignancy, presence of bronchus sign, and position of probe in relation to the lesion. The diagnostic yield is around 55–60% for lesions ≤2 cm and 70–80% for lesions >2 cm size. The diagnostic yield was 52% when the probe was adjacent to the lesion compared to 78.7% when RP-EBUS probe could reach within the lesion [42]. Similarly, the diagnostic yield was 76.5% for the lesions with and 52.4% for the lesions without a positive bronchus sign on CT imaging. Overall complication rate is reported to vary from 1% to 2.8%.

An important observation is a high heterogeneity in the diagnostic sensitivity in different studies included in meta-analysis on RP-EBUS. Although this could reflect the patient selection criteria, the lower yield could also be due to lack of experience and learning curve issues. Interestingly, AQuIRE registry, which has better external validity, reported a 57% diagnostic yield with RP-EBUS for peripheral lesions [22]. It must also be pointed out that negative likelihood ratio of RP-EBUS in a meta-analysis was 0.28 [40]. Therefore, a nondiagnostic bronchoscopy that utilized RP-EBUS technique cannot be accepted as an evidence of absence of malignancy.

Not uncommonly, the screening CT detects lesions that are predominantly or entirely ground glass in appearance. Ground glass opacities (GGO) cannot be visualized on fluoroscopy. This seriously limits the usefulness of conventional bronchoscopy in these patients. Several recent reports suggest that RP-EBUS could assist the operators in identifying these lesions during bronchoscopy. In an earlier study, the diagnostic yield of RP-EBUS was 65% in 40 patients with predominant GGO peripheral pulmonary lesions [43]. In a more recent study, there was a diagnostic yield of 69% for pure GGO or part solid, part GGO lesions using RP-EBUS and VBN [44].

RP-EBUS images in pure or predominant GGO demonstrate blizzard sign seen as subtle but noticeable white acoustic shadows around the ultrasound probe (Fig. 3.8a–c). This appearance differs from snowstorm appearance of normal lung parenchyma. In contrast, lesions with a greater proportion of solid component disclose a mixed blizzard sign on RP-EBUS images in which hyper-echoic dots, linear arcs, and vessels are seen to be irregularly distributed within a blizzard. Identification

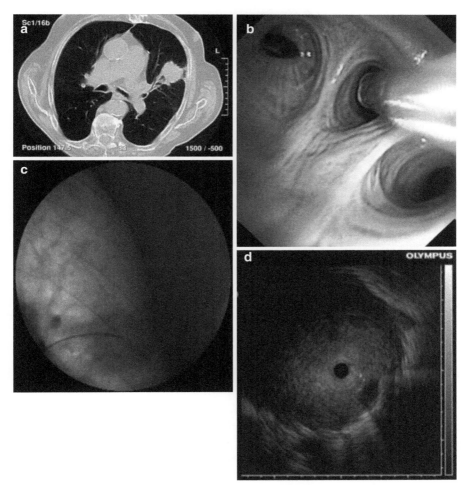

Fig. 3.7 An example of use of radial probe endobronchial ultrasound technology to obtain tissue specimen from left upper lobe lesion (**a**). Radial probe ultrasound within the guide sheath is navigated towards the target (**b**). The distal end of the radial probe ultrasound is seen within the lesion on fluoroscopy images (**c**). Ultrasound images confirm the presence of tumor surrounding the probe (**d**). At this time, the probe is removed leaving the guide sheath in place and biopsies are performed under fluoroscopy guidance (**e**). (Reproduced with permission from Eberhardt [100])

Fig. 3.7 (continued)

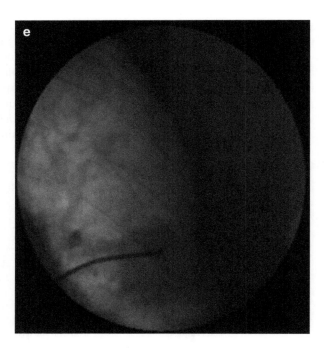

of blizzard and mixed blizzard sign may improve the ability of the operator to locate and biopsy such peripheral opacities not visible on fluoroscopy [45].

Radial probe EBUS is radiation neutral and simple to learn. It does not require special or expensive accessories. It compliments other navigational technologies by providing real-time confirmation of target localization. The application of this technique to assist in biopsy of peripheral pulmonary opacities is strongly recommended.

Bronchoscopic Trans-Parenchymal Access (BTPNA)

Numerous studies and meta-analyses have reported a higher diagnostic yield of bronchoscopy when a bronchus sign is present in lung nodule on CT [42, 46]. The obvious explanation is that a leading bronchus in such cases provides a direct endo-bronchial path for the biopsy instrument to reach the peripheral lesion. Unfortunately, not all peripheral lesions have a positive bronchus sign on pre-procedure chest CT. For example, in NAVIGATE study, a bronchus sign was detectable only in 48.8% of all peripheral lesions [32]. A newer technique called bronchoscopic trans-parenchymal access (BTPNA) technique has been used to approach lesions that do not have a bronchus sign (Fig. 3.9). In a preliminary study, Herth and associates described application of this technique in 12 patients [47]. Lesion sizes varied from

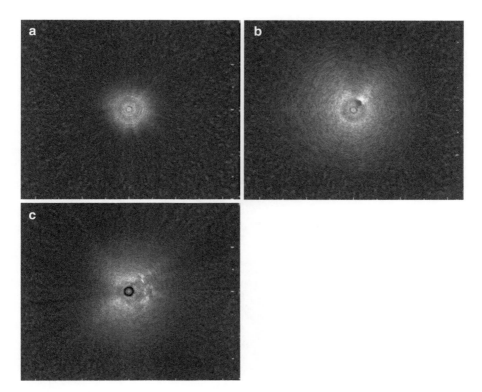

Fig. 3.8 Endobronchial ultrasound images of normal lung and ground glass nodules. Normal lung (**a**) has a snow-storm appearance. Pure ground glass nodules have a mixed blizzard appearance with a diffuse hyperintense shadow without any low echoic areas (**b**). The lesions which are part solid and part ground glass disclose a mixed blizzard sign on RP-EBUS images in which hyper-echoic dots, linear arcs, and vessels are seen to be irregularly distributed within a blizzard (**c**). (Reproduced with permission from Fielding [99])

17 mm to 40 mm. CT data was reconstructed into virtual bronchoscopy using Archimedes™ Virtual Bronchoscopy Navigation system. The system allowed the operator to identify two most appropriate point of entry (POE) on airway wall and the most vessel free direct path from this point to the lesion. During bronchoscopy, the operators introduced a coring needle through the airway wall at POE, dilated the point of entry with a balloon dilator, and then passed a sheath with blunt dilator to create a tunnel in lung parenchyma from POE to the lesion. Biopsies were obtained by passing biopsy instruments through the sheath. The procedure was technically feasible in 10 of 12 patients. Adequate material for histology was obtained in all ten successful procedures. Every study patient underwent surgical resection after the procedure. The trans-pulmonary path was accurate and final histology matched with surgical findings in all cases. There were no major complications. Same group of investigators have reported additional six patients [48]. Successful biopsies could be obtained in five patients. However, pneumothorax developed in two of six patients.

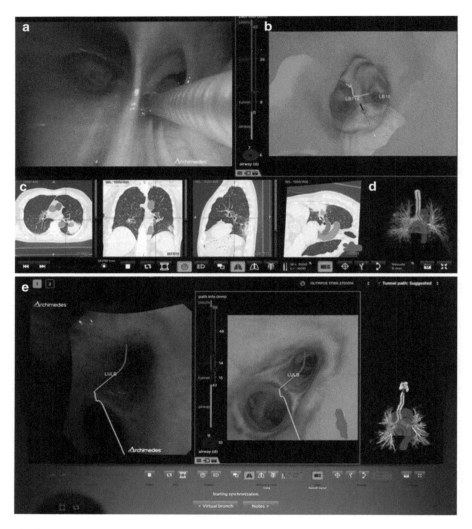

Fig. 3.9 Bronchoscopic transparenchymal nodule access (BTNA). Bronchoscopic image showing the point of entry (**a**). Virtual image showing target lesion in green and overlaid point of entry (**b**). CT images showing the target lesion (green) and blood vessels (blue and red) in relation to airway (**c**). The screen also depicts three-dimensional reconstruction of airways (**d**). The most recent platform helps bronchoscopist to avoid pathway that is likely to encounter blood vessels and cause parenchymal bleeding (**e**). (Reproduced with permission from Bronchus Archimedes ™)

These studies establish the feasibility of accessing and obtaining biopsies with a higher success from small nodules without a leading bronchus. Although no major complications were noted in the preliminary studies, on face value, it appears more invasive with a higher potential for complications. More experience is needed before BTPNA is adopted in everyday practice. An ongoing multicenter trial is looking at the safety and usefulness of this technique.

Electromagnetic-Guided Transthoracic Needle Aspiration (EMTTNA)

There is recent interest in performing percutaneous biopsy under electromagnetic navigation guidance without needing real-time CT imaging. The procedure is performed using SPiN Perc™ system offered by Veran Medical. The system uses a 19G needle with a stylet. The electromagnetic field and sensor on stylet guide the operator to the target [49]. In a small study involving 24 patients, EMTTNA had a diagnostic yield of 83%. The average size of lesions was 20.3 mm. The procedure was complicated by pneumothorax in 21% of patients [50].

This procedure cannot be performed for lesions that require a posterior approach. Since there is no real-time guidance, the issue of how navigation error affects the accuracy of the procedure needs to be clarified. More data is needed before this procedure can be adopted in daily practice.

Cone-Beam CT

Despite optimal use of advanced bronchoscopic techniques, another major challenge in successful biopsy of a small peripheral nodule is inability of the operator to be certain that biopsy instrument has reached its intended target in real time. RP-EBUS is helpful in this regard as discussed above. An alternative emerging technique for this purpose is cone-beam CT technology.

Interventional radiologists have used cone-beam CT technology for quite some time to perform percutaneous biopsy and angiographic procedures. It is also used extensively in the field of orthodontics. Several investigators have reported use of cone-beam CT during bronchoscopy. Basically, the C-arm of cone-beam CT is rotated around the patient to acquire imaging data which is reconstructed and superimposed on live fluoroscopy to confirm the location of biopsy instrument in relation to the target. The software allows the operator to choose the most appropriate path to the lesion on fluoroscopy using a method called segmentation. In a pilot study, cone-beam-assisted biopsy was performed in 33 incidental pulmonary nodules. Cone-beam CT-assisted bronchoscopy using conventional methods achieved an overall 70% diagnostic yield and 82% diagnostic yield for malignant lesions [51].

A logical extension is to apply this technique with ENB. Ng and associates were the first to explore that idea and successfully obtained diagnostic specimen from an 8 mm nodule with cone-beam CT-assisted ENB [52]. A recent series has reported a high success with application of cone-beam CT technology with ENB for biopsy of peripheral nodules [35]. In this study, the authors performed a cone-beam CT during bronchoscopy and fused CT images with live fluoroscopy. This allowed operators to confirm the appropriate position of locatable guide in relation to the target in real time. Additional cone-beam CT was performed when necessary. Radial probe ultrasound was not used in any case. A total of 93 suspicious lung nodules were biopsied in 75 patients. The median size of the lesion was 1.6 cm (range 0.7–5.5 cm).

Importantly, only 49% of lesions were visible on standard fluoroscopy, and bronchus sign on pre-procedure CT was present only in 39% of lesions. The diagnostic yield was 83.7%. An average of 1.5 CT was performed per case and effective radiation dose per CT was estimated to be 2 mSV. No significant complications were reported. High success has also been reported with combination of cone-beam CT and the transbronchial access tool in 14 patients with peripheral pulmonary opacities. The overall diagnostic yield was 71% [53].

The encouraging results from these studies strongly suggest improved ability to obtain representative tissue from peripheral lesions by combining cone-beam CT with ENB and other similar methods. Performing cone-beam CT and confirming accurate placement of biopsy instruments in real time appears to provide a practical solution to the problem of registration/navigation error that has traditionally plagued the otherwise robust ENB technology. However, the majority of these studies come from a few experienced centers. These data need independent confirmation by others. A randomized study comparing ENB yields with cone-beam CT versus radial probe EBUS confirmation is now imminently needed.

Since cone-beam CT involves radiation, it is important to know how much additional patient exposure may be expected if cone-beam technology is routinely applied during bronchoscopy for peripheral nodules. In a phantom study, radiation exposure during a 20-minute bronchoscopy using fluoroscopy and cone-beam CT was estimated to be 0.98–1.5 mSV [54]. Such radiation exposure is safe and is not likely to cause a major harm to the patient. Therefore, radiation safety issues are not likely to pose a major roadblock to future application of this important emerging technology in bronchoscopy.

Therapeutic Contributions of Interventional Pulmonology

Managing lung nodule is a complex undertaking, and a team approach provides more streamlined, appropriate, cost-effective, and patient-centered care. In this setting, advanced bronchoscopic techniques can assist thoracic surgeons as well as radiation oncologists in several different ways. In the following sections, we briefly discuss how interventional pulmonologists can assist in appropriate management of lung nodules.

Assistance During Video-Assisted Thoracoscopic Surgery (VATS)

VATS or robotic approaches have replaced thoracotomy for surgical resection of lung nodules and are associated with less morbidity and pain and shorter length of stay as compared to thoracotomy. However, in many instances, palpation of the subcentimeter nodules is not possible due to its location, consistency, or patient's body habitus. A careful planning is essential in such cases. The most important step in this context is to review the preoperative imaging. When a CT shows that the nodule is limited to a pulmonary segment, a VATS or robotic pulmonary segmentectomy will successfully remove the nodule along with an appropriate lymph node dissection. However, when the nodule is not confined to one segment and when a wedge resection is intended, inability to palpate the nodule may require conversion to open thoracotomy. Such conversion to thoracotomy has been reported in 1–7.5% of patients initially scheduled to undergo VATS procedure [55, 56].

Thoracic surgeons have used many techniques to locate lung nodules during VATS or robotic-assisted thoracic surgery (RATS). A common method is CT-guided transthoracic placement of a hook wire or injection of methylene blue. Complications of this approach include pneumothorax and bleeding, which were reported in 24.5% and 2.4%, respectively, in a VATS study [57]. Additional limitations include inability to recognize methylene blue dye and dislodgement of hook wire. In one series, dislodgement of hook wire occurred in 12% of patients without associated pneumothorax and 33% of patients with pneumothorax. Another issue of practical importance is scheduling conflicts that cause difficulty in coordinating the localization procedure in interventional radiology with the surgical procedure in the operating room [58]. Due to these reasons, a need is felt for a more practical localization procedure for these patients.

Interventional bronchoscopy provides an important alternative for accurate localization of small lung nodules during VATS procedure. A major advantage of this approach is that localization is done immediately before the surgical procedure without needing to move the patient from radiology department to the operating room. Several studies have report high success with navigation bronchoscopy-guided injection of methylene blue to assist surgeons with visual localization of small nodules during VATS. Awais and associates performed ENB-guided localization and VATS resection in 29 patients with lung nodules [59]. The median size of the lesions was 10 mm and the median distance from visceral pleura was 13 mm. The nodule could be localized and removed with VATS in all 29 (100%) of cases. In another study, Marino and associates marked 72 nodules in 70 patients with methylene blue using ENB [60]. The median size of nodules was 8 mm (range 4–17 mm) and the median distance from pleural surface was 6 mm (range 1–19 mm). Tattooing of nodules was successful in 70 of 72 (97.2%), and no patient required conversion to thoracotomy. Injection of methylene blue was harmless to patients, and it did not seem to interfere with pathological interpretation of the specimen. No major adverse effects from bronchoscopy were reported in this study. Decreased downtime between localization procedure and surgery with ENB for this purpose clearly improves the workflow and efficiency in the operating room [61].

The same goal can be achieved with other bronchoscopic techniques. In a recent study, RP-EBUS and VBN were used to localize peripheral nodules before VATS procedure in 25 patients [62]. The median size of lung nodules was 8 mm. The dye was visible on pleural surface in 24 patients. Cancer-free margin resection could be accomplished in all cases without needing conversion to open thoracotomy in any patient. The endoscopic procedure needed 10 min of additional time, but no major complications were encountered.

Assistance with Stereotactic Radiation Therapy

Although surgery remains the gold standard for the treatment of early-stage lung cancer, stereotactic body radiation therapy (SBRT) is an acceptable alternative treatment option for some patients with clinical stage I lung cancer. In a recent meta-analysis of 23 studies, surgery was associated with superior overall survival in both unmatched and matched cohorts with better cancer-specific survival, disease-free survival, and freedom from locoregional recurrence [63]. SBRT is the current standard of care for early-stage lung cancer patients who are medically inoperable or decline surgical treatment. A careful analysis of current literature indicates better local control and overall survival with SBRT than with conventional radiation therapy [64].

The basic principle behind stereotactic radiation is the ability to deliver high biologic effective dose of radiation to the tumor with minimal irradiation of healthy surrounding tissues. Rapid dose fall-off from tumor to surrounding tissues reduces overall high-dose treatment volume, thereby reducing treatment-related toxicity. Entire radiation therapy can be accomplished in 3–5 fractions over 1–2-week period. However, accurate target delineation, which is central to SBRT, requires meticulous treatment planning with strict attention to tumor motion with breathing during the therapy. There are several motion management strategies [65]. Placement of fiducials is one such strategy to track tumor in real time. To be an effective strategy, three conditions must be met: (1) the fiducial markers must be placed in accurate location, close to the tumor, (2) markers must not move significantly from the time of placement to the time of radiation therapy, and (3) procedure-related complications should be low. Gold fiducials can be placed via transthoracic or bronchoscopic approaches. CT-guided percutaneous placement of fiducial markers is complicated by pneumothorax in 13–60% of cases [66–69]. Chest tube is needed in 3–44% of cases. Such high complication rate is unacceptable. Bronchoscopic placement of fiducials provides a safer alternative (Fig. 3.10). Several investigators have reported high success rates with fiducial placement using navigation bronchoscopy. Typically, a combination of ENB, or virtual bronchoscopy navigation, and radial probe ultrasound is used for accurate bronchoscopic placement of fiducials [70, 71].

Nabavizadeh and associates placed 105 embolization coil fiducials in 34 lung nodules under ENB guidance [72]. Average size of lung nodule was 2.27 cm. CT imaging showed 86% of fiducial markers to be within 1 cm of lung nodule. Retention rate was 98%. Bronchoscopic placement of fiducials is safe and can be accomplished during initial diagnostic bronchoscopy [73]. Biopsy of peripheral nodule, mediastinal staging, and fiducial placement in a single sitting may require a prolonged bronchoscopy but was well tolerated in a study involving 21 patients [74].

Pneumothorax rate with ENB-guided placement is considerably lower than with percutaneous approach, ranging from 0% to 6%. The choice of fiducial marker appears to a matter of personal preference, but many investigators have found that coil spring markers are less likely to move from their original position than linear or gold seed fiducials [75, 76].

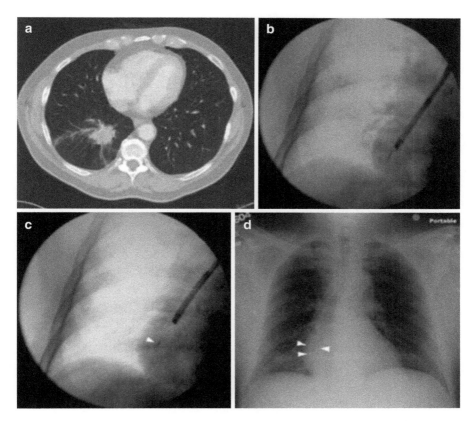

Fig. 3.10 Bronchoscopic placement of fiducials in and around the tumor. (**a**) shows the tumor on chest CT. The fluoroscopic image shows a microbiology brush preloaded with fiducial marker close to the target (**b**). Fiducial markers can be seen after placement on fluoroscopy image (**c**). Chest radiograph shows three fiducial markers around the tumor (**d**). (Reproduced with permission from Mayse [101])

Bronchoscopic Treatments of Early Lung Cancer

Interventional pulmonology procedures such as laser photo-resection, argon plasma coagulation, cryotherapy, photodynamic therapy, and brachytherapy have an established role in palliative treatment of advanced central airway tumors [77]. In recent years, with more accurate ability to locate peripheral lung nodules, there is emerging role of bronchoscopy in treatment of early-stage peripheral lung cancer [78, 79].

One such technique is radiofrequency ablation. The basic premise of radiofrequency ablation is to expose tumor to electromagnetic energy and inflict thermal injury to the tumor. An active electrode placed within the tumor and the radiofrequency generator sends high-frequency alternating current from this electrode to the dispersive electrodes placed on body surface. The heat generated around the tumor causes coagulative necrosis.

Traditionally, radiofrequency ablation for peripheral lung nodule is performed via transthoracic approach in which electrode is placed into tumor under CT guidance. Several studies have shown technical feasibility and efficacy of RFA in treatment of early-stage lung cancer. However, pneumothorax has been reported in as many as 20% of patients undergoing the procedure. With better ability to navigate to the tumor, there is interest in exploring possibility of performing radiofrequency ablation of tumor using electrode placed through bronchoscopy. Koizumi and associates used CT-guided bronchoscopy to place a cooled radiofrequency ablation catheter to treat 28 peripheral lung tumors in 20 medically inoperable patients using this technique [80]. Median size of lesions was 24 mm with a range of 12–45 mm. Local control was achieved in 82.6% of tumors. Median progression-free survival was 35 months, and 5-year survival was 61.5%. No major adverse effects were encountered. Xie and associates have reported navigation bronchoscopy-guided radiofrequency ablation in two patients with nonsurgical stage IA lung cancer and one patient with solitary metastasis [81]. Electromagnetic navigation bronchoscopy was used to reach the lesions. Radial probe ultrasound was used to confirm appropriate positioning of extended working channel in relation to the tumor. One patient achieved complete response and two patients achieved partial response 3 months after the procedure. No complications were noted.

Although these reports establish technical feasibility of bronchoscopic radiofrequency ablation, many issues need to be clarified before this technique finds its way into mainstream treatment of early-stage lung cancer. To start, the most fundamental question is to decide who should receive radiofrequency ablation. Current standards of treatment are surgery or SBRT for early-stage lung cancer. Radiofrequency ablation cannot be considered a frontline therapy for these patients. Studies are needed to compare long-term outcome with surgery or SBRT and radiofrequency ablation. Such studies will clarify the role of RFA in treatment of early peripheral lung cancer. Until then, RFA can be considered as an alternative treatment option for early-stage peripheral lung cancer patients who are poor surgical candidates and have already received maximally tolerable radiation therapy. In such patients, bronchoscopic radiofrequency ablation may provide additional local control of tumor. Solitary metastasis can also be treated using this technique once primary tumor is controlled.

Better ability to navigate to the lesion with bronchoscopy is also paving way to explore other therapeutic modalities for peripheral lung cancer, which have been used in the past for centrally located lung cancer. In one report, ten patients with peripheral lung cancer were treated with ENB-guided brachytherapy [82]. All patients achieved clinical remission.

Several ongoing studies are also looking at possibility of ENB-guided photodynamic therapy for early-stage lung cancer. In one report, ENB-guided lung interstitial PDT was performed in three patients with malignant nodule [83]. The size of lesions varied from 8 mm to 36 mm. Patients underwent ENB bronchoscopy 48 hours after receiving intravenous Photofrin. A PDT probe was placed through extended working channel. Accurate positioning of PDT probe was confirmed using intra-procedural cone-beam CT. After successful placement, the peripheral tumor was exposed to 630 nm light. Evaluation with chest CT 3 months after the procedure revealed complete response in one patient and partial response in two patients. There were no procedure-related complications.

As with bronchoscopic RFA, brachytherapy and PDT are not likely to replace current standard therapies for malignant nodules, but they provide valuable therapeutic options for local control of tumors for patients who cannot undergo surgery and can no longer receive additional radiation therapy.

Emerging Techniques

The diagnostic yield of navigational bronchoscopy with or without application of radial probe ultrasound has remained significantly lower than that of CT-guided biopsy. There is great interest in further refinement in existing techniques and developing innovative technologies to improve diagnostic yield of bronchoscopy in small pulmonary nodules.

As discussed in prior sections, in many instances, the operators are able to navigate to the lesion, as confirmed with RP-EBUS, but the biopsies fail to provide tissue diagnosis. Navigational success notwithstanding, the inability to obtain diagnostic tissue makes bronchoscopy procedure unhelpful for the clinician and certainly a futile test for the patient. There is a need to narrow the gap between navigational success and diagnostic yield. There is a potential role for peripheral cryobiopsies in improving diagnostic yield in this situation. For example, in one study, Kho and associates compared the diagnostic yield of peripheral cryobiopsies and standard biopsies from peripheral nodules after a successful navigation, confirmed with RP-EBUS. For the lesions adjacent to airways on RP-EBUS, the diagnostic yield of cryobiopsies (75%) was significantly higher than that of standard forceps (49%). The diagnostic yield was similar when the bronchus was in the center of the lesion. Moderate bleeding was encountered in 8% of patients undergoing cryobiopsies [84].

Another major issue that limits the diagnostic yield of bronchoscopy is navigational error due to CT to body divergence. Improvements in existing guided navigational bronchoscopy platforms and introduction of newer platforms such as LungVision™ is an area of great interest to interventional pulmonologists. For example, superDimension™ has recently introduced a tomosynthesis-based fluoroscopic navigation system in which the lesion is located in real time with fluoroscopy, and local registration is performed to improve the accuracy of navigation to intended target. In a recent retrospective study, Aboudara and associates reported a 25% increase in diagnostic yield using this digital tomosynthesis-based platform compared with standard electromagnetic navigation technique. These results are encouraging, especially considering that 64% of the nodules in this study were smaller than 2 cm [85].

In addition to augmented fluoroscopy and tomosynthesis to correct for CT-body diversion, the new Illumisite™ platform from Medtronic has an additional feature. The catheter used during the procedure has a sensor embedded in it tips that continues to provide positional feedback to the operator even after the locatable guide is removed. Any movement of catheter tip away from the target can be detected and corrective actions may be taken before obtaining biopsies. This movement of catheter tip during the biopsy procedure was a significant problem with prior systems. This feature has the potential to reduce discrepancy between navigational success and actual diagnostic yield. Although clinical experience is limited, continuous guidance during an actual biopsy procedure makes intuitive sense. Illumisite™ platform has also introduced crossCountry™ transbronchial tool that allows the operator to approach and biopsy lesions that are outside the bronchus and cannot be reached with standard needles and biopsy forceps.

LungVision™ (Body Vision Medical LTD, Ramat HaSharon, Israel) is another recent platform that pairs 3-D map of the lung using pre-procedure chest CT with real-time fluoroscopic information to generate a path on fluoroscopy screen that a bronchoscopist can follow to navigate to the lesion. RP-EBUS is performed once the LungVision™ catheter tip reaches the augmented target. In a recent study, navigational success was 93% and diagnostic yield was 75% in 57 nodules with a median size of 2.0 cm [86].

Technical advances in navigational techniques are likely to improve the diagnostic yield of bronchoscopy in small nodules, but more prospective studies are needed to confirm these results. Bronchoscopists must also consider potential for excessive radiation exposure to patients and operators when using these techniques.

Another area of great excitement in this field is introduction of robotic bronchoscopy for biopsy of peripheral lung nodules [87]. Robotic bronchoscopy systems are said to have better maneuverability, more precise navigation, ability to reach deeper, and improved ability to navigate through tight corners and bends and stability of the tip during introduction of biopsy instruments. A major advantage of robotic system over EMN bronchoscopy is its ability to visualize airways directly as the operator is negotiating through smaller peripheral airways. Better control over distal tip of bronchoscope is another advantage that may serve to narrow the gap between navigational and diagnostic yields. Two Food and Drug Administration (FDA)-approved robotic bronchoscopy systems are Monarch™ (MA; Auris Health, Redwood City, CA) and Ion™ endoluminal platform (IEP; Intuitive, Sunnydale, CA). The Monarch™ system uses electromagnetic navigation along with 4.2 mm inner bronchoscope and 5.9 mm outer sheath that can be independently controlled by the robotic arms. The inner bronchoscope has a working channel of 2.1 mm. Initially, both outer sheath and inner bronchoscope are navigated toward the nodule. The outer sheath is firmly wedged into a segmental or sub-segmental bronchus, and the inner scope is advanced further toward the lesion. A cadaver study has reported a greater reach of robotic bronchoscope compared to a comparable-sized thin bronchoscope. Robotic bronchoscope performed much better than traditional bronchoscope in RB1 and LB 1 + 2 in this study [88]. A biopsy success of 97% was reported in a cadaver study in which biopsies were performed using this system on artificially implanted nodules of 10–30 mm diameter [89].

The Ion™ robotic system has a single bronchoscope with an outer diameter of 3.5 mm and a working channel of 2 mm. This system uses a unique shape-sensing technology to navigate toward the nodule following the path generated by the pre-procedure chest CT. Apart from usual accessories, a special flexible needle (Flexision™) can be used to obtain the tissue specimens.

Clinical studies using these systems have started to emerge and initial experience is encouraging. In a single center study from Costa Rica, Monarch system was used to obtain biopsy from 15 lung nodules [90]. Mean size of nodules was 2.6 cm. Cancer was confirmed in 9 of 15 (60%) patients. No significant adverse effects were encountered. In a recent post-marketing study of Monarch™ robotic endoscopic system that included 165 patients from 4 centers, the navigational success was 88.6% and biopsy yield was 69–77%. The average size of lesion was 2.5 cm and 71% were located in the peripheral third of the lung. Pneumothorax and pulmonary hemorrhage occurred in 3.6% and 2.4% of procedures, respectively [91]. Similar results have been reported in a recent multicenter trial in which Monarch™ robotic system was used in 54 patients with peripheral lung opacities from 1 to 5 cm in size. Navigation success based on RP-EBUS finding was 96.2%. Diagnostic yield was 74.1%. All procedures were performed under general anesthesia and pneumothorax occurred in 3.7% of cases [92]. Monarch™ robotic system has also been used for visceral pleural marking prior to surgical resection in 17 patients with 100% success [93].

Initial human experience with Ion™ robotic system is also encouraging. Fielding and associates used this system to obtain biopsies from 30 lesions with the mean size of 12.3 mm. The overall diagnostic yield was 80% and yield for malignancy was 88%. No major procedure-related complications were noted [94]. A large ongoing multicenter study (PRECISE trial) is currently studying the usefulness of this system for obtaining tissue diagnosis from peripheral lung nodules.

More data is needed to define the exact role of robotic bronchoscopy systems in small peripheral nodules. The technology is expensive, and it still falls short in dealing with the issue of CT to body diversion. Navigation still needs confirmation with complementary techniques such as RP-EBUS or cone-beam CT. An unbiased direct comparison with existing and other emerging techniques is needed before it can be recommended for a wider use. Certainly, there is potential for this technique to become a component of a modern hybrid theater for the appropriate and timely management of lung nodules as discussed below.

Future Directions

It is clear that the burden of CT-detected nodules will continue to increase and challenge pulmonologists, thoracic and interventional radiologists, radiation oncologists, and thoracic surgeons. Every time a lung nodule is detected, the primary goal is to identify and treat a malignant nodule with a curative intent while minimizing the invasive testing and surgical interventions for a benign nodule. This goal has not changed in the past several decades [6]. What has changed is how we approach these nodules to achieve the stated goal. The traditional piecemeal and territorial diagnostic and therapeutic approach to lung nodules is inefficient and is not patient centered. There is a clear need for paradigm shift. Several advanced healthcare facilities have recognized this need and have developed hybrid theaters to offer a more comprehensive and streamlined diagnostic and therapeutic approach to lung nodules [95]. The basic principle is to have advanced bronchoscopy techniques, real-time on-table cone-beam CT imaging, percutaneous intervention, and thoracic surgery expertise under the same roof. This allows all required services to be provided at the same time without requiring separate procedures and multiple visits to hospital. Despite high initial cost and commitment, such care can be very efficient, patient centered, safe, and cost-effective. Advanced bronchoscopy is a critical component of hybrid theaters. This allows interventional pulmonologists and thoracic surgeons to work closely for appropriate management of lung nodules. For instance, several studies have shown ENB-guided dye injection prior to video-assisted thoracoscopic surgery in hybrid theaters to be highly successful in localizing small peripheral nodules and ground glass opacities [96]. Compared to percutaneous hook wire placement, this approach obviates the need to transport the patient from the radiology department to the operating room, lowers the risk of pneumothorax, reduces operative time, and increases success of single-port video-assisted thoracoscopic surgery for peripheral lung nodules. In medically inoperable cases, broad capabilities of the hybrid theater can be used for diagnostic and staging procedures, for placement fiducials to facilitate SBRT, and for navigation bronchoscopy-guided therapies for lung cancer in appropriate candidates [97].

Approaching the lung nodules in such multidisciplinary fashion is no longer an option but is rapidly becoming a necessity. Hybrid theaters with broad capabilities and expertise are also proving to be an ideal venue for high-quality studies, innovations, and novel approaches [98]. It is certain that technical advances in the near future will further streamline the approach to the management of small lung nodules and bring interventional pulmonologists, interventional radiologists, radiation oncologists, and thoracic surgeons to work more closely than ever before.

References

1. National Lung Screening Trial Research Team, Aberle DR, Adams AM, Berg CD, et al. Reduced lung cancer mortality with low dose computed tomographic screening. N Engl J Med. 2011;365:395–409.
2. National Lung Screening Trial Research Team, Church TR, Black WC, Aberle DR, et al. Results of initial low-dose computed tomographic screening for lung cancer. N Engl J Med. 2013;368:1980–91.
3. Koning H, Aalst CM, Jong PA, et al. Reduced lung-cancer mortality with volume CT screening in a randomized trial. N Engl J Med. 2020;382:503–13.
4. Goodman DM. Initiatives focus on limiting radiation exposure to patients during CT scan. JAMA. 2013;309:647–8.
5. Hadique S, Jain P, Hadi Y, et al. Utility of FDG PET/CT for assessment of lung nodules identified during low dose computed tomography screening. BMC Med Imaging. 2020;20:69.
6. Jain P, Kathawalla SA, Arroliga AC. Managing solitary pulmonary nodules. Cleve Clin J Med. 1998;65:315–26.
7. Heo EY, Lee KW, Jheon S, et al. Surgical resection of highly suspicious lung nodules without a tissue diagnosis. Jpn J Clin Oncol. 2011;41:1017–22.

8. Cho J, Ko SJ, Kim SJ, et al. Surgical resection of nodular-ground glass opacity without percutaneous needle aspiration or biopsy. BMC Cancer. 2014;14:838.
9. National Comprehensive Network Guidelines on Non-small lung cancer version 2.2021. Online/html.
10. Mudambi L, Ost DE. Advanced bronchoscopic techniques for the diagnosis of peripheral pulmonary lesions. Curr Opin Pulm Med. 2016;22:309–18.
11. Khan KA, Nardelli P, Jaeger A, et al. Navigational bronchoscopy for early lung cancer: a road to therapy. Adv Ther. 2016;33:580–96.
12. DiBardino DM, Yarmus LB, Semann RW. Transthoracic needle biopsy of the lung. J Thorac Dis. 2015;7(Suppl4):S304–16.
13. Ohno Y, Hatabu H, Takenka D, et al. CT-guided transthoracic needle aspiration biopsy of small (< or = 20 mm) solitary pulmonary nodules. AJR Am J Roentgenol. 2003;180:1665–9.
14. Hiraki T, Mimura H, Gobara H, et al. CT fluoroscopy guided biopsy of 1000 pulmonary lesions performed with 20-gauge coaxial cutting needles: diagnostic yield and risk factors for diagnostic failure. Chest. 2009;136:1612–7.
15. Kim TJ, Lee JH, Lee CT, et al. Diagnostic accuracy of CT-guided core biopsy of ground glass opacity pulmonary lesions. AJR Am J Roentgenol. 2008;190:234–9.
16. Laurent F, Michel P, Latrabe V, et al. Pneumothoraces and chest tube placement after CT-guided transthoracic lung biopsy using a coaxial technique: incidence and risk factors. AJR Am J Roentgenol. 1999;172:1049–53.
17. Rivera MP, Mehta AC. Initial diagnosis of lung cancer. ACCP evidence-based clinical practice guidelines. 2nd edition. Chest. 2007;132(3 suppl):131S–48S.
18. Bilaceroglu S, Kumcuoglu Z, Alper H, et al. CT-bronchus sign guided bronchoscopic multiple diagnostic procedures in carcinomatous pulmonary nodules and masses. Respiration. 1998;65:49–55.
19. Gaeta M, Pandolfo I, Volta S, et al. Bronchus sign on CT in peripheral carcinoma of the lung. Value in predicting results of transbronchial biopsy. AJR Am J Roengenol. 1991;157:1181–5.
20. Gaeta M, Russi EG, La Spada F, et al. Small bronchogenic carcinomas presenting as solitary pulmonary nodules. Bioptic approach guided by CT-positive bronchus sign. Chest. 1992;102:1167–70.
21. Mazzone P, Jain P, Arroliga AC, Matthay RA. Bronchoscopic and needle biopsy techniques for diagnosis and staging of lung cancer. Clin Chest Med. 2002;23:137–58.
22. Ost DE, Ernst A, Lei X, et al. Diagnostic yield and complications of bronchoscopy for peripheral lung lesions. Results of the AQuIRE registry. Am J Respir Crit Care Med. 2016;193:68–77.
23. Asano F, Eberhardt R, Herth FJF. Virtual bronchoscopy navigation for peripheral pulmonary lesions. Respiration. 2014;88:430–40.
24. Ishida T, Asano F, Yamazaki K, et al. Virtual bronchoscopic navigation combined with endobronchial ultrasound to diagnose small peripheral pulmonary lesions: a randomized trial. Thorax. 2011;66:1072–7.
25. Oki M, Saka H, Ando M, et al. Ultrathin bronchoscopy with multimodal devices for peripheral pulmonary lesions. A randomized trial. Am J Respir Crit Care Med. 2015;192:468–76.
26. Asano F, Shinagawa N, Ishida T, et al. Virtual bronchoscopy navigation combined with ultrathin bronchoscopy. A randomized clinical trial. Am J Respir Crit Care Med. 2013;188:327–33.
27. Mehta AC, Hood KL, Schwarz Y, Solomon SB. The evolutionary history of electromagnetic navigation bronchoscopy. State of the art. Chest. 2018;154:935–47.
28. Kalanjeri S, Gildea TR. Electromagnetic navigational bronchoscopy for peripheral pulmonary nodules. Thorac Surg Clin. 2016;26:203–13.
29. Gildea TR, Mazzone PJ, Karnak D, et al. Electromagnetic navigation diagnostic bronchoscopy: a prospective study. Am J Respir Crit Care Med. 2006;174:982–9.
30. Gex G, Pralong JA, Combescure C, et al. Diagnostic yield and safety of electromagnetic navigation bronchoscopy for lung nodules: a systemic review and meta-analysis. Respiration. 2014;87:165–76.

31. Folch EF, Pritchett MA, Nead MA, et al. Electromagnetic bronchoscopy for peripheral pulmonary lesions: one year results of the prospective multicenter NAVIGATE study. J Thorac Oncol. 2019;14:445–58.
32. Khandhar SJ, Bowling MR, Flandes J, et al. Electromagnetic navigation bronchoscopy to access lung lesions in 1000 subjects: first results of the prospective, multicenter NAVIGATE study. BMC Pulm Med. 2017;17:59.
33. Bowling MR, Kohan MW, Walker P, Efird J, Or SB. The effect of general anesthesia versus intravenous sedation on diagnostic yield and success in electromagnetic navigation bronchoscopy. J Bronchol Intervent Pulmonol. 2015;22:5–13.
34. Eberhardt R, Anantham D, Ernst A, et al. Multimodality bronchoscopic diagnosis of peripheral lung lesions: a randomized controlled trial. Am J Respir Crit Care Med. 2007;176:36–41.
35. Pritchett MA, Schampaert S, de Groot JAH, Schirmer CC, van der Bom I. Cone-beam CT with augmented fluoroscopy combined with electromagnetic navigation bronchoscopy for biopsy of pulmonary nodules. J Bronchol Intervent Pulmonol. 2018;25:274–82.
36. Chenna P, Chen AC. Radial probe endobronchial ultrasound and novel navigation biopsy techniques. Semin Respir Crit Care Med. 2014;35:645–54.
37. Zhang L, Wu H, Wang G. Endobronchial ultrasonography using a guide sheath technique for diagnosis of peripheral pulmonary lesions. Endosc Ultrasound. 2017;6:292–9.
38. Oki M, Saka H, Kitagawa C, et al. Randomized study of endobronchial ultrasound guided transbronchial biopsy. Thin bronchoscopic method versus guide sheath method. J Thorac Oncol. 2012;7:535–41.
39. Chen A, Chenna P, Loiselle A, et al. Radial probe endobronchial ultrasound for peripheral pulmonary lesions. A 5-year institutional experience. Ann Am Thorac Soc. 2014;11:578–82.
40. Steinfort DP, Khor YH, Manser RL, Irving LB. Radial probe endobronchial ultrasound for the diagnosis of peripheral lung cancer: systematic review and meta-analysis. Eur Respir J. 2011;37:902–10.
41. Wang Memoli JS, Nietert PJ, Silvestri GA. Meta-analysis of guided bronchoscopy for the evaluation of the pulmonary nodule. Chest. 2012;142:385–93.
42. Ali MS, Trick W, Mba BI. Radial endobronchial ultrasound for the diagnosis of peripheral pulmonary lesions: a systematic review and meta-analysis. Respirology. 2017;22:443–53.
43. Izumo T, Sasada S, Chavez C, Tsuchida T. The diagnostic utility of endobronchial ultrasonography with a guide sheath and tomosynthesis images for ground glass opacity pulmonary lesions. J Thorac Dis. 2013;5:745–50.
44. Ikezawa Y, Shinagawa N, Sukoh N, et al. Usefulness of endobronchial ultrasonography with a guide sheath and virtual bronchoscopic navigation for ground-glass opacity lesions. Ann Thorac Surg. 2017;103:470–5.
45. Izumo T, Sasada S, Chavez C, et al. Radial endobronchial ultrasound images for ground glass opacity pulmonary lesions. Eur Respir J. 2015;45:1661–8.
46. Seijo LM, de Torres JP, Lozano MD, et al. Diagnostic yield of electromagnetic navigation bronchoscopy is highly dependent on the presence of a Bronchus sign on CT imaging: results from a prospective study. Chest. 2010;138:1316–21.
47. Herth FJF, Eberhardt R, Sterman D, Silvestri GA, Hoffmann H, Shah PL. Bronchoscopic transparenchymal nodule access (BTPNA): first in human trial of a novel procedure for sampling solitary pulmonary nodules. Thorax. 2015;70:326–32.
48. Harzheim D, Sterman D, Shah PL, Eberhardt R, Herth FJF. Nodule access: feasibility and safety in an endoscopic unit. Respiration. 2016;91:302–6.
49. Arias S, Yarmus L, Argento AC. Navigational transbronchial needle aspiration, percutaneous needle aspiration and its future. J Thorac Dis. 2015;7(Suppl 4):S317–28.
50. Yarmus LB, Arias S, Feller-Kopman D, et al. Electromagnetic navigation transthoracic needle aspiration for the diagnosis of pulmonary nodules: a safety and feasibility pilot study. J Thorac Dis. 2016;8:186–94.
51. Hohenforst-Schmidt W, Zarogoulidis P, Vogl T, et al. Cone beam computer tomography (CBCT) in interventional chest medicine – high feasibility for endobronchial realtime navigation. J Cancer. 2014;5:231–41.

52. Ng CHS, Yu SCH, Lau RWH, Yim APC. Hybrid DynaCT-guided electromagnetic navigational bronchoscopic biopsy. Eur J Cardiothorac Surg. 2016;49(suppl 1):i87–8.
53. Bowling MR, Brown C, Anciano CJ. Feasibility and safety of the transbronchial access tool for peripheral pulmonary nodule and mass. Ann Thorac Surg. 2017;104:443–9.
54. Hohenforst-Schmidt W, Banckwitz R, Zarogoulidis P, et al. Radiation exposure of patients by cone beam CT during endobronchial navigation - a phantom study. J Cancer. 2014;5:192–202.
55. Mack MJ, Hazelrigg SR, Landreneau RJ, Acuff TE. Thoracoscopy for the diagnosis of the indeterminate solitary pulmonary nodule. Ann Thorac Surg. 1993;56:825–30.
56. Bernard A. Resection of pulmonary nodules using video-assisted thoracic surgery. Thorax Group Ann Thorac Surg. 1996;61:202–4.
57. Chen S, Zhou J, Zhang J, et al. Video-assisted thoracoscopic solitary pulmonary nodule resection after CT-guided hookwire localization: 43 cases report and literature review. Surg Endosc. 2011;25:1723–9.
58. Thaete FL, Peterson MS, Plunkett MB, Ferson PF, Keenan RJ, Landreneau RJ. Computed tomography-guided wire localization of pulmonary lesions before thoracoscopic resection: results in 101 cases. J Thorac Imaging. 1999;14:90–8.
59. Awais O, Reidy MR, Mehta K, et al. Electromagnetic navigation bronchoscopy-guided dye marking for thoracoscopic resection of pulmonary nodules. Ann Thorac Surg. 2016;102:223–9.
60. Marino KA, Sullivan JL, Weksler B. Electromagnetic navigation bronchoscopy for identifying lung nodules for thoracoscopic resection. Ann Thorac Surg. 2016;102:454–7.
61. Bolton WD, Cochran T, Ben-Or S, et al. Electromagnetic navigational bronchoscopy reduces the time required for localization and resection of lung nodules. Innovations (Phila). 2017;12:333–7.
62. Lachkar S, Baste JM, Thiberville L, et al. Pleural dye marking using radial endobronchial ultrasound and virtual bronchoscopy before sublobar pulmonary resection for small peripheral nodules. Respiration. 2018;95:354–61.
63. Cao C, Wang D, Chung C, et al. A systemic review and meta-analysis of stereotactic body radiation therapy versus surgery for patients with non-small cell lung cancer. J Cardiovasc Thor Surg. 2019;157:362–73.
64. Sebastian NT, Xu-Welliver M, Williams TM. Stereotactic body radiation therapy (SBRT) for early stage non-small cell lung cancer (NSCLC): contemporary insights and advances. J Thorac Dis. 2018;10(suppl 21):S2451–64.
65. Molitoris JK, Diwanji T, Snider JW 3rd, et al. Advances in the use of motion management and image guidance in radiation therapy treatment for lung cancer. J Thorac Dis. 2018;10(Suppl 21):S2437–50.
66. Yousefi S, Collins BT, Reichner CA, et al. Complications of thoracic computed tomography-guided fiducial placement for the purpose of stereotactic body radiation therapy. Clin Lung Cancer. 2007;8:252–6.
67. Bhagat N, Fidelman N, Durack JC, et al. Complications associated with the percutaneous insertion of fiducial markers in the thorax. Cardiovasc Intervent Radiol. 2010;33:1186–91.
68. Ohta K, Shimohira M, Iwata H, et al. Percutaneous fiducial marker placement under CT fluoroscopic guidance for stereotactic body radiotherapy of the lung: an initial experience. J Radiat Res. 2013;54:957–61.
69. Whyte RI, Crownover R, Murphy MJ, et al. Stereotactic radiosurgery for lung tumors: preliminary report of a phase I trial. Ann Thorac Surg. 2003;75:1097–101.
70. Anantham D, Feller-Kopman D, Shanmugham L, et al. Electromagnetic navigation bronchoscopy—guided fiducial placement for robotic stereotactic radiosurgery of lung tumors: a feasibility study. Chest. 2007;132:930–5.
71. Harley DP, Krimsky WS, Sarkar S, et al. Fiducial marker placement using endobronchial ultrasound and navigational bronchoscopy for stereotactic radiosurgery: an alternative strategy. Ann Thorac Surg. 2010;89:368–74.
72. Nabavizadeh N, Zhang J, Elliott DA, et al. Electromagnetic navigational bronchoscopy-guided fiducial markers for lung stereotactic body radiation therapy: analysis of safety, feasibility, and interfraction stability. J Bronchology Interv Pulmonol. 2014;21:123–30.

73. Steinfort DP, Siva S, Kron T, et al. Multimodality guidance for accurate bronchoscopic insertion of fiducial markers. J Thorac Oncol. 2015;10:324–30.
74. Kular H, Mudambi L, Lazarus D, et al. Safety and feasibility of prolonged bronchoscopy involving diagnosis of lung cancer, systematic nodal staging, and fiducial marker placement in a high-risk population. J Thorac Dis. 2016;8:1132–8.
75. Schroeder C, Hejal R, Linden PA. Coil spring fiducial markers placed safely using navigation bronchoscopy in inoperable patients allows accurate delivery of CyberKnife stereotactic radiosurgery. J Thorac Cardiovasc Surg. 2010;140:1137–42.
76. Minnich DJ, Bryant AS, Wei B, et al. Retention rate of electromagnetic navigation bronchoscopic placed fiducial markers for lung radiosurgery. Ann Thorac Surg. 2015;100:1163–5.
77. Hadique S, Jain P, Mehta AC. Therapeutic bronchoscopy for central airway obstruction. In: Mehta AC, Jain P, editors. Interventional bronchoscopy. New York: Humana Press; 2013. p. 143–76.
78. Krimsky WS, Pritchett MA, Lau KK. Towards an optimization of bronchoscopic approaches to the diagnosis and treatment of the pulmonary nodules: a review. J Thorac Dis. 2018;10(Suppl 14):S1637–44.
79. Vieira T, Stern JB, Girard P, Caliandro R. Endobronchial treatment of peripheral tumors: ongoing development and perspectives. J Thorac Dis. 2018;10(Suppl 10):S1163–7.
80. Koizumi T, Tsushima K, Tanabe T, et al. Bronchoscopy-guided cooled radiofrequency ablation as a novel intervention therapy for peripheral lung cancer. Respiration. 2015;90:47–55.
81. Xie F, Zheng X, Xiao B, et al. Navigation bronchoscopy-guided radiofrequency ablation for nonsurgical peripheral pulmonary tumors. Respiration. 2017;94:293–8.
82. Harms W, Krempien R, Grehn C, et al. Electromagnetically navigated brachytherapy as a new treatment option for peripheral pulmonary tumors. Strahlenther Onkol. 2006;182:108–11.
83. Chen KC, Lee JM. Photodynamic therapeutic ablation for peripheral pulmonary malignancy via electromagnetic navigation bronchoscopy localization in a hybrid operating room (OR): a pioneering study. J Thorac Dis. 2018;10(suppl 6):S725–30.
84. Kho SS, Chan SK, Yong MC, Tie ST. Performance of transbronchial cryobiopsy in eccentrically and adjacent oriented radial endobronchial ultrasound lesions. ERJ Open Res. 2019;5:000135–2019.
85. Aboudara M, Roller L, Rickman O, et al. Improved diagnostic yield for lung nodules with digital tomosynthesis-correlated navigational bronchoscopy: initial experience with a novel adjunct. Respirology. 2020;25:206–13.
86. Cicenia J, Bhadra K, Sethi S, et al. Augmented fluoroscopy. A new and novel navigation platform for peripheral bronchoscopy. J Bronchol Intervent Pulmonol. 2020. https://doi.org/10.1097/LBR.0000000000000722. Online ahead of print.
87. Agrawal A, Hogarth DK, Murgu S. Robotic bronchoscopy for pulmonary lesions: a review of existing technologies and clinical data. J Thorac Dis. 2020;12:3279–86.
88. Chen AC, Gillespie CT. Robotic endoscopic airway challenge: REACH assessment. Ann Thorac Surg. 2018;106:293–7.
89. Chen AC, Pastis NJ, Machuzak MS, et al. Accuracy of a robotic endoscopy system in cadaver models with simulated tumor targets: ACCESS study. Respiration. 2020;99:56–61.
90. Rojas-Solano JR, Ugaldee-Gambao L, Machuzak M. Robotic bronchoscopy for diagnosis of suspected lung cancer. A feasibility study. J Bronchol Intervent Pulmonol. 2018;25:168–75.
91. Chaddha U, Kovacs SP, Manley C, Hogarth DK, et al. Robotic assisted bronchoscopy for pulmonary lesion diagnosis: result from the initial multicenter experience. BMC Pulm Med. 2019;19:243.
92. Chen AC, Pastis Jr NJ, Mahajan AK, et al. Robotic bronchoscopy for peripheral pulmonalry lesions: a multicenter pilot and feasibility study (BENEFIT). Chest. 2020;S0012-3692(20)34233-1. https://doi.org/10.1016/j.chest.2020.08.2047.
93. Chhaya R, Lam GT, Egan JP, Cumbo-Nacheli G. The use of robotic bronchoscopy for visceral pleural marking prior to surgical resection of pulmonary nodules. J Pulm Respir Med. 2020;10:4.

94. Fielding DIK, Bashirzadeh F, Son JH, et al. First human use of a new robotic-assisted fiber optic sensing navigation system for small peripheral pulmonary nodules. Respiration. 2019;98:142–50.
95. Zhao ZR, Lau RW, Yu PS, et al. Image-guided localization of small lung nodules in video-assisted thoracic surgery. J Thorac Dis. 2016;8(Suppl 9):S731–7.
96. Obeso A, Ng CSH. Electromagnetic navigation bronchoscopy in the thoracic hybrid operating room: a powerful tool for a new era. J Thorac Dis. 2018;10(Suppl 6):S764–8.
97. Schroeder C, Chung JM, Mitchell A, et al. Using the hybrid operating room in thoracic surgery: a paradigm shift. Innovations (Phila). 2018;13:372–7.
98. Ujiie H, Effat A, Yasufuku K. Image-guided thoracic surgery in the hybrid operation room. J Visc Surg. 2017;3:148.
99. Fielding D. Technologies for targeting the peripheral pulmonary nodule including robotics. Respirology. 2020;25:914–23.
100. Eberhardt R. Endobronchial ultrasound for peripheral lesions. In: Ernst A, Herth FJF, editors. Endobronchial ultrasound. New York: Springer Science+Business Media LLC; 2009. p. 103–17.
101. Mayse ML. Radiation therapy and techniques for fiducial placement. In: Ernst A, Herth FJF, editors. Principles and practice of interventional pulmonology. New York: Springer Science+Business Media; 2013. p. 391–407.

Chapter 4
Mediastinoscopy: Surgical Versus Medical

Kasia Czarnecka-Kujawa and Kazuhiro Yasufuku

Introduction

Mediastinal staging is a key component in evaluations of patient with lung cancer as it determines prognosis and guides management. Presence of mediastinal nodal metastasis signifies advanced disease and higher possibility of distant metastasis. For that reason, with some exceptions, patients with mediastinal nodal metastasis are offered nonsurgical therapy, while surgical management is reserved for patients without mediastinal nodal metastasis.

Mediastinal staging consists of preoperative and intraoperative assessments. Preoperative evaluation has a noninvasive component consisting of computerized tomography (CT) and positron emission tomography (PET) [1]. There is also an emerging data on the use of diffusion-weighted magnetic resonance imaging (DWI) in noninvasive lung cancer staging [2]. Invasive preoperative and operative staging includes surgical approaches of cervical mediastinoscopy (Med), anterior mediastinotomy, extended cervical mediastinoscopy, and more recently, video-assisted thoracoscopic surgery (VATS) and "supermediastinoscopies"- transcervical extended mediastinal lymphadenectomy (TEMLA), video-assisted mediastinal

K. Czarnecka-Kujawa
Division of Respirology, Toronto General Hospital, University Health Network, University of Toronto, Toronto, ON, Canada

Division of Thoracic Surgery, Toronto General Hospital, University Health Network, University of Toronto, Toronto, ON, Canada
e-mail: kasia.czarnecka@uhn.ca

K. Yasufuku (✉)
Division of Thoracic Surgery, Toronto General Hospital, University Health Network, University of Toronto, Toronto, ON, Canada
e-mail: kazuhiro.yasufuku@uhn.ca

© The Author(s), under exclusive license to Springer Nature Switzerland AG 2021
J. F. Turner, Jr. et al. (eds.), *From Thoracic Surgery to Interventional Pulmonology*, Respiratory Medicine,
https://doi.org/10.1007/978-3-030-80298-1_4

lymphadenectomy (VAMLA), and lymphadenectomy performed at the time of planned surgical resection.

Over the past decade, minimally invasive needle-based techniques of endobronchial ultrasound-guided transbronchial needle aspiration (EBUS-TBNA) and endoscopic ultrasound-guided fine needle aspiration (EUS-FNA) have become available and are now considered tests of first choice for invasive mediastinal staging [1, 3]. Pathological confirmation of nodal status is an important step in assessment of patients with lung cancer because the noninvasive techniques of CT chest and PET-CT lack diagnostic accuracy to guide clinical decision-making. ^{18}F-fluododeoxygluose (FDG)-avid lymph nodes (LN) are truly positive in 75–85% of patients. Only 60% of enlarged LNs (more than 1 cm in short axis) on CT chest harbor metastasis. This means that if there is no pathological confirmation of the noninvasive staging results, 15–40% of patients could be denied a curative surgical management of cancer because of false-positive noninvasive tests [1, 4].

In this chapter, we plan to discuss the clinical importance and mediastinal LN staging in lung cancer and the basic diagnostic approach to noninvasive mediastinal LN staging and its limitations, address the indications for invasive mediastinal LN staging, provide a historical perspective on the approaches to invasive mediastinal LN staging in lung cancer, outline the advantages and limitations of surgical and nonsurgical strategies, discuss the paradigm shift in mediastinal LN staging toward the use of minimally invasive techniques of EBUS-TBNA and EUS-FNA, and discuss the new technologies in mediastinal LN staging.

Scope of the Problem

Lung cancer is the leading cause of cancer mortality worldwide [5]. Despite evolving knowledge of lung cancer and its molecular genetics and improved ways of detection, the overall 5-year survival is still poor at approximately 18% [5]. Survival in lung cancer is driven by the stage of disease at presentation, with over 90% 5-year survival in patients with clinical stage IA disease to only 10% in stage IVA and 0% in stage IVB [6]. Presence of mediastinal nodal metastasis is associated with significant reduction in 5-year survival (~36% for stage IIIA disease vs. 53% for stage IIB disease) [6]. Mediastinal LN involvement signifies advanced disease and increased risk of distant metastasis with reported disease progression at 16 weeks of 70% in patients with N2 and N3 disease [7]. This most likely reflects presence of distant micrometastasis in patients with mediastinal nodal involvement that may not be apparent at the time of original evaluation. Since benefit of surgery in lung cancer has been limited to patients in whom complete resection, including sterilization of all mediastinal involvement, can be accomplished, with few exceptions, patients with mediastinal nodal metastasis are treated with chemotherapy and radiation, rather than with curative surgery. Accurate preoperative mediastinal staging is, therefore, crucial to avoid noncurative resection.

From management perspective, mediastinal LN involvement can be divided into three distinct categories: (1) incidental/occult, micrometastatic disease (detected either at the time of curative resection during intraoperative "quick section" or in the final surgical specimen in patients with clinical N0 and N1 disease on preoperative staging, (2) discrete but potentially resectable, and (3) bulky unresectable or infiltrative disease [8]. In patients with occult mediastinal metastasis, complete resection with systematic mediastinal LN evaluation is recommended as these patients have been shown to have improved survival as compared with patients with N2 nodal disease detected on preoperative staging. This could be related to different lung cancer biology in patients with nodal disease detected on preoperative staging as compared to those with occult metastatic disease (i.e., higher disease burden, more rapid progression of metastasis, and overall more advanced disease at the time of original assessment). Different management strategies are possible for patients with resectable or potentially resectable disease including surgical resection with a combination of chemotherapy and radiation. Current guidelines recommend multi-disciplinary approach to management of this patient population [9]. Patients with clearly unresectable disease should be managed medically with chemotherapy and radiation as numerous prospective trails have demonstrated that adjuvant therapy does not increase resectability and incomplete resection does not result in survival benefit [8].

Data on natural history of lung cancer is sparse given that most patients receive some sort of therapy. Data from patients who are not candidates for any type of therapy because of medical comorbidities is confounded by multiple medical comorbidities that can contribute to decreased survival. For medically inoperable patients with stage I and II disease, one study reported overall 14-month survival for patients who did not receive any therapy vs. 21-month and 46-month survival in stage-matched patients treated with radiotherapy and surgery, respectively [10]. Diagnostic workup in lung cancer can take a significant amount of time with some studies quoting an over 100-day delay between disease detection and initiation of treatment [11]. However, delay in diagnostic assessment and management in patients with lung cancer has been associated with disease progression [7]. Clinical disease progression rates of 13%, 21%, and 46% at 4, 8, and 16 weeks, respectively, have been reported. Overall, stage advancement of 13% and 21% at 8 and 16 weeks, respectively, have been reported [7]. Prompt patient evaluation, including noninvasive and invasive mediastinal staging, and management are key in ensuring success of the selected management modality and curability. The British Thoracic Society and Canadian Society of Surgical Oncology and Canadian Association of Thoracic Surgery recommend that curative surgery be performed within 4 weeks of patient evaluation except for patients selected for induction therapy. If there is a delay in access to surgical management of more than 8 weeks, restaging imaging is strongly recommended [12, 13].

Routine evaluation of patients with suspected lung cancer includes CT of the chest. PET scan is recommended in all but peripheral stage IA tumors and pure ground glass lesions [4]. CT chest is the first assessment modality that allows for evaluation of intrathoracic disease extent and guides further diagnostic interventions. Systematic review and meta-analysis of studies evaluating CT chest performance in mediastinal LN staging in patients with lung cancer showed sensitivity ranging between 55% and 64% with specificity of 81% [4, 14]. Due to low CT sensitivity, as many as 20–25% of patients with clinical N0-N1 disease based on CT chest assessment will have N2 or N3 disease on subsequent surgical LN sampling [1]. Conversely, as many as 20% of patients suspected of having nodal metastasis on CT chest will not in fact harbor metastatic disease.

High accuracy of PET in differentiation between malignant and benign lesions, as well as detection of distant and mediastinal metastasis, has made it a crucial diagnostic modality in evaluation of patients with suspected lung cancer. PET has much higher than CT sensitivity and specificity in mediastinal LN staging with multiple randomized controlled trials, systematic reviews, and meta-analysis available. The first study to assess utility of PET in assessment of patients with lung cancer showed that staging with PET reduces rate of unnecessary thoracotomies by correct identification of mediastinal nodal disease and distant metastasis (19/92 [21%] in the PET arm vs. 39/96 [41%] in the conventional staging) which corresponded to 51% relative risk reduction in futile thoracotomies with the use of PET staging [15]. Studies in early lung cancer (predominantly stage I disease) showed that the use of PET results in stage change in 18% of patients and management change in 13% predominantly due to identification of N2 disease [16]. A meta-analysis on PET demonstrated pooled sensitivity of 74% (90% CI, 69–79%) and specificity of 85% (95% CI, 82–88%). Development of PET/CT has brought the presumed advantage of making a correlation between the anatomic location and metabolic activity of the tissues. Integrated PET/CT shows improved CT chest and PET diagnostic accuracy in mediastinal LN staging in lung cancer with multiple single center, randomized controlled studies, meta-analysis, and recently a Cochrane database review. Overall sensitivity, specificity, PPV, and NPV were 77.4% (95% CI 65.3–86.1), 90.1% (95% CI 85.3–93.5), 65% (95% CI 43–80), and 95% (95% CI 90–98), respectively [17–22]. Integrated PET/CT decreases the rate of futile thoracotomies (resections in patients with N2/3 disease [stage IIIA disease or higher] or benign disease). Preventing 1 unnecessary thoracotomy per five PET/CT scans [18]. However, PET/CT is associated with a significant false-positive rate ranging between 5% and 15% [20, 21]. False-positive results may occur in inflammatory, nonmalignant lesions (pneumonia, sarcoidosis, chronic, smoking-related bronchitis). For that reason, positive PET/CT findings should always be confirmed pathologically.

False-negative PET/CT results may occur in micrometastatic disease, in smaller lesions (<1 cm) and in well-differentiated, low-grade malignancies (including adenocarcinomas) [22]. PET/CT has shown high diagnostic accuracy in assessment of T1N0 lesions with documented prevalence of mediastinal metastasis in patients with clinical T1N0M0 (stage IA) disease and peripheral tumors of 4%, suggesting that invasive mediastinal staging in this patient population can be omitted [1].

Based on this evidence, international thoracic and pulmonology associations, including the American College of Chest Physicians (ACCP), European Society of Thoracic Surgeons (ESTS), and Cancer Care Ontario (CCO), independently devised mediastinal LN staging guidelines in patients with NSLC, showing concordance in their recommendations (Table 4.1) [4, 23, 24]. Invasive mediastinal LN staging is not

Table 4.1 Indications for invasive mediastinal staging in NSCLC

American College of Chest Physicians (ACCP) Mediastinal Staging Guidelines [1]
Absence of extrathoracic disease and any of:
Mediastinal lymphadenopathy (short axis of >1 cm) with or without LN FDG avidity
Mediastinal lymphadenopathy and FDG-avid in any mediastinal (N2–N3), hilar, or interlobar (N1–N3) LNs
Central tumor (inner 2/3 of the lung) with or without mediastinal lymphadenopathy or FDG avidity in N1-N3 LNs
European Society of Thoracic Surgeons (ESTS) Guidelines [2]
Abnormal LNs on CT chest
FDG-avid LNs on PET
Central tumors (inner 2/3 of the lung)
Suspicion on N1 disease (based on CT or PET findings)
Low FDG avidity of the primary tumor
Tumors >3 cm in size
Cancer Care Ontario Guidelines [3]
Mediastinal lymphadenopathy (CT chest)
FDG-avid LNs on PET
Central tumors (inner 2/3 of the lung)
Clinical N1 disease
Tumors >3 cm in size

recommended for peripheral (outer 1/3 of the lung), stage IA tumors and no suspicion of mediastinal disease (based on CT and PET assessment) [1, 23, 24]. In infiltrative mediastinal disease diagnostic, rather than staging mediastinal assessment is suggested, using the mediastinal staging technique with the best diagnostic performance (based on the local availability and local test performance characteristics) [1, 25].

Traditional Approach to Mediastinal Lymph Node Staging

Until just over two decades ago, invasive mediastinal staging was performed with the use of surgical invasive techniques including mediastinoscopy, specifically cervical mediastinoscopy [Med], and less commonly, left anterior mediastinotomy (aka Chamberlain's procedure). In addition, extended cervical mediastinoscopy and, more recently, video-assisted thoracoscopic surgery (VATS) and "supermediastinoscopies"- transcervical extended mediastinal lymphadenectomy (TEMLA) and video-assisted mediastinal lymphadenectomy (VAMLA) have become available [26, 27].

Cervical Mediastinoscopy [Med]

Med is a surgical technique that allows for exploration of the mediastinum along the tracheobronchial structures, from the sternal notch to the subcarinal space and along both main bronchi [28]. Procedure is performed under general anesthesia and orotracheal intubation. Three to 5 cm incision is made over the sternal notch with

Fig. 4.1 Finger palpation of the superior mediastinum through the collar incision for mediastinoscopy. The innominate artery is palpated anteriorly

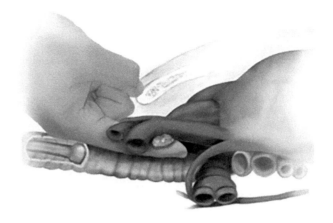

patient in supine position. Incision is extended through the subcutaneous tissues and the platysma muscle. Pretracheal muscles are separated to expose the trachea and pretracheal fascia is incised with scissors to develop pretracheal plane. The mediastinum is explored by blunt finger dissection as far caudally as possible (Fig. 4.1). Mediastinoscope is inserted into the space created by the finger dissection for the biopsies to be performed (full technique is described elsewhere) [29]. Med allows access to the pretracheal (station 1), upper paratracheal (stations 2R and 2L), lower paratracheal (stations 4R and 4L), anterior subcarinal (station 7), as well as hilar (stations 10R and 10L) LNs. Med cannot access the pulmonary ligament (station 9), paraesophageal (station 8), posterior subcarinal (station 7), and aortopulmonary window (stations 5 and 6) LNs. The video-assisted Med has now replaced the traditional Med in majority of thoracic surgery centers, increasing procedure safety and diagnostic performance in lung cancer staging. In mediastinal LN staging of primary lung cancer, Med yield depends on LN location and operator skills [30, 31]. Recently reported systematic review of conventional (26 studies reviewed between 1983 and 2011 with 9267 patients included) and video-assisted Med (7 studies reviewed between 2003 and 2011, with 995 patients included) performance in NSCLC staging showed median sensitivity and NPV of conventional and video-assisted Med of 0.78 and 0.91 and 0.89 and 0.92, respectively [1].

Generally, Med is a safe procedure, performed in outpatient setting. Reported complication rate is up to 3%, including a pneumothorax, infection, and injury to the major mediastinal vessels (which can lead to a life-threatening bleeding), peripheral nerves (which can result in vocal cord palsy), bronchi, and esophagus. Mortality has been reported at 0.08% in relation to vascular injury [32–35]. The procedure is contraindicated in patients with tracheostomy, severe cervical spine arthritis, or instability that prohibits neck extension. Mediastinal adhesions may make a repeat Med challenging [32, 36, 37].

Variants of Mediastinoscopic Lymphadenectomy

Video-assisted mediastinoscopic lymphadenectomy (VAMLA) and transcervical extended mediastinal lymphadenectomy (TEMLA) are surgical procedures performed from collar incision used to perform Med, but the objective of these procedures is not to take LN biopsies but to perform systematic lymphadenectomy [29].

VAMLA is performed with a two-blade separable mediastinoscope. Subcarinal (station 7) and right inferior paratracheal (4R) LNs are removed en block. Station 4L is removed separately [38]. VAMLA sensitivity in lung cancer staging is 0.96 (95% CI, 0.81–99.3); specificity, 1 (95% CI, 0.97–1); PPV, 1 (95% CI, 0.87–1); NPV, 0.99 (95% CI, 0.95–0.99); and diagnostic accuracy, 0.99 (95% CI, 0.96–0.99).

In contrast to the VAMLA, transcervical extended mediastinal lymphadenectomy (TEMLA) is an open technique performed with the use of videomediastinoscope or videothoracoscope allowing access to stations 1, 2R, 2L, 3a, 4R, 4L, 5, 6, 7, and 8 LNs. Large number of nodes can be removed with this technique (mean, 43; range, 26–85) [26, 27]. Reported sensitivity and NPV of TEMLA for detection of mediastinal LN metastases are 0.9 and 0.95, respectively. In contrast to other surgical mediastinal sampling methods, TEMLA and VAMLA offer complete lymphadenectomy [38]. However, the high rate of complications (6.0–13.2%) including recurrent laryngeal nerve palsy, respiratory decompensation, arrhythmia, pneumothorax, vascular injury requiring an open repair complicated by persistent severe neurological deficit and mortality rate of 1.2% (TEMLA), post-procedure clinical status deterioration preventing surgical management in as many as 20% of qualifying patients, and a long procedure time (mean 161 min, range 80–330 min) (TEMLA) makes use of both, VAMLA and TEMLA, unpopular given development of endoscopic techniques with comparable diagnostic yield but much better safety profile and shorter procedure duration [26, 27, 38–40].

Parasternal Mediastinotomy

Parasternal mediastinotomy allows access to the subaortic (station 5), para-aortic (station 6) (L sided), and prevascular (station 3a) LNs [41]. Four to 7 cm transverse incision is made over the second costal cartilage on the R or on the L down to the pectoralis major muscle. The cartilage may be excised or alternatively, the procedure may be performed thorough intercostal space. Internal mammary vessels need to be ligated or retraced. Mediastinal pleura needs to be separated laterally with finger dissection to expose the anterior mediastinum (Fig. 4.2). The L subaortic and para-aortic space may be assessed directly or with the use of mediastinoscope (anterior mediastinotomy, aka Chamberlain's procedure). On the R, prevascular LNs can be reached. Parasternal mediastinoscopy is a versatile procedure, not only allowing for the exploration of the anterior mediastinum but also allowing for the opening of the mediastinal pleura, exploration of the hilum and the pleural space, and opening

Fig. 4.2 Digital
exploration of subaortic
space during combined
cervical and anterior
mediastinotomy.
(Reprinted with permission
from Shields [46])

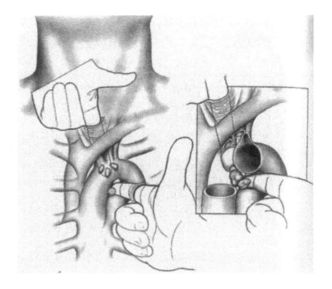

of the pericardium to assess for possible tumor invasion. Additionally, lung biopsies can be performed this way (single lung ventilation is optimal for these additional procedures) [29]. Reported sensitivity and NPV of anterior mediastinotomy in assessment of AP window LNs are 78% and 91%, respectively [1]. Complications of this technique are rare and include injury to the phrenic and recurrent laryngeal nerve, mediastinitis, and pneumothorax. Given technical challenges in accessing the anterior mediastinum (i.e., navigation around great vessels) and a convenient and relatively simple access to the AP window LNs via L VATS approach, VATS has been increasingly replacing this technique for staging purposes in patients with indications to sample AP window LNs.

Extended Cervical Mediastinoscopy

Extended cervical mediastinoscopy, introduced by Kirschner in 1971 and popularized by Ginsburg, allows access to the AP window LNs, stations 2, 4, and 7 [42–44]. The technique starts with standard mediastinoscopy, and once that is completed, a passage is created by finger dissection over the aortic arch between the innominate and the L carotid arteries. Mediastinoscope is inserted over the aortic arch either anterior or posterior to the L innominate vain [29] (Fig. 4.3). Reported sensitivity of extended mediastinoscopy ranges from 71% to 81%, while NPV is 91% [41]. Complications are uncommon (2.3%) including pneumothorax, mediastinitis, ventricular fibrillation, and minor bleeding controlled with compression [38, 45]. One intraoperative death has been reported from aortic injury [29]. Just like parasternal mediastinoscopy, extended cervical mediastinoscopy is performed infrequently with VATS being used increasingly more commonly for access to the subaortic LNs given limited maneuverability of the mediastinoscope in the anterior mediastinum.

Fig. 4.3 Extended cervical
mediastinoscopy. From the
cervical incision used for
mediastinoscopy, the
mediastinoscope is
advanced obliquely over
the aortic arch

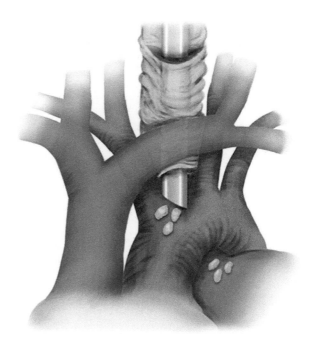

VATS and Thoracoscopy

VATS and video-thoracoscopy have been used for mediastinal LN staging allowing
for exploration of the ipsilateral mediastinum (stations 2 and 4), hilar [10], interlobar [11], and inferior mediastinal LNs (stations 8 and 9). VATS has progressively
replaced anterior mediastinotomy and extended cervical mediastinoscopy in
patients who need sampling of the para-aortic (station 6) and subaortic (station 5)
LNs. Because of access to the thoracic cavity from the lung apex to the diaphragm,
video-thoracoscopy and VATS not only can be used for mediastinal staging but also
can help with the T and M components of lung cancer staging given the access to
pericardial cavity and pleura. Techniques have been described elsewhere [46].
VATS sensitivity and PPV in mediastinal LN staging in a series of four studies
including 246 patients were 0.95 and 0.96, respectively [1]. Video-thoracoscopy
done before the planned lung resection can prevent futile resections in 4.4% of
patients (mainly due to identification of mediastinal invasion [1.4%], pleural dissemination [2.1%], or involvement of adjacent structures in non-pneumonectomy
candidates. Video-thoracoscopy has nigh NPV in excluding unresectability (0.97)
[47]. Procedure-related complications are rare (~5%) and include air leak, subcutaneous emphysema, chest pain, bleeding, surgical wound infection, and empyema
[29]. Comparison of intrathoracic LN access by all surgical techniques is provided
in Table 4.2.

Table 4.2 Intrathoracic LN access by different surgical and endoscopic techniques

LN station	Staging techniques							
	Med	VAMLA	TEMLA	Anterior mediastinotomy	Extended cervical mediastinoscopy	VATS	EBUS-TBNA	EUS-FNA
1	✓	✗	✓	✗	✓	✗	✗	✗
2R	✓	✓	✓	✗	✓	✓[a]	✓	✓
2L	✓	✓	✓	✗	✓	✓[a]	✓	✓
3A	✗	✗	✓	✗	✗	✗	✗	✗
3P	✗	✗	✗	✗	✗	✓	✓	✗
4R	✓	✓	✓	✗	✓	✓[a]	✓	✓
4L	✓	✓	✓	✗	✓	✓[a]	✓	✓
5	✗	✗	✓	✓	✓	✓[b]	✗	✗
6	✗	✗	✓	✓	✓	✓[b]	✗	✗
7	✓	✓	✓	✗	✓	✓[a]	✓	✓
8	✗	✗	✓	✗	✗	✓[a]	✗	✓
9	✗	✗	✗	✗	✗	✓[a]	✗	✓
10	✓	✓	✓	✗	✗	✓[a]	✓	✗
11	✗	✗	✗	✗	✗	✓[a]	✓[c]	✗
12	✗	✗	✗	✗	✗	✓[a]	✓[c]	✗

Abbreviations: *Med* cervical mediastinoscopy, *VAMLA* video-assisted mediastinoscopic lymphadenectomy, *TEMLA* transcervical extended mediastinal lymphadenectomy, *VATS* video-assisted thoracoscopic surgery, *EBUS-TBNA* endobronchial ultrasound-guided transbronchial needle aspiration, *EUS-FNA* endoscopic ultrasound-guided fine needle aspiration
Symbols: [a]ipsilateral, [b]left-sided only, [c]some, no access to the upper lobe N1 lymph nodes

Role of Interventional Pulmonology Procedures in Mediastinal LN Staging in NSCLC

The idea of nonsurgical mediastinal LN staging in lung cancer was born with the introduction of radial probe endobronchial ultrasound (RP-EBUS) in the early 1990s [48–51]. Beside its role in diagnosis of peribronchial lesions [52, 53], RP-EBUS has been used to guide transbronchial needle aspiration (TBNA) in patients with mediastinal lymphadenopathy and in lung cancer mediastinal LN staging. Diagnostic yield of RP-EBUS-guided TBNA of mediastinal LNs ranged between 72% and 80% (in a population with high prevalence of mediastinal nodal metastasis [86%]) [51, 54]. But RP-EBUS has not been able to provide the same systematic mediastinal LN assessment Med has. For that reason, for decades, Med had been considered the test of first choice for mediastinal LN staging in lung cancer. However, introduction of endobronchial ultrasound-guided transbronchial needle aspiration (EBUS-TBNA) and esophageal ultrasound-guided fine needle aspiration (EUS-FNA), showing equivalent or better performance than Med in mediastinal LN staging in primary lung cancer, has led to paradigm shift. Currently, multiple international thoracic surgery and pulmonology and cancer organizations recommend the needle-based techniques as tests of first choice in mediastinal LN staging in primary lung cancer [1, 24, 32, 55, 56].

CP-EBUS is a flexible bronchoscope integrated with a convex transducer at the tip which scans parallel to the insertion direction of the bronchoscope. Insertion tube distal end outer and scope outer diameters are 6.9 mm and 6.3 mm, respectively (Table 4.3).

Table 4.3 Comparison of the endoscopes, EBUS-TBNA, *thin EBUS-TBNA, prototype, tested in animal and ex vivo models; EUS-FNA scopes

Endoscope	EBUS-TBNA	Thin EBUS-TBNA*	EUS-FNA
Tip diameter (mm)	6.9	5.9	13–14.6
Endoscope diameter (mm)	6.3	5.7	11.8–12.8
Scanning range (degree)	50	60	120–180
Channel size (mm)	2.2	1.7	2.8–3.7
Needle sizes for use (gauge)	19, 21, 22, 25	25	19, 21, 22, 25

Refs. [1, 23, 24]

Incorporation of EBUS at the tip of a flexible bronchoscope allows for real-time TBNA of the visualized structures (LNs, tumors). The ultrasound probe has B-mode and power color Doppler capabilities, allowing differentiation of LNs from vascular structures.

Like Med, CP-EBUS can access stations 2R, 2L, 4R, 4L, and 7 LNs. Posteriorly and deep located station 7 LNs may not be readily accessible to Med, resulting in false-negative results, but can be easily assessed with EBUS-TBNA [30, 57]. EBUS-TBNA can reach N1 LNs, including the hilar (station 10), interlobar (station 11), and some of the lobar LNs (station 12) which are not accessible to Med. However, not all interlobar and lobar LN locations are accessible to the currently commercially available CP-EBUS because of its size and flexion angle. A new thin CP-EBUS (BF-Y0046, Olympus, Japan) is currently under development with the goal of improving EBUS-TBNA capabilities in the interlobar and lobar regions [58, 59]. Some groups access station 5 LN using trans-pulmonary approach. Given the procedure risks (major artery puncture at a non-compressible site), this approach is not routinely recommended given safer alternative (L VATS) [60].

Neither EBUS-TBNA nor Med can access prevascular (3A), para-aortic (station 6), paraesophageal (station 8), and pulmonary ligament (station 9) nodes.

Bronchoscopic examination of the airway should be performed with a regular flexible bronchoscope before EBUS-TBNA. After administration of local anesthesia and conscious sedation, the CP-EBUS is inserted orally and passed through the vocal cords by visualizing the anterior angle of the glottis. Once the bronchoscope is introduced into the airway until the desired LN station is reached (Fig. 4.4a), the balloon is inflated with normal saline to achieve a maximum contact with the tissue of interest. The tip of the CP-EBUS is flexed and gently pressed against the airway (Fig. 4.4b). Ultrasonically visible vascular landmarks are used to identify the specific LN stations as per the International Lymph Node Map devised by the International Association for the Study of Lung Cancer (IASLC) [61]. The Doppler

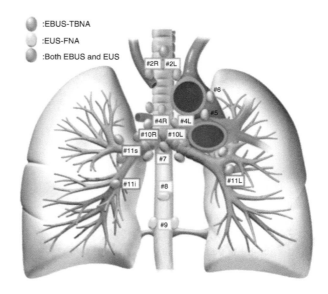

Fig. 4.4 Regional lymph node map for lung cancer staging. Most mediastinal lymph nodes can routinely be assessed with a combination of endobronchial ultrasound-guided transbronchial needle aspiration (EBUS-TBNA) and endoscopic ultrasound-guided fine needle aspiration (EUS-FNA) with the exception of stations 5 and 6. EBUS-TBNA can also sample some N1 nodes. (Reprinted with permission from Yasufuku [62])

mode is used to confirm and identify surrounding vessels as well as the blood flow within lymph nodes. After identifying the lesion of interest, bronchoscopic image of the airway is simultaneously visualized to localize the insertion point of the needle. Once the point of entry is decided using airway landmarks, the TBNA needles are attached to the working channel of the scope, and the sheath is protruded to the desired length by loosening the sheath knob adjustor (Fig. 4.4c, d). The scope is then flexed up to visualize the LN on the ultrasonic image. Location of the needle insertion point is chosen between the cartilage rings by following the white light image (Fig. 4.4f). Needle is protruded out of the sheath at the desired location, and once the needle position within the lymph node is conformed with the ultrasound image, internal stylet is used to clear the needle channel of debris, and removed. TBNA is performed using cutting motion of the needle within the LN (Fig. 4.4g) [62].

EBUS-TBNA is a safe procedure, with an average complication rate of 1.23% (95% CI 0.97–1.48%). Reported complications include hemorrhage (0.68%), infection (0.19%) (mediastinitis, pneumonia, pericarditis, cyst infection, sepsis), and pneumothorax (0.03%). EBUS-TBNA reported mortality is 0.01% [63–65]. EBUS-TBNA is a day procedure that can be performed safely in an endoscopy suite, under conscious sedation [66].

EUS-FNA

EUS-FNA is performed by using a side-viewing dedicated videogastroscope with a curved linear-array transducer attached on the tip. Different companies manufacture EUS scopes. The outer diameter of the EUS scope insertion tube ranges from 11.8 to 12.8 mm, and that of the tip is 13–14.6 mm. Instrument channel inner diameter measures 2.8–3.7 mm. The dedicated 22-gauge needles are usually used, but smaller (25-gauge) and larger (19-gauge) needles are also available (Table 4.3). The ultrasonographic image is processed by connecting the EUS scope to either the dedicated ultrasound scanner (EU-C60; Olympus), the universal endoscopic ultrasound scanner (EU-ME1; Olympus), or the Aloka Prosound Alpha5 (Aloka), enabling tissue visualization at a radius of 2–10 cm around the esophagus [62]. After introduction, the EUS scope is advanced into the distal esophagus and then slowly withdrawn while making circular movements. Anatomic landmarks such as the inferior vena cava, right and left atrium, azygos vein, main pulmonary artery, and aorta are identified. If present, LNs are described and numbered as per the International Lymph Node Map devised by the IASLC [61]. Lymph nodes are then usually biopsied with a 22-gauge needle under real-time ultrasound guidance with monitoring of the needle during insertion and aspiration. EUS can access the pulmonary ligament (station 9), paraesophageal (station 8), subcarinal (station 7), and paratracheal (stations 2, 4) lymph nodes. In addition, EUS-FNA can access L adrenal, celiac axis LNs, and L lobe of the liver, which can be useful in ruling out stage IV disease. EUS usually cannot access the perivascular (station 3a), subaortic (station 5), para-aortic (station 6), and N1 lymph nodes. EUS is a safe procedure with most of the complications related only to FNA. The complications include bleeding (0–1.3%), perforation (0–0.4%), and infection (0.3%). The risk of bacteremia is low and prophylactic antibiotics are not recommended except for EUS-FNA of pancreatic cystic lesions [67–69]. Comparison of intrathoracic LN access among surgical and endoscopic techniques is provided in Table 4.2.

Endoscopic Techniques: Performance in Mediastinal LN Staging

First study reporting on EBUS-TBNA in mediastinal LN staging in lung cancer showed sensitivity of 94.5%, specificity and PPV of 100%, NPV of 89.5%, and diagnostic accuracy of 96.3% [55]. The prevalence of mediastinal nodal metastasis was 63%. In 19% of patients, in addition to offering staging information, EBUS-TBNA provided diagnostic information, eliminating the need for further invasive tests. EBUS-TBNA staging prevented 29 mediastinoscopies, 8 thoracotomies, 4 thoracoscopies, and 9 percutaneous LN biopsies, streamlining the diagnostic workup [55]. Another study of EBUS-TBNA staging in a population with high prevalence of mediastinal nodal metastasis (98.2%) and mediastinal lymphadenopathy confirmed high diagnostic performance of EBUS-TBNA with sensitivity, specificity, diagnostic yield, and accuracy of 94%, 100%, 93%, and 94%, respectively. However, NPV was only 11%, suggesting that in a population of patients with high pretest probability of mediastinal nodal metastasis, confirmatory Med or other staging procedure should be performed to exclude false negatives [70].

EBUS-TBNA can accurately distinguish between the pathological N0 and N1 disease with sensitivity, specificity, diagnostic accuracy, and NPV of 73%, 100%, 96.6%, and 96.2%, respectively [71]. Overall, EBUS-TBNA can correctly identify mediastinal nodal metastasis in ~one out of three patients with clinical N0 disease. Given EBUS-TBNA safety profile and the advantage of access to N1 LNs, staging with EBUS-TBNA may become an important step in workup of patients with early lung cancer.

To date, systematic reviews and four meta-analyses evaluated performance of EBUS-TBNA in lung cancer staging [1, 72–75]. Populations with different prevalence of mediastinal nodal metastasis were included (prevalence range 33.7–99.3%). Data from nearly 3000 patients were analyzed, 36 studies, spanning 12 years (from 2002 to 2012). Overall, EBUS-TBNA demonstrated excellent sensitivity and specificity of 0.88–0.93 (95% CI 0.79–0.94) and 1.00 (95% CI 0.92–1.00), respectively, and an NPV of 91% (range 83–96%) [1, 72–74].

EBUS-TBNA performance in mediastinal LN staging in lung cancer has also been compared to that of Med, in prospective studies [30, 31, 57] and recently in a meta-analysis [76]. Populations with moderate and high prevalence of mediastinal nodal metastasis were assessed (prevalence ranged from 32% to 89%). Yasufuku et al. performed a first head-to-head comparison of EBUS-TBNA and Med staging in a cohort of 153 patients with potentially resectable lung cancer. Sensitivity, NPV, and diagnostic accuracy of EBUS-TBNA and Med were 81%, 91%, and 93% and 79%, 90%, and 93%, respectively. Specificity and the PPV for both staging procedures were 100%. This study demonstrated that in expert hands and controlled setting, EBUS-TBNA is equivalent to Med in mediastinal LN staging [57]. Ernst et al.'s study showed similar results [31]. Ninety three percent vs. 82% of patients with lung cancer evaluated by EBUS-TBNA and Med, respectively, had their pathological stage correctly identified ($p = 0.083$). Overall, sensitivity and NPV of EBUS-TBNA and Med were 89% vs. 68% and 78% vs. 59%, respectively. However, per LN analysis showed that EBUS-TBNA had higher diagnostic accuracy (91%) than Med (78%, $p = 0.007$). There was a discrepancy in diagnostic yield at station 7 (79% for Med vs. 98% for EBUS-TBNA, $p = 0.007$). Recently, Um et al. demonstrated, superior to Med, per patient performance of EBUS-TBNA in lung cancer staging in a cohort of patients with biopsy-proven lung cancer [30]. EBUS-TBNA and Med sensitivity and diagnostic accuracy were 88% vs. 81.3% and 92.9% vs. 89%, respectively ($p = 0.005$). No difference was demonstrated between the procedures in specificity (100% for both), PPV (100% EBUS-TBNA vs. 89% Med), and NPV (EBUS-TBNA 85.2% vs. 78.8% Med). Similar to Ernst et al.'s study, there was a discrepancy between the modalities in disease detection at station 7 LN, with a nonsignificant trend toward inferior yield with Med than EBUS-TBNA, 75% vs. 82% ($p = 0.0614$). However, Med yield at station 4L was significantly lower than that of EBUS-TBNA (52.4% vs. 81%, $p = 0.0270$) [30].

Recently, a large meta-analysis was conducted comparing indirectly diagnostic yield of mediastinal staging with EBUS-TBNA to that of Med [76]. Ten EBUS-TBNA and seven Med studies were included. Outcomes of nearly 1000 patients staged were analyzed and compared. Overall, sensitivity for detection of mediastinal metastasis was equivalent between EBUS-TBNA and Med at 0.84 (95% CI 0.79–0.88) and 0.86 (95% CI 0.82–0.90), respectively ($P = 0.6321$). Med was associated with fewer false negatives, which in both staging modalities were attributed to metastasis in inaccessible LNs (stations 5 and 6) and inadequate sampling at accessible LNs. Med was associated with more complications (17 vs. 4). EBUS-TBNA-related complications were minor and resolved without intervention.

Neither Med nor EBUS-TBNA can access stations 5, 6, 8, and 9 nodes. Some authors have advocated for a combined approach, and adding EUS-FNA to EBUS-TBNA (combined ultrasonography (CUS)) for mediastinal LN staging in lung cancer [77, 78]. EUS-FNA is complimentary to EBUS-TBNA and Med in terms of mediastinal LN access (Fig. 4.4). It allows access to stations 2R, 2L, 4L, 4R, 5, 7, 8, and 9 LNs. EUS-FNA can also access L adrenal, left lobe of the liver, and celiac axis, some of which are common sites of metastasis from lung cancer. However, due to intervening airways, right-sided upper paratracheal (2R, 2L) and lower paratracheal (4R) LNs may be more challenging to access. EUS-FNA performance in mediastinal LN staging in lung cancer has reported sensitivity, specificity, PPV, and NPV equivalent to that of EBUS-TBNA at 89%, 100%, 100%, and 86%, respectively [1].

CUS has been shown to improve access to the mediastinum [79], and the extended LN sampling that occurs with both modalities combined may improve diagnostic yield as compared to EBUS-TBNA alone, thanks to detection of additional metastatic foci [79–81]. The concept of CUS was first presented by Vilmann et al. [80]. Thirty-one patients with suspected or proven lung cancer underwent CUS. A total of 119 lesions were sampled by EUS-FNA ($n = 59$) and EBUS-TBNA ($n = 60$). Cancer diagnosis was made in 26 EUS-FNA and 28 EBUS-TBNA sampled lesions, respectively. Eleven additional cancer diagnoses and three samples with suspicious cells were obtained by EBUS-TBNA that had not been detected by the EUS-FNA. Conversely, 12 additional cancer diagnoses, one suspicious and one specific benign diagnosis (sarcoidosis), were found by EUS-FNA that had not been picked up by EBUS-TBNA. Mediastinal involvement was confirmed in 20 of the 28 patients in whom a final diagnosis was obtained. The accuracy of CUS, for diagnosis of mediastinal metastasis, was 100% (95% CI, 83–100%).

Diagnostic yield of CUS has been shown to be equivalent to that of EBUS-TBNA regardless of whether one (CP-EBUS-TBNA scope used in the airways [EBUS-TBNA] and the esophagus [EBUS-transesophageal-guided needle aspiration [EBUS-TENA]) [82] or two scopes (a dedicated CP-EBUS-TBNA scope and a dedicated EUS-FNA scopes) are used. Diagnostic performance of EBUS-TBNA compared to CUS showed sensitivity, NPV, and diagnostic accuracy of 84.4%, 93.3%, and 95.1%; 91.1%, 96.1%, and 97.2%; and $p = 0.332$, $p = 0.37\ 9$, and $p = 0.360$, respectively [79, 81, 83]. However, one-scope CUS significantly reduced procedure time as compared to the two-scope approach (25 ± 4.4 min vs. 14.9 ± 2.3 min, $p = 0.001$) [82–84].

Based on these results, some authors suggest to use CUS in mediastinal LN staging in all patients with lung cancer and promote the use of EBUS-TENA over EBUS-TBNA and EUS-FNA for time-saving purposes [81, 85–87]. However, some important aspects of these studies need to be considered before CUS can be recommended routinely. Herth et al. reported only three cases where positive results were obtained exclusively by EBUS-TENA from stations 2L, 10L, and 7, all of which are accessible by EBUS-TBNA [81]. In another study, three exclusively positive cases determined by EBUS-TENA (2.1% of patients) were from stations 4L and 5 (frequently involved together with station 4L which is accessible to EBUS-TBNA). Stations 8 and 9 LNs did not contribute to increased diagnostic yield by EBUS-TENA in that study [79]. Overall, prevalence of mediastinal LN metastasis in stations inaccessible to EBUS-TBNA is low, ranging between 0.19% and 1.2% for station 8 and 0.83% and 2.2% in stations 5 and 6 [57, 78, 86]. The low prevalence of mediastinal metastasis in exclusively EUS-accessible LNs, limitations of EUS in assessment of R-sided mediastinal LNs (described below), and given the equivalent to Med yield of EBUS-TBNA in the hands of a skilled operator may be the reasons behind the lack of statistically significant difference in diagnostic yield when adding EUS-FNA to EBUS-TBNA staging, while a statistically significant increase in diagnostic yield has been achieved by adding EBUS-TBNA to EUS-FNA [82, 88]. The use of EBUS through the esophagus to increase the yield further or CUS using two scopes may not be justifiable from the health economics perspective, and instead a selective use of CUS should be implemented if there is a high index of suspicion of metastasis in EBUS-TBNA-inaccessible LNs.

A recent prospective study of mediastinal staging in patients with lung cancer compared the yield of combined EBUS-EUS and Med with the results of surgical lymphadenectomy [86]. CUS and Med approach diagnosed additional N2/N3 and M1 disease in 14% of study patients that had not been detected by the Med approach, preventing inappropriate surgical resections. CUS sensitivity, NPV, and diagnostic accuracy were 91%, 100%, 96%, and 97%, respectively. Interestingly, NPV and diagnostic accuracy of EBUS alone, CUS, and Med compared with mediastinal lymphadenectomy at thoracotomy were quite similar (~90%, 95% CI ~0.84–0.95) [86].

Positive result of mediastinal LN staging with needle-based techniques has a significant impact on patient management and may result in improved survival [1, 48, 89–91]. However, if the endoscopic staging is negative, the question remains whether there is a role for a confirmatory Med in this setting, and if so, which patients should it be offered to.

For EBUS-TBNA, performance depends on the operator's skill and prevalence of mediastinal metastasis in the studied population. In skilled hands, performance of EBUS-TBNA has been shown to be equivalent or better than that of Med [30, 57]. In a population with intermediate prevalence of mediastinal metastasis (35%), Yasufuku et al. showed sensitivity and NPV of EBUS-TBNA of 81% and 91%, respectively. Combined EBUS-TBNA and Med improved sensitivity to 91% and NPV to 96%. This represents an overall 5% increase in NPV and number needed to treat of 9. In a patient population with clinical N0 disease, surgical staging may not contribute significantly to improving diagnostic yield. Szlubowski et al. demonstrated CUS sensitivity, specificity, diagnostic accuracy, PPV, and NPV of 68% (95% CI: 48–84), 98% (95% CI: 92–100), 91% (95% CI: 86–96), 91% (95% CI: 70–99), and 91% (95% CI: 83–96). TEMLA was performed in 99 patients whose CUS was negative detecting nine additional cases of mediastinal metastatic disease (8%) [92].

Therefore, in a patient population with clinical N0 disease and low prevalence of mediastinal nodal metastasis, confirmatory Med following negative EBUS-TBNA staging may not be justifiable. Annema et al. compared the yield of CUS and Med combined to that of Med in a population of patients with high prevalence of mediastinal nodal metastasis (49%). Sensitivity for detecting N2 and N3 disease was 79% (95% CI 66–88%) in Med arm, 85% (95% CI 74–92%) in CUS arm ($p = 0.47$), and 94% (62/66; 95% CI 85–98%) for the CUS strategy followed by Med ($p = 0.02$). Evaluating sonography (CUS) and surgical components (Med) separately showed sensitivity and NPV of 85% and 85% for CUS and 79% and 86% for Med. This demonstrated that Med and CUS staging may be equivalent but that CUS approach followed by Med in CUS negative cases in a patient population with high prevalence of mediastinal nodal metastasis has higher than Med alone sensitivity and results in fewer unnecessary surgeries (7% in CUS and Med arm vs. 18% in the Med alone arm, $p = 0.02$). Adding Med to CUS increased sensitivity and NPV of staging by 9% (94%) and 11% (93%), respectively, indicating that with rising prevalence of mediastinal nodal metastasis, confirmatory Med may be of value and that the decision about confirmatory testing should be made on a case-by-case basis. (Post hoc analysis of survival data from this trial has recently been reported, showing no survival advantage in the CUS and Med arm as compared with the Med alone arm. This may be explained by insufficient powering of the study to detect survival difference.) [93]

Limitations of Endoscopic Mediastinal LN Staging

Needle-based techniques have offered a safe and accurate alternative to invasive mediastinal LN staging in patients with lung cancer. However, it is important to realize limitations of these techniques as used for this indication, to ensure they are used only when the procedure yield and patient benefits are maximized.

Even when combined, EBUS-TBNA and EUS-FNA cannot access majority of the intrathoracic LNs. EBUS-TBNA cannot access mediastinal stations 5, 6, 8, and 9. EUS-FNA tends to underdiagnose N3 disease in left-sided tumors, and N2 disease in right-sided tumors (due to decreased diagnostic yield resulting from higher rate of false negatives in the R-sided LNs due to reduced LN visualization through the air-filled trachea) [82, 88]. EUS-FNA cannot access any of the interlobar/lobar and segmental LNs, while EBUS-TBNA can access some interlobar and segmental LNs in the lower lobes, but not N1 lymph nodes adjacent to the upper lobe airways. While invasive sampling of N1 LNs may not be relevant in surgical candidates, many patients are unable to undergo curative surgery. For these patients, local therapies like stereotactic body radiation (SBRT) or radiofrequency ablation (RFA) are available. In addition, tissue-sparing surgery (wedge, sublobar resection) has become more popular and may be the treatment of choice for patients [94] or the only surgical option for patients with limited pulmonary reserve. High post-SBRT local failure (15%) may be due to undetected nodal metastasis in patients undergoing treatment under presumption that the clinical stage correlates with the pathological stage [1, 95–103].

All of these recent developments stress the growing need for invasive nodal staging that extends beyond the mediastinum and into the hilar, interlobar, and perhaps even the lobar LNs including in patients with clinical N0 disease [104] . Performance of EBUS-TBNA and EUS-FNA has been assessed in patients with clinical N0 disease. EBUS-TBNA and EUS-FNA have varying performance in patients with clinical N0 disease. For EBUS-TBNA, some studies report sensitivity and NPV ranging between 89% and 92.3% and 96.3% and 98.9%, respectively [99, 100], while others show sensitivity and NPV ranging between 35% and 60% and 88.4% and 93.4% [96, 98]. Reported EUS-FNA sensitivity and NPV in patients with clinical N0 range between 45% and 61% and 79% and 88%, respectively [92, 105, 106].

There may be a variety of reasons for this wide discrepancy aside from clinical expertise of the operator: (1) presence of multiple LNs at a station, but only selective LN sampling is possible with both techniques; (2) LNs inaccessible for sampling due to intervening structures (i.e., vascular structures in the needle path, or air-filled trachea in case of EUS-FNA); (3) micrometastasis in LNs not sampled (i.e., in many studies, the lower limit of LN size considered for TBNA was 5 mm, with LNs smaller than that not sampled); and (4) micrometastasis in small LNs which may be more challenging to sample (some authors reported higher percentage of nondiagnostic results from LNs smaller than 5 mm in size, suggesting that this may represent the lower limit of needle technique accessibility beyond which adequate tissue sampling may be challenging and negative results should be interpreted with caution) [57]. Reported performance of surgical techniques including Med and VATS may not be affected by the prevalence of mediastinal nodal metastasis (sensitivity of 89% in cN0–3) to the same extent as the performance of the needle-based techniques [1]. Development of the new thin EBUS scope can circumvent some of the N1 LN access challenges but not necessarily the LN size and related diagnostic yield issues [58, 59]. Until then, surgical staging may be necessary for some of the patients requiring sublobar resections.

While the endoscopic techniques can assess for mediastinal invasion in bulky tumors and prevent unnecessary thoracotomies and futile resections [78], this assessment is nonspecific, and if there is a high degree of suspicion of mediastinal invasion with negative needle-based technique assessment, surgical staging (Med or VATS) is a sensitive way of assessment in such patients with the VATS ability to safely access stations 5 and 6 LNs [1].

Patient survival is related to the T component of the tumor. Patients with lower T stage have a better survival [107]. Unlike surgical techniques (VATS), endoscopic techniques cannot assess mobility of the tumor, or the presence or the degree of direct invasion into the chest wall or the mediastinum [78, 108]. Aside from EUS-FNA ability to access L adrenal, the left lobe of the liver, and celiac axis LNs, needle-based techniques cannot assess the M component of the tumor in relation to pleural and pericardial disease, while VATS, by direct visualization of the pleura and pericardium, can diagnose unexpected stage IV disease (reported in 4–6% of patients in some series) [109, 110].

Another challenge in the application for the needle-based techniques is the access to training and endoscopy resources [111]. Needle-based techniques have become more popular over the past two decades, and many academic centers have implemented the use of EBUS-TBNA and/or EUS-FNA into the armamentarium of tests available. This allows both thoracic surgery and pulmonology trainees to gain access to training. However, training access is an issue for physicians already in practice. The number of supervised procedures to achieve proficiency in endobronchial ultrasound is unknown. Previous guidelines suggested 40–50 supervised procedures [112]. However, recent studies show that individual physician learning curves vary, and a median of 212 and 163 procedures may be needed to achieve an "expert" performance and to correctly identify nodal stations, respectively [113, 114]. These statistics, however, do not pertain to performance in systematic mediastinal LN sampling of not only large but also subcentimeter LNs, needed in mediastinal staging, which may be one of the most challenging procedures performed using the needle-based techniques. Individual physician learning curves vary with as many as 33% of trainees not gaining an expert level within their fellowship training time (usually 1 year) [113]. Many physicians already in practice gain their needle-based techniques training through a 1- or a 2-day course. Post-course surveys suggest that as many as 77.5% of attendants may not feel confident about their needle-based technique skills after course completion [115]. Access to technology even for trained physicians is another issue, with technology being less available in nonacademic centers (only 54% of former endoscopy training course attendees reporting access to EBUS at their centers) [111], with cost of equipment, high per procedure cost, and access to support staff identified as other challenges in the use of needle-based techniques [116].

Neoadjuvant chemoradiation followed by surgery in lung cancer patients with N2 disease may offer survival advantage over definitive chemoradiation, if the mediastinum can be downstaged to N0/N1 preoperatively [117–119]. Sensitivity and NPV of EBUS-TBNA and EUS-FNA for mediastinal restaging have shown to be lower than in initial mediastinal staging, ranging between 50% and 77% for EBUS-TBNA [120–123] and 42–91% and 53–91% for EUS-FNA [124–126]. This is thought to be attributable to LN necrosis and fibrosis. Given a wide range of NPV of the needle-based technique assessment in this group of patients (~40–90%), surgical staging with Med may offer a better alternative [127, 128]. Even though the yield of Med in lung cancer restaging is lower than in staging, multiple studies have reported feasibility of repeated Med for restaging with 98–100% planned procedures completed [127, 128] and low morbidity (1.9%) [127] but unfortunately also a death reported in one study due to perioperative bleeding [128]. One of the largest series was reported by De Waele et al. [128]. One hundred four patients were restaged with Med after neoadjuvant therapy. Med sensitivity, specificity, and diagnostic accuracy were 71%, 100%, and 84%, respectively [128]. Med prevented 20 futile thoracotomies by detection of persistent N2/3 disease. Patients without nodal metastasis proceeded to surgical resection with median survival of 28 months (95% confidence interval 15–41). Survival in patients with positive- and false-negative Med was 14 months (95% confidence interval 8–20) and 24 months (95% confidence interval 3–45), respectively. This suggests that Med is also able to provide a prognostic information. Other studies reported similar performance characteristics for Med with sensitivity of 61–83%, diagnostic accuracy of 84–91%, and NPV of 85% [127–130]. One study, however, showed very low sensitivity and diagnostic accuracy of Med, 29% and 60%, respectively, which was presumed to be due to inadequate sampling of station 7 LN in majority of patients [131]. The choice of restaging procedure should be based on local expertise and having weighted in the diagnostic test performance characteristic based on the location of suspected metastasis.

Recommendations

Current evidence confirms that both needle-based techniques and Med have similar performance in mediastinal LN staging in lung cancer, with the EBUS-TBNA and EUS-FNA being less invasive, better tolerated, and with fewer complications. These findings led to a recent recommendation by the American College of Chest

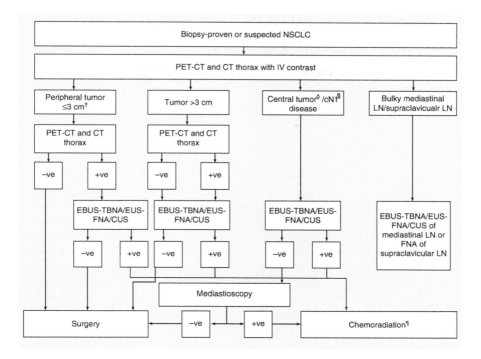

Fig. 4.5 The algorithm for mediastinal assessment in patients with non-small cell lung cancer. †Implies stage IA: T1N0M0 (T1: primary tumor diameter 3 cm or smaller and surrounded by lung or visceral pleura, or endobronchial tumor distal to the lobar bronchus). ‡Tumor in the central third of the hemithorax is considered central. A tumor in the distal two-thirds of the hemithorax is considered peripheral. §cN1: clinical N1 disease = interlobar LN involved. In some patients with mediastinal LN metastasis, surgical management may be considered following neoadjuvant chemoradiation depending on patient status and institutional expertise. CT computed tomography, CUS combined ultrasonography, EBUS endobronchial ultrasound, EUS endoscopic ultrasound, FNA fine needle aspiration, M0 no metastases, N0 no lymph nodes involved, NSCLC non-small cell lung cancer, +ve/−ve pertains to mediastinal LN involvement, PET positron emission tomography. (Reprinted with permission from Czarnecka and Yasufuku [48])

Physicians (ACCP) and the European Society of Thoracic Surgeons (ESTS) that the endoscopic mediastinal staging be the tests of first choice in invasive mediastinal LN staging, and that they be followed by Med in case of negative results if the index of suspicion for metastatic disease is high [1, 3] (Fig. 4.5).

At present, there is insufficient evidence to clearly define the role of surgical and endoscopic modalities in patients with advanced lung cancer and considered for trimodality therapy and in setting of suspected recurrent lung cancer. However, recently, literature has emerged on cost-effectiveness of mediastinal LN staging in this patient population [25]. In a population with high prevalence of mediastinal nodal metastasis, EBUS-TBNA followed by Med has been shown to be the most cost-effective strategy, suggesting a clear role for confirmatory Med in some patients while advocating for EBUS-TBNA as the test of first choice for invasive staging

[25]. Studies demonstrate that EBUS-TBNA sensitivity and prevalence of mediastinal nodal metastasis are important factors in deciding on the most cost-effective staging modality. Recent study showed that if the EBUS-TBNA sensitivity of at least 25% cannot be achieved, Med should be the preferred staging strategy, proving that the previous "gold standard" is still preferred over poorly performed endoscopic staging [25, 132].

Given better and safer performance of Med when performed for the first time, and equivalent performance of Med and endoscopic staging in primary mediastinal staging, it appears that "saving" Med for restaging after neoadjuvant therapy and staging initially endoscopically might be the most cost-effective staging approach in lung cancer patients considered for a curative resection. However, if endoscopic staging is performed for restaging, a confirmatory Med should follow in the event of negative endoscopic staging [3].

Surgical mediastinal staging techniques are routinely available at thoracic surgery centers managing lung cancer, although the number of surgical staging performed may be reduced at the academic centers due to introduction of needle-based techniques. With a paradigm shift and implementation of needle-based techniques more frequently for mediastinal LN staging in lung cancer, it will be important to ensure that current and future thoracic surgery trainees gain access to training in Med, to ensure high-quality performance, given an important role surgical techniques play in invasive staging of patients with lung cancer.

Conclusion and Future Directions

Lung cancer diagnosis and management have undergone significant changes over the past decade with introduction of the minimally invasive endoscopic techniques. Endoscopic staging offers an accurate and cost-effective means of mediastinal evaluation in primary lung cancer. Quality data on performance of EBUS-TBNA in mediastinal LN staging in lung cancer led to a recent recommendation from the ACCP and ESTS to use the needle-based techniques for the initial mediastinal staging [1, 3]. When combined with EUS-FNA, EBUS-TBNA offers nearly complete assessment of the mediastinum and may have higher diagnostic accuracy than the previous gold standard, Med, in patients with metastatic disease in EBUS-TBNA-inaccessible LNs.

Practice of medicine has evolved in many specialities with focus on minimally invasive diagnosis and treatment as well as personalized treatments of disease. At present, lung cancer is being treated not only with surgery but also with therapies like RFA and SBRT. Sublobar resections may become standard of care for T1a tumors [94] and are the only surgical option for patients with significantly impaired lung function [95]. In this setting, development of a thin CP-EBUS scope opens up a possibility of not only reaching further into the airways and sampling the more distant and upper lobe N1 LNs but also personalized therapy where a tumor-specific treatment could be delivered to a metastatic LN or a primary lung tumor, using a real-time ultrasound imaging [133, 134]. In addition, it will be important to continue work on improving the endoscopic staging technologies, to increase their diagnostic yield. The new EU-ME2 processor (Olympus, Japan) is equipped with the elastography function which may offer a useful noninvasive adjunct to endo-sonograpic LN assessment, pointing out the areas which are more likely to be involved with tumor, for a more directed TBNA [135]. Analysis of the unique spectral features of the LNs may be another useful way allowing to differentiate between malignant and noninvolved LNs, further increasing diagnostic accuracy of the endoscopic staging [136].

Even though many centers globally have acquired endoscopic ultrasound technology, it is unlikely that Med will be eliminated from the armamentarium of invasive tests used in lung cancer patients. Instead, a combination of endoscopic and surgical assessments will become the standard of care, depending on the unique clinical scenario. This will allow highest diagnostic yield at all stages of the disease and optimal patient management. For example, Med is recommended as a confirmatory test in patients with negative needle-based staging in patients with high pretest probability of mediastinal metastasis, and it should be the test of first choice for mediastinal restaging, following neoadjuvant therapy (especially if needle-based technique was used to stage mediastinum initially). In addition, despite the recent change in the guidelines and a shift to the minimally invasive endoscopic staging, acquisition of this technology in many thoracic surgery and pulmonology centers is hindered by the lack of EBUS-TBNA expertise and limited resources. Therefore, Med is still the test of first choice in many thoracic surgery programs worldwide for mediastinal staging, restaging, and diagnosis of disease recurrence. For these reasons, it is important that thoracic surgeons get adequate training in both Med and the needle-based techniques like EBUS-TBNA or EUS-FNA and that the focus of lung cancer diagnosis and treatment be on a multidisciplinary approach with a close collaboration of the radiologists, thoracic surgeons, pulmonologists, pathologists, and oncologists to ensure the optimal patient management at all stages of the disease.

References

1. Silvestri GA, Gonzalez AV, Jantz MA, Margolis ML, Gould MK, Tanoue LT, et al. Methods for staging non-small cell lung cancer: diagnosis and management of lung cancer, 3rd ed: American College of Chest Physicians evidence-based clinical practice guidelines. Chest. 2013;143(5 Suppl):e211S–50S.
2. Wu LM, Xu JR, Gu HY, Hua J, Chen J, Zhang W, et al. Preoperative mediastinal and hilar nodal staging with diffusion-weighted magnetic resonance imaging and fluorodeoxyglucose positron emission tomography/computed tomography in patients with non-small-cell lung cancer: which is better? J Surg Res. 2012;178(1):304–14.
3. De Leyn P, Dooms C, Kuzdzal J, Lardinois D, Passlick B, Rami-Porta R, et al. Preoperative mediastinal lymph node staging for non-small cell lung cancer: 2014 update of the 2007 ESTS guidelines. Transl Lung Cancer Res. 2014;3(4):225–33.
4. Silvestri GA, Gould MK, Margolis ML, Tanoue LT, McCrory D, Toloza E, et al. Noninvasive staging of non-small cell lung cancer: ACCP evidenced-based clinical practice guidelines (2nd edition). Chest. 2007;132(3 Suppl):178s–201s.

5. Siegel RL, Miller KD, Jemal A. Cancer statistics, 2016. CA Cancer J Clin. 2016;66(1):7–30.
6. Goldstraw P, Chansky K, Crowley J, Rami-Porta R, Asamura H, Eberhardt WE, et al. The IASLC lung Cancer staging project: proposals for revision of the TNM stage groupings in the forthcoming (eighth) edition of the TNM classification for lung cancer. J Thorac Oncol. 2016;11(1):39–51.
7. Mohammed N, Kestin LL, Grills IS, Battu M, Fitch DL, Wong CY, et al. Rapid disease progression with delay in treatment of non-small-cell lung cancer. Int J Radiat Oncol Biol Phys. 2011;79(2):466–72.
8. Donington JS, Pass HI. Surgical resection of non-small cell lung cancer with N2 disease. Thorac Surg Clin. 2014;24(4):449–56.
9. Ramnath N, Dilling TJ, Harris LJ, Kim AW, Michaud GC, Balekian AA, et al. Treatment of stage III non-small cell lung cancer: diagnosis and management of lung cancer, 3rd ed: American College of Chest Physicians evidence-based clinical practice guidelines. Chest. 2013;143(5 Suppl):e314S–40S.
10. McGarry RC, Song G, des Rosiers P, Timmerman R. Observation-only management of early stage, medically inoperable lung cancer: poor outcome. Chest. 2002;121(4):1155–8.
11. Saint-Jacques N, Rayson D, Al-Fayea T, Virik K, Morzycki W, Younis T. Waiting times in early-stage non-small cell lung cancer (NSCLC). J Thorac Oncol. 2008;3(8):865–70.
12. Darling GE, Maziak DE, Clifton JC, Finley RJ. The practice of thoracic surgery in Canada. Canadian journal of surgery Journal canadien de chirurgie. 2004;47(6):438–45.
13. BTS recommendations to respiratory physicians for organising the care of patients with lung cancer. The Lung Cancer Working Party of the British Thoracic Society Standards of Care Committee. Thorax. 1998;53 Suppl 1:S1–8.
14. Gould MK, Kuschner WG, Rydzak CE, Maclean CC, Demas AN, Shigemitsu H, et al. Test performance of positron emission tomography and computed tomography for mediastinal staging in patients with non-small-cell lung cancer: a meta-analysis. Ann Intern Med. 2003;139(11):879–92.
15. van Tinteren H, Hoekstra OS, Smit EF, van den Bergh JH, Schreurs AJ, Stallaert RA, et al. Effectiveness of positron emission tomography in the preoperative assessment of patients with suspected non-small-cell lung cancer: the PLUS multicentre randomised trial. Lancet (London, England). 2002;359(9315):1388–93.
16. Viney RC, Boyer MJ, King MT, Kenny PM, Pollicino CA, McLean JM, et al. Randomized controlled trial of the role of positron emission tomography in the management of stage I and II non-small-cell lung cancer. J Clin Oncol. 2004;22(12):2357–62.
17. Cerfolio RJ, Ojha B, Bryant AS, Raghuveer V, Mountz JM, Bartolucci AA. The accuracy of integrated PET-CT compared with dedicated PET alone for the staging of patients with nonsmall cell lung cancer. Ann Thorac Surg. 2004;78(3):1017–23; discussion −23.
18. Fischer B, Lassen U, Mortensen J, Larsen S, Loft A, Bertelsen A, et al. Preoperative staging of lung cancer with combined PET-CT. N Engl J Med. 2009;361(1):32–9.
19. Fischer BM, Lassen U, Hojgaard L. PET-CT in preoperative staging of lung cancer. N Engl J Med. 2011;364(10):980–1.
20. Maziak DE, Darling GE, Inculet RI, Gulenchyn KY, Driedger AA, Ung YC, et al. Positron emission tomography in staging early lung cancer: a randomized trial. Ann Intern Med. 2009;151(4):221–8, w-48.
21. Darling GE, Maziak DE, Inculet RI, Gulenchyn KY, Driedger AA, Ung YC, et al. Positron emission tomography-computed tomography compared with invasive mediastinal staging in non-small cell lung cancer: results of mediastinal staging in the early lung positron emission tomography trial. J Thorac Oncol. 2011;6(8):1367–72.
22. Schmidt-Hansen M, Baldwin DR, Hasler E, Zamora J, Abraira V, Roque IFM. PET-CT for assessing mediastinal lymph node involvement in patients with suspected resectable non-small cell lung cancer. Cochrane Database Syst Rev. 2014;(11):Cd009519.
23. Darling GE, Dickie AJ, Malthaner RA, Kennedy EB, Tey R. Invasive mediastinal staging of non-small-cell lung cancer: a clinical practice guideline. Curr Oncol (Toronto, Ont). 2011;18(6):e304–10.

24. De Leyn P, Dooms C, Kuzdzal J, Lardinois D, Passlick B, Rami-Porta R, et al. Revised ESTS guidelines for preoperative mediastinal lymph node staging for non-small-cell lung cancer. Eur J Cardiothorac Surg. 2014;45(5):787–98.
25. Czarnecka-Kujawa K, Rochau U, Siebert U, Atenafu E, Darling G, Waddell TK, et al. Cost-effectiveness of mediastinal lymph node staging in non-small cell lung cancer. J Thorac Cardiovasc Surg. 2017;153:1567–78.
26. Kuzdzal J, Zielinski M, Papla B, Szlubowski A, Hauer L, Nabialek T, et al. Transcervical extended mediastinal lymphadenectomy--the new operative technique and early results in lung cancer staging. Eur J Cardiothorac Surg. 2005;27(3):384–90; discussion 90.
27. Kuzdzal J, Szlubowski A, Grochowski Z, Czajkowski W. Current evidence on transcervical mediastinal lymph nodes dissection. Eur J Cardiothorac Surg. 2011;40(6):1470–3.
28. Carlens E. Mediastinoscopy: a method for inspection and tissue biopsy in the superior mediastinum. Dis Chest. 1959;36:343–52.
29. Pass HI, Ball David, Scagliotti Giorgio V, The IASCL multidisciplinary approach to thoracic oncology. Pass HI, editor. Aurora: International Association for the Study of Lung Cancer; 2014.
30. Um SW, Kim HK, Jung SH, Han J, Lee KJ, Park HY, et al. Endobronchial ultrasound versus mediastinoscopy for mediastinal nodal staging of non-small-cell lung cancer. J Thorac Oncol. 2015;10(2):331–7.
31. Ernst A, Anantham D, Eberhardt R, Krasnik M, Herth FJ. Diagnosis of mediastinal adenopathy-real-time endobronchial ultrasound guided needle aspiration versus mediastinoscopy. J Thorac Oncol. 2008;3(6):577–82.
32. Toloza EM, Harpole L, Detterbeck F, McCrory DC. Invasive staging of non-small cell lung cancer: a review of the current evidence. Chest. 2003;123(1 Suppl):157s–66s.
33. Hammoud ZT, Anderson RC, Meyers BF, Guthrie TJ, Roper CL, Cooper JD, et al. The current role of mediastinoscopy in the evaluation of thoracic disease. J Thorac Cardiovasc Surg. 1999;118(5):894–9.
34. Kirschner PA. Cervical mediastinoscopy. Chest Surg Clin N Am. 1996;6(1):1–20.
35. Urschel JD. Conservative management (packing) of hemorrhage complicating mediastinoscopy. Ann Thorac Cardiovasc Surg. 2000;6(1):9–12.
36. Pearson G, Cooper J, Deslauriers J, et al. Mediastinoscopy. In: Thoracic surgery. 2nd ed. New York: Churchill Livingstone; 2002. p. 98–103.
37. Lemaire A, Nikolic I, Petersen T, Haney JC, Toloza EM, Harpole DH Jr, et al. Nine-year single center experience with cervical mediastinoscopy: complications and false negative rate. Ann Thorac Surg. 2006;82(4):1185–9; discussion 9-90.
38. Call S, Obiols C, Rami-Porta R, Trujillo-Reyes JC, Iglesias M, Saumench R, et al. Video-assisted mediastinoscopic lymphadenectomy for staging non-small cell lung cancer. Ann Thorac Surg. 2016;101(4):1326–33.
39. Kuzdzal J, Zielinski M, Papla B, Urbanik A, Wojciechowski W, Narski M, et al. The transcervical extended mediastinal lymphadenectomy versus cervical mediastinoscopy in non-small cell lung cancer staging. Eur J Cardiothorac Surg. 2007;31(1):88–94.
40. Witte B, Wolf M, Hillebrand H, Kriegel E, Huertgen M. Extended cervical mediastinoscopy revisited. Eur J Cardiothorac Surg. 2014;45(1):114–9.
41. Passlick B. Initial surgical staging of lung cancer. Lung Cancer (Amsterdam, Netherlands). 2003;42 Suppl 1:S21–5.
42. Ginsberg RJ, Rice TW, Goldberg M, Waters PF, Schmocker BJ. Extended cervical mediastinoscopy. A single staging procedure for bronchogenic carcinoma of the left upper lobe. J Thorac Cardiovasc Surg. 1987;94(5):673–8.
43. Freixinet Gilart J, Garcia PG, de Castro FR, Suarez PR, Rodriguez NS, de Ugarte AV. Extended cervical mediastinoscopy in the staging of bronchogenic carcinoma. Ann Thorac Surg. 2000;70(5):1641–3.
44. Semik M, Netz B, Schmidt C, Scheld HH. Surgical exploration of the mediastinum: mediastinoscopy and intraoperative staging. Lung Cancer (Amsterdam, Netherlands). 2004;45 Suppl 2:S55–61.

45. Obiols C, Call S, Rami-Porta R, Iglesias M, Saumench R, Serra-Mitjans M, et al. Extended cervical mediastinoscopy: mature results of a clinical protocol for staging bronchogenic carcinoma of the left lung. Eur J Cardiothorac Surg. 2012;41(5):1043–6.
46. Shields TW. General thoracic surgery. In: Shields TW, editor. . 7th ed. Philadelphia: Wolters Klumer/Lippincott Williams and Wilkins; 2009. p. 1.
47. Almeida FA, Casal RF, Jimenez CA, Eapen GA, Uzbeck M, Sarkiss M, et al. Quality gaps and comparative effectiveness in lung cancer staging: the impact of test sequencing on outcomes. Chest. 2013;144(6):1776–82.
48. Czarnecka K, Yasufuku K. The role of endobronchial ultrasound/esophageal ultrasound for evaluation of the mediastinum in lung cancer. Expert Rev Respir Med. 2014;8(6):763–76.
49. Czarnecka K, Yasufuku K. Interventional pulmonology: focus on pulmonary diagnostics. Respirology (Carlton, Vic). 2013;18(1):47–60.
50. Yasufuku K. Current clinical applications of endobronchial ultrasound. Expert Rev Respir Med. 2010;4(4):491–8.
51. Herth F, Becker HD, Ernst A. Conventional vs endobronchial ultrasound-guided transbronchial needle aspiration: a randomized trial. Chest. 2004;125(1):322–5.
52. Herth FJ, Ernst A, Becker HD. Endobronchial ultrasound-guided transbronchial lung biopsy in solitary pulmonary nodules and peripheral lesions. Eur Respir J. 2002;20(4):972–4.
53. Paone G, Nicastri E, Lucantoni G, Dello Iacono R, Battistoni P, D'Angeli AL, et al. Endobronchial ultrasound-driven biopsy in the diagnosis of peripheral lung lesions. Chest. 2005;128(5):3551–7.
54. Herth FJ, Becker HD, Ernst A. Ultrasound-guided transbronchial needle aspiration: an experience in 242 patients. Chest. 2003;123(2):604–7.
55. Yasufuku K, Chiyo M, Sekine Y, Chhajed PN, Shibuya K, Iizasa T, et al. Real-time endobronchial ultrasound-guided transbronchial needle aspiration of mediastinal and hilar lymph nodes. Chest. 2004;126(1):122–8.
56. Yasufuku K, Chhajed PN, Sekine Y, Nakajima T, Chiyo M, Iyoda A, et al. Endobronchial ultrasound using a new convex probe: a preliminary study on surgically resected specimens. Oncol Rep. 2004;11(2):293–6.
57. Yasufuku K, Pierre A, Darling G, de Perrot M, Waddell T, Johnston M, et al. A prospective controlled trial of endobronchial ultrasound-guided transbronchial needle aspiration compared with mediastinoscopy for mediastinal lymph node staging of lung cancer. J Thorac Cardiovasc Surg. 2011;142(6):1393–400.e1.
58. Wada H, Hirohashi K, Nakajima T, Anayama T, Kato T, Grindlay A, et al. Assessment of the new thin convex probe endobronchial ultrasound bronchoscope and the dedicated aspiration needle: a preliminary study in the porcine lung. J Bronchology Interv Pulmonol. 2015;22(1):20–7.
59. Patel P, Wada H, Hu HP, Hirohashi K, Kato T, Ujiie H, et al. First evaluation of the new thin convex probe endobronchial ultrasound scope: a human ex vivo lung study. Ann Thorac Surg. 2017;103(4):1158–64.
60. Folch E, Santacruz JF, Fernandez-Bussy S, Gangadharan S, Kent MS, Jantz M, et al. The feasibility of EBUS-guided TBNA through the pulmonary artery in highly selected patients. J Bronchology Interv Pulmonol. 2016;23(1):7–13.
61. Rusch VW, Asamura H, Watanabe H, Giroux DJ, Rami-Porta R, Goldstraw P. The IASLC lung cancer staging project: a proposal for a new international lymph node map in the forthcoming seventh edition of the TNM classification for lung cancer. J Thorac Oncol. 2009;4(5):568–77.
62. Yasufuku K. Relevance of endoscopic ultrasonography and endobronchial ultrasonography to thoracic surgeons. Thorac Surg Clin. 2013;23(2):199–210.
63. Asano F, Aoe M, Ohsaki Y, Okada Y, Sasada S, Sato S, et al. Complications associated with endobronchial ultrasound-guided transbronchial needle aspiration: a nationwide survey by the Japan Society for Respiratory Endoscopy. Respir Res. 2013;14:50.
64. von Bartheld MB, Annema JT. Endosonography-related mortality and morbidity for pulmonary indications: a nationwide survey in the Netherlands. Gastrointest Endosc. 2015;82(6):1009–15.

65. Caglayan B, Yilmaz A, Bilaceroglu S, Comert SS, Demirci NY, Salepci B. Complications of convex-probe endobronchial ultrasound-guided transbronchial needle aspiration: a multicenter retrospective study. Respir Care. 2016;61(2):243–8.
66. Yarmus LB, Akulian JA, Gilbert C, Mathai SC, Sathiyamoorthy S, Sahetya S, et al. Comparison of moderate versus deep sedation for endobronchial ultrasound transbronchial needle aspiration. Ann Am Thorac Soc. 2013;10(2):121–6.
67. Wiersema MJ, Vilmann P, Giovannini M, Chang KJ, Wiersema LM. Endosonography-guided fine-needle aspiration biopsy: diagnostic accuracy and complication assessment. Gastroenterology. 1997;112(4):1087–95.
68. Iqbal S, Friedel D, Gupta M, Ogden L, Stavropoulos SN. Endoscopic-ultrasound-guided fine-needle aspiration and the role of the cytopathologist in solid pancreatic lesion diagnosis. Patholog Res Int. 2012;2012:317167.
69. O'Toole D, Palazzo L, Arotcarena R, Dancour A, Aubert A, Hammel P, et al. Assessment of complications of EUS-guided fine-needle aspiration. Gastrointest Endosc. 2001;53(4):470–4.
70. Herth FJ, Eberhardt R, Vilmann P, Krasnik M, Ernst A. Real-time endobronchial ultrasound guided transbronchial needle aspiration for sampling mediastinal lymph nodes. Thorax. 2006;61(9):795–8.
71. Yasufuku K, Nakajima T, Waddell T, Keshavjee S, Yoshino I. Endobronchial ultrasound-guided transbronchial needle aspiration for differentiating N0 versus N1 lung cancer. Ann Thorac Surg. 2013;96(5):1756–60.
72. Adams K, Shah PL, Edmonds L, Lim E. Test performance of endobronchial ultrasound and transbronchial needle aspiration biopsy for mediastinal staging in patients with lung cancer: systematic review and meta-analysis. Thorax. 2009;64(9):757–62.
73. Gu P, Zhao YZ, Jiang LY, Zhang W, Xin Y, Han BH. Endobronchial ultrasound-guided transbronchial needle aspiration for staging of lung cancer: a systematic review and meta-analysis. Eur J Cancer (Oxford, England: 1990). 2009;45(8):1389–96.
74. Dong X, Qiu X, Liu Q, Jia J. Endobronchial ultrasound-guided transbronchial needle aspiration in the mediastinal staging of non-small cell lung cancer: a meta-analysis. Ann Thorac Surg. 2013;96(4):1502–7.
75. Sehgal IS, Dhooria S, Aggarwal AN, Behera D, Agarwal R. Endosonography versus mediastinoscopy in mediastinal staging of lung cancer: systematic review and meta-analysis. Ann Thorac Surg. 2016;102:1747–55.
76. Ge X, Guan W, Han F, Guo X, Jin Z. Comparison of endobronchial ultrasound-guided fine needle aspiration and video-assisted mediastinoscopy for mediastinal staging of lung cancer. Lung. 2015;193(5):757–66.
77. Hu LX, Chen RX, Huang H, Shao C, Wang P, Liu YZ, et al. Endobronchial ultrasound-guided transbronchial needle aspiration versus standard bronchoscopic modalities for diagnosis of sarcoidosis: a meta-analysis. Chin Med J (Engl). 2016;129(13):1607–15.
78. Annema JT, van Meerbeeck JP, Rintoul RC, Dooms C, Deschepper E, Dekkers OM, et al. Mediastinoscopy vs endosonography for mediastinal nodal staging of lung cancer: a randomized trial. JAMA. 2010;304(20):2245–52.
79. Hwangbo B, Lee GK, Lee HS, Lim KY, Lee SH, Kim HY, et al. Transbronchial and transesophageal fine-needle aspiration using an ultrasound bronchoscope in mediastinal staging of potentially operable lung cancer. Chest. 2010;138(4):795–802.
80. Vilmann P, Puri R. The complete "medical" mediastinoscopy (EUS-FNA + EBUS-TBNA). Minerva Med. 2007;98(4):331–8.
81. Herth FJ, Krasnik M, Kahn N, Eberhardt R, Ernst A. Combined endoscopic-endobronchial ultrasound-guided fine-needle aspiration of mediastinal lymph nodes through a single bronchoscope in 150 patients with suspected lung cancer. Chest. 2010;138(4):790–4.
82. Czarnecka-Kujawa K, Yasufuku K. The role of endobronchial ultrasound versus mediastinoscopy for non-small cell lung cancer. J Thorac Dis. 2017;9(Suppl 2):S83–s97.
83. Szlubowski A, Soja J, Kocon P, Talar P, Czajkowski W, Rudnicka-Sosin L, et al. A comparison of the combined ultrasound of the mediastinum by use of a single ultrasound bronchoscope versus ultrasound bronchoscope plus ultrasound gastroscope in lung cancer staging: a prospective trial. Interact Cardiovasc Thorac Surg. 2012;15(3):442–6; discussion 6.

84. Rintoul RC, Skwarski KM, Murchison JT, Wallace WA, Walker WS, Penman ID. Endobronchial and endoscopic ultrasound-guided real-time fine-needle aspiration for mediastinal staging. Eur Respir J. 2005;25(3):416–21.
85. Hegde PV, Liberman M. Mediastinal staging: endosonographic ultrasound lymph node biopsy or mediastinoscopy. Thorac Surg Clin. 2016;26(3):243–9.
86. Liberman M, Sampalis J, Duranceau A, Thiffault V, Hadjeres R, Ferraro P. Endosonographic mediastinal lymph node staging of lung cancer. Chest. 2014;146(2):389–97.
87. Vilmann P, Clementsen PF, Colella S, Siemsen M, De Leyn P, Dumonceau JM, et al. Combined endobronchial and esophageal endosonography for the diagnosis and staging of lung cancer: European Society of Gastrointestinal Endoscopy (ESGE) guideline, in cooperation with the European Respiratory Society (ERS) and the European Society of Thoracic Surgeons (ESTS). Endoscopy. 2015;47(6):545–59.
88. Kang HJ, Hwangbo B, Lee GK, Nam BH, Lee HS, Kim MS, et al. EBUS-centred versus EUS-centred mediastinal staging in lung cancer: a randomised controlled trial. Thorax. 2014;69(3):261–8.
89. Yang CF, Kumar A, Gulack BC, Mulvihill MS, Hartwig MG, Wang X, et al. Long-term outcomes after lobectomy for non-small cell lung cancer when unsuspected pN2 disease is found: a National Cancer Data Base analysis. J Thorac Cardiovasc Surg. 2016;151(5):1380–8.
90. Aggarwal C, Li L, Borghaei H, Mehra R, Somaiah N, Turaka A, et al. Multidisciplinary therapy of stage IIIA non-small-cell lung cancer: long-term outcome of chemoradiation with or without surgery. Cancer Control J Moffitt Cancer Center. 2014;21(1):57–62.
91. Darling GE, Li F, Patsios D, Massey C, Wallis AG, Coate L, et al. Neoadjuvant chemo-radiation and surgery improves survival outcomes compared with definitive chemoradiation in the treatment of stage IIIA N2 non-small-cell lung cancer. Eur J Cardiothorac Surg. 2015;48(5):684–90; discussion 90.
92. Szlubowski A, Zielinski M, Soja J, Annema JT, Sosnicki W, Jakubiak M, et al. A combined approach of endobronchial and endoscopic ultrasound-guided needle aspiration in the radiologically normal mediastinum in non-small-cell lung cancer staging--a prospective trial. Eur J Cardiothorac Surg. 2010;37(5):1175–9.
93. Kuijvenhoven JC, Korevaar DA, Tournoy KG, Malfait TL, Dooms C, Rintoul RC, et al. Five-year survival after endosonography vs mediastinoscopy for mediastinal nodal staging of lung cancer. JAMA. 2016;316(10):1110–2.
94. Koike T, Kitahara A, Sato S, Hashimoto T, Aoki T, Koike T, et al. Lobectomy versus segmentectomy in radiologically pure solid small-sized non-small cell lung cancer. Ann Thorac Surg. 2016;101(4):1354–60.
95. Crabtree TD, Denlinger CE, Meyers BF, El Naqa I, Zoole J, Krupnick AS, et al. Stereotactic body radiation therapy versus surgical resection for stage I non-small cell lung cancer. J Thorac Cardiovasc Surg. 2010;140(2):377–86.
96. Shingyoji M, Nakajima T, Yoshino M, Yoshida Y, Ashinuma H, Itakura M, et al. Endobronchial ultrasonography for positron emission tomography and computed tomography-negative lymph node staging in non-small cell lung cancer. Ann Thorac Surg. 2014;98(5):1762–7.
97. Choi YS, Shim YM, Kim J, Kim K. Mediastinoscopy in patients with clinical stage I non-small cell lung cancer. Ann Thorac Surg. 2003;75(2):364–6.
98. Ong P, Grosu H, Eapen GA, Rodriguez M, Lazarus D, Ost D, et al. Endobronchial ultrasound-guided transbronchial needle aspiration for systematic nodal staging of lung cancer in patients with N0 disease by computed tomography and integrated positron emission tomography-computed tomography. Ann Am Thorac Soc. 2015;12(3):415–9.
99. Herth FJ, Ernst A, Eberhardt R, Vilmann P, Dienemann H, Krasnik M. Endobronchial ultrasound-guided transbronchial needle aspiration of lymph nodes in the radiologically normal mediastinum. Eur Respir J. 2006;28(5):910–4.
100. Herth FJ, Eberhardt R, Krasnik M, Ernst A. Endobronchial ultrasound-guided transbronchial needle aspiration of lymph nodes in the radiologically and positron emission tomography-normal mediastinum in patients with lung cancer. Chest. 2008;133(4):887–91.

101. Coughlin M, Deslauriers J, Beaulieu M, Fournier B, Piraux M, Rouleau J, et al. Role of mediastinoscopy in pretreatment staging of patients with primary lung cancer. Ann Thorac Surg. 1985;40(6):556–60.
102. Luke WP, Pearson FG, Todd TR, Patterson GA, Cooper JD. Prospective evaluation of mediastinoscopy for assessment of carcinoma of the lung. J Thorac Cardiovasc Surg. 1986;91(1):53–6.
103. Hoffmann H. Invasive staging of lung cancer by mediastinoscopy and video-assisted thoracoscopy. Lung Cancer (Amsterdam, Netherlands). 2001;34 Suppl 3:S3–5.
104. Czarnecka-Kujawa K, Yasufuku K. Invited commentary. Ann Thorac Surg. 2017;103(5):1605–6.
105. LeBlanc JK, Devereaux BM, Imperiale TF, Kesler K, DeWitt JM, Cummings O, et al. Endoscopic ultrasound in non-small cell lung cancer and negative mediastinum on computed tomography. Am J Respir Crit Care Med. 2005;171(2):177–82.
106. Fernandez-Esparrach G, Gines A, Belda J, Pellise M, Sole M, Marrades R, et al. Transesophageal ultrasound-guided fine needle aspiration improves mediastinal staging in patients with non-small cell lung cancer and normal mediastinum on computed tomography. Lung Cancer (Amsterdam, Netherlands). 2006;54(1):35–40.
107. Uy KL, Darling G, Xu W, Yi QL, De Perrot M, Pierre AF, et al. Improved results of induction chemoradiation before surgical intervention for selected patients with stage IIIA-N2 non-small cell lung cancer. J Thorac Cardiovasc Surg. 2007;134(1):188–93.
108. Sebastian-Quetglas F, Molins L, Baldo X, Buitrago J, Vidal G. Clinical value of video-assisted thoracoscopy for preoperative staging of non-small cell lung cancer. A prospective study of 105 patients. Lung Cancer (Amsterdam, Netherlands). 2003;42(3):297–301.
109. Roberts JR, Blum MG, Arildsen R, Drinkwater DC Jr, Christian KR, Powers TA, et al. Prospective comparison of radiologic, thoracoscopic, and pathologic staging in patients with early non-small cell lung cancer. Ann Thorac Surg. 1999;68(4):1154–8.
110. Landreneau RJ, Hazelrigg SR, Mack MJ, Fitzgibbon LD, Dowling RD, Acuff TE, et al. Thoracoscopic mediastinal lymph node sampling: useful for mediastinal lymph node stations inaccessible by cervical mediastinoscopy. J Thorac Cardiovasc Surg. 1993;106(3):554–8.
111. Sabur NF, Stather D, MacEachern P, Chee A, Tremblay A. Endobronchial ultrasound knowledge, implementation, and perceived barriers after attendance at a dedicated hands-on course. J Bronchology Interv Pulmonol. 2011;18(2):138–43.
112. Lamb CR, Feller-Kopman D, Ernst A, Simoff MJ, Sterman DH, Wahidi MM, et al. An approach to interventional pulmonary fellowship training. Chest. 2010;137(1):195–9.
113. Stather DR, Chee A, MacEachern P, Dumoulin E, Hergott CA, Gelberg J, et al. Endobronchial ultrasound learning curve in interventional pulmonary fellows. Respirology (Carlton, Vic). 2015;20(2):333–9.
114. Stather DR, Maceachern P, Rimmer K, Hergott CA, Tremblay A. Assessment and learning curve evaluation of endobronchial ultrasound skills following simulation and clinical training. Respirology (Carlton, Vic). 2011;16(4):698–704.
115. Woo L, Panteno J, Goetz J, Lamb CR. Assessing efficacy of a one-day course in EBUS Transbronchial Needle Aspiration Training. Chest. 2010;138(4_MetingAbstracts):588A.
116. Sabur NF, Chee A, Stather DR, Maceachern P, Amjadi K, Hergott CA, et al. The impact of tunneled pleural catheters on the quality of life of patients with malignant pleural effusions. Respiration Int Rev Thorac Dis. 2013;85(1):36–42.
117. Zielinski M, Hauer L, Hauer J, Nabialek T, Szlubowski A, Pankowski J. Non-small-cell lung cancer restaging with transcervical extended mediastinal lymphadenectomy. Eur J Cardiothorac Surg. 2010;37(4):776–80.
118. Van Meerbeeck JP, Van Schil PE, Senan S. Reply: randomized controlled trial of resection versus radiotherapy after induction chemotherapy in stage IIIA-N2 non-small cell lung cancer. J Thorac Oncol. 2007;2(12):1138–9.
119. Betticher DC, Hsu Schmitz SF, Totsch M, Hansen E, Joss C, von Briel C, et al. Mediastinal lymph node clearance after docetaxel-cisplatin neoadjuvant chemotherapy is prognostic of survival in patients with stage IIIA pN2 non-small-cell lung cancer: a multicenter phase II trial. J Clin Oncol. 2003;21(9):1752–9.

120. Herth FJ, Annema JT, Eberhardt R, Yasufuku K, Ernst A, Krasnik M, et al. Endobronchial ultrasound with transbronchial needle aspiration for restaging the mediastinum in lung cancer. J Clin Oncol. 2008;26(20):3346–50.
121. Nasir BS, Bryant AS, Minnich DJ, Wei B, Dransfield MT, Cerfolio RJ. The efficacy of restaging endobronchial ultrasound in patients with non-small cell lung cancer after preoperative therapy. Ann Thorac Surg. 2014;98(3):1008–12.
122. Shingyoji M, Nakajima T, Nishimura H, Ishikawa A, Itakura M, Kaji S, et al. Restaging by endobronchial ultrasound-guided transbronchial needle aspiration in patients with inoperable advanced lung cancer. Intern Med (Tokyo, Japan). 2010;49(8):787–90.
123. Kunst PW, Lee P, Paul MA, Senan S, Smit EF. Restaging of mediastinal nodes with transbronchial needle aspiration after induction chemoradiation for locally advanced non-small cell lung cancer. J Thorac Oncol. 2007;2(10):912–5.
124. Varadarajulu S, Eloubeidi M. Can endoscopic ultrasonography-guided fine-needle aspiration predict response to chemoradiation in non-small cell lung cancer? A pilot study. Respiration Int Rev Thorac Dis. 2006;73(2):213–20.
125. Annema JT, Veselic M, Versteegh MI, Willems LN, Rabe KF. Mediastinal restaging: EUS-FNA offers a new perspective. Lung Cancer (Amsterdam, Netherlands). 2003;42(3):311–8.
126. Stigt JA, Oostdijk AH, Timmer PR, Shahin GM, Boers JE, Groen HJ. Comparison of EUS-guided fine needle aspiration and integrated PET-CT in restaging after treatment for locally advanced non-small cell lung cancer. Lung Cancer (Amsterdam, Netherlands). 2009;66(2):198–204.
127. Marra A, Hillejan L, Fechner S, Stamatis G. Remediastinoscopy in restaging of lung cancer after induction therapy. J Thorac Cardiovasc Surg. 2008;135(4):843–9.
128. De Waele M, Serra-Mitjans M, Hendriks J, Lauwers P, Belda-Sanchis J, Van Schil P, et al. Accuracy and survival of repeat mediastinoscopy after induction therapy for non-small cell lung cancer in a combined series of 104 patients. Eur J Cardiothorac Surg. 2008;33(5):824–8.
129. De Waele M, Hendriks J, Lauwers P, Ortmanns P, Vanroelen W, Morel AM, et al. Nodal status at repeat mediastinoscopy determines survival in non-small cell lung cancer with mediastinal nodal involvement, treated by induction therapy. Eur J Cardiothorac Surg. 2006;29(2):240–3.
130. Rami-Porta R, Mateu-Navarro M, Serra-Mitjans M, Hernandez-Rodriguez H. Remediastinoscopy: comments and updated results. Lung Cancer (Amsterdam, Netherlands). 2003;42(3):363–4.
131. De Leyn P, Stroobants S, De Wever W, Lerut T, Coosemans W, Decker G, et al. Prospective comparative study of integrated positron emission tomography-computed tomography scan compared with remediastinoscopy in the assessment of residual mediastinal lymph node disease after induction chemotherapy for mediastinoscopy-proven stage IIIA-N2 Non-small-cell lung cancer: a Leuven Lung Cancer Group Study. J Clin Oncol. 2006;24(21):3333–9.
132. Steinfort DP, Liew D, Conron M, Hutchinson AF, Irving LB. Cost-benefit of minimally invasive staging of non-small cell lung cancer: a decision tree sensitivity analysis. J Thorac Oncol. 2010;5(10):1564–70.
133. Celikoglu F, Celikoglu SI, Goldberg EP. Bronchoscopic intratumoral chemotherapy of lung cancer. Lung Cancer (Amsterdam, Netherlands). 2008;61(1):1–12.
134. Mehta HJ, Begnaud A, Penley AM, Wynne J, Malhotra P, Fernandez-Bussy S, et al. Restoration of patency to central airways occluded by malignant endobronchial tumors using intratumoral injection of cisplatin. Ann Am Thorac Soc. 2015;12(9):1345–50.
135. http://www.olympus-europa.com. September 17 2016.
136. Nakajima T, Shingyoji M, Anayama T, Kimura H, Yasufuku K, Yoshino I. Spectrum analysis of endobronchial ultrasound radiofrequency of lymph nodes in patients with lung cancer. Chest. 2016;149(6):1393–9.

Chapter 5
Airway Foreign Bodies: Rigid vs Flexible Approach

Inderpaul Singh Sehgal, Sahajal Dhooria, Rajiv Goyal, and Ritesh Agarwal

Introduction

Foreign body (FB) aspiration can present as a medical emergency. FB aspiration generally has a bimodal distribution, and is more commonly encountered in children <3 years and in the elderly population [1–6]. In adults, FB aspiration is uncommon, and the proportion of flexible bronchoscopies performed with airway FB as an indication range from 0.2% to 0.3% across various centres [1, 7]. The presentation of FB aspiration may be acute with respiratory failure or subacute-to-chronic with non-specific respiratory symptoms. The diagnosis requires a high index of clinical suspicion, especially in patients without a history of FB aspiration and in those with a normal chest radiograph. In this review, we discuss the clinical and radiological manifestation of FB aspiration. We also discuss the various tools that are used for removing airway foreign body. In addition, we provide practical tips in handling and removing different types of airway foreign bodies.

I. S. Sehgal · S. Dhooria · R. Agarwal (✉)
Department of Pulmonary Medicine, Postgraduate Institute of Medical Education and Research (PGIMER), Chandigarh, India

R. Goyal
Department of Pulmonary Medicine, Jaipur Golden Hospital, New Delhi and Rajiv Gandhi Cancer Institute, New Delhi, India

© The Author(s), under exclusive license to Springer Nature Switzerland AG 2021
J. F. Turner, Jr. et al. (eds.), *From Thoracic Surgery to Interventional Pulmonology*, Respiratory Medicine, https://doi.org/10.1007/978-3-030-80298-1_5

What Are the Types of Airway FB?

Airway foreign bodies (FBs) are broadly classified as organic, inorganic, mineral and endogenous [1, 3, 7, 8]. The inorganic FBs include metallic (coins, pins, needles, screws, nails and others), plastic (pen cap, buttons, whistle and others), tablets and magnetic objects. The organic FBs include food particles, vegetables, seeds, nuts and others. The minerals include the dental prosthesis, tooth and bones, while the endogenous foreign bodies include broncholiths. Besides, the airway FB can also be described based on its characteristics (small or large, smooth or uneven surface, brittle or hard, sharp or blunt).

Practical point While planning bronchoscopy for an airway FB, it is a good practice to characterize the type of FB as it enables selection of the instruments required for its removal (flexible or rigid bronchoscope, type of forceps). This information can be obtained from the history, thoracic imaging (in case of a radio-opaque FB) and endoscopic findings during flexible bronchoscopy.

What Is the Clinical Presentation of Airway FB?

FB aspiration occurs due to the failure of airway protective mechanisms. In children, it is due to the immature swallowing coordination, while in adults, it occurs due to secondary causes. The risk factors for FB aspiration in adults include altered sensorium, drug intoxication, old age, neurological disorders, psychiatric illness and occasionally accidental during laughing, crying or sneezing [3]. The clinical presentation of FB aspiration depends on the age, the type of FB, the location of FB impaction and others. An acute presentation is more common in children than adults [8]. This is due to the smaller size of airways in children that causes the FB to lodge in the more proximal airways (subglottic region and trachea), with resultant acute airway obstruction and asphyxiation [5, 9–11]. In adults, the presentation is generally more innocuous as the FB gets impacted in the distal airways. The most common site of FB aspiration in adults is the right bronchial tree, which is in direct continuation of the trachea, and is straighter and shorter compared to the left bronchial tree [6, 7, 12]. A clear history of aspirating a FB is not always forthcoming and is present in up to 30–50% of cases [13, 14]. The common presenting symptoms are recent onset cough, a choking episode, wheezing, breathlessness and occasionally hemoptysis. In long-standing foreign bodies, patients may present with symptoms of non-resolving pneumonia, bronchitis or bronchiectasis (chronic productive cough, fever, hemoptysis and others) [1, 15–18].

Clinical examination may reveal features of central airway obstruction such as stridor or monophonic wheeze or can be unrevealing in the case of a distally placed FB [6, 19]. Occasionally, there may be features of collapse (decreased intensity of breath sounds, impaired percussion note with or without a monophonic wheeze). In those with long-standing FB aspiration, there may be features of non-resolving pneumonia or bronchiectasis. The findings on chest imaging depend on the type of FB. Chest imaging is mostly normal especially in case of organic foreign bodies [20]. Imaging is diagnostic in cases of a metallic (pins, needles, nails and others) FB or dentures (Figs. 5.1, 5.2 and 5.3). There may also be indirect signs of airway FB (unilateral hyperinflation, collapse, consolidation or bronchiectasis) [20]. Computed tomography (CT) of the thorax is more sensitive than the chest radiographs for identifying tracheobronchial foreign bodies [21, 22]. CT thorax with virtual bronchoscopy can not only pinpoint the location but can also help in planning the procedure for retrieval of the FB [22].

Practical tips A history of FB aspiration is absent in almost 50% of the patients; thus, diagnosis requires a high index of clinical suspicion. Chest imaging (especially CT chest) helps in locating the airway FB and helps in planning the subsequent procedure.

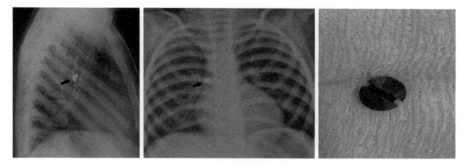

Fig. 5.1 Chest radiograph (lateral view and postero-anterior view) demonstrating a radio-opaque foreign body (arrow) in the right intermediate bronchus. The foreign body (screw-head) was successfully removed using the flexible bronchoscope

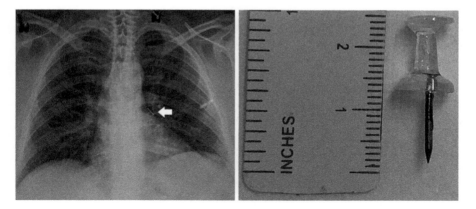

Fig. 5.2 Chest radiograph demonstrating a sharp (pin) foreign body with its pointed edge facing upwards in the left main bronchus. The board pin (right panel) was removed during flexible bronchoscopy

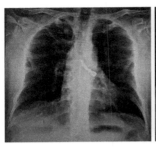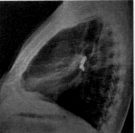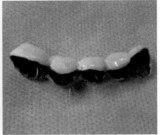

Fig. 5.3 Chest radiograph (postero-anterior and lateral view) demonstrating a denture in the left main bronchus that was successfully removed during flexible bronchoscopy

How to Select Between Flexible and Rigid Bronchoscopy in the Management of Airway FB?

Before the advent of bronchoscopy, the morbidity and the mortality of FB aspiration were high [23]. The first description of airway FB removal was by Gustav Killian using the rigid bronchoscope [24]. Subsequently, Jackson et al. demonstrated a decrease in mortality with successful removal of airway foreign bodies using rigid bronchoscopy [25]. The flexible bronchoscope was developed by Ikeda in 1968 [26]. Animal studies demonstrated that foreign bodies could be successfully removed during flexible bronchoscopy [5, 12, 27, 28]. Thereafter, several case series have described the successful removal of airway foreign bodies in adults [6, 29–31]. Flexible bronchoscopy is now the initial procedure of choice in the diagnostic evaluation of tracheobronchial FB, especially in adults and older children [7]. It helps to visualize the FB, confirm the location, size and disposition within the airways, and the presence of granulation and oedema around the FB. This information is invaluable for planning the procedure, selecting the appropriate instruments and the need for rigid bronchoscopy. Thus, flexible bronchoscopy is not only diagnostic but can also be therapeutic in most cases. In a recent meta-analysis, flexible bronchoscopy was found to help in successfully retrieving airway FB in 90% (95% confidence interval, 86–93%) of the cases in adults [7].

Flexible bronchoscopy offers several advantages. It is a day care procedure performed under conscious sedation. The flexible bronchoscope is widely available and is associated with low morbidity and mortality. It enables a comprehensive airway examination, including that of the upper lobes and distal airways that cannot be negotiated with rigid bronchoscopy. However, flexible bronchoscopy does not provide a secure airway and cannot protect the glottis during the retrieval of a FB. In children <3 years of age, rigid bronchoscopy is the preferred modality for FB extraction as they are more likely to present with respiratory distress and need a secure airway. In adults, the use of rigid bronchoscopy is rarely required for FB removal, except in case of an asphyxiating FB, large foreign bodies with smooth margins or where flexible bronchoscopy was unsuccessful in removing the FB [32]. Rigid bronchoscopy offers several benefits. It provides a secure airway and protects the glottis during FB extraction [32, 33]. Rigid bronchoscopy, however, requires general anaesthesia and may not be available at all centres. Also, one cannot visualize the upper lobes and the distal airways with rigid bronchoscopy alone; however, a flexible bronchoscope can always be inserted through the rigid bronchoscope for distal visualization [33].

Practical tips Flexible bronchoscopy is the preferred initial modality for diagnosis in patients with FB aspiration. At the authors' centres, flexible bronchoscopy is the first procedure for FB visualization and removal. It is generally performed using local anaesthesia and moderate conscious sedation. In case flexible bronchoscopy is unsuccessful, the procedure is then performed using rigid bronchoscopy. Patients with asphyxiating FBs and younger children are taken up for rigid bronchoscopy directly [6, 7, 34, 35].

What Are the Basic Principles in Removal of Foreign Body?

The first step in the management of an airway FB is to assess the patency of the patient's airway and any compromise in the ventilation. In patients who are asphyxiated, rigid bronchoscopy is the procedure of choice. In case it is not immediately available, ventilation may be ensured using non-invasive ventilation. Inserting an endotracheal tube is an individualized decision based on the patient's condition, as it may displace the FB more distally in the airway. Another option is to use a laryngeal mask airway (a supraglottic device) to secure the airways for performing flexible bronchoscopy. For patients who are maintaining a patent airway allowing sufficient ventilation, flexible bronchoscopy may be performed first. Flexible bronchoscopy is performed using the oral route. The entire tracheobronchial tree is examined to locate the FB. Once the FB is localized, the removal of airway FB involves three steps (Mehta's technique), namely, dislodgement of, securing and removing the FB [1]. For dislodging an airway FB, the FB has to be grasped using the appropriate forceps and a Fogarty balloon has to be placed distal to the FB and inflated [36–38]. Occasionally, the Fogarty balloon is then gently pulled to bring the FB in more proximal airways (main bronchi or the trachea). Sometimes the granulation tissue may cover the foreign body, and dislodgement in such instances requires removal of the granulation using either argon plasma coagulation or electrocautery. Once the FB is dislodged, it is secured by grasping it with a suitable forceps. After securing the FB with a suitable forceps, the entire assembly, namely, the bronchoscope, the forceps and the FB, is withdrawn *en bloc* via the transoral route [1, 7]. All the three steps may not be required in all cases. In case a FB allows an easy hold, it can be grasped with suitable forceps and retrieved instantly. After removing the FB, the airways should always be re-examined to ensure complete removal of the FB and to remove the pooled secretions.

Practical tips The removal of airway FB involves three basic steps (dislodgement, securing and retrieval). The airways should always be re-examined to ensure complete removal of the FB.

What Are the Instruments for Grasping and Removing the FB Through the Flexible Bronchoscope?

The common instruments used for removing a tracheobronchial FB include forceps, snare, baskets and the cryoprobe (Fig. 5.4).

Forceps are the most commonly used instrument for removing tracheobronchial foreign bodies. The commonly used forceps include the alligator jaw grasping forceps (for small objects), rat tooth grasping forceps (for soft and flat objects), rat

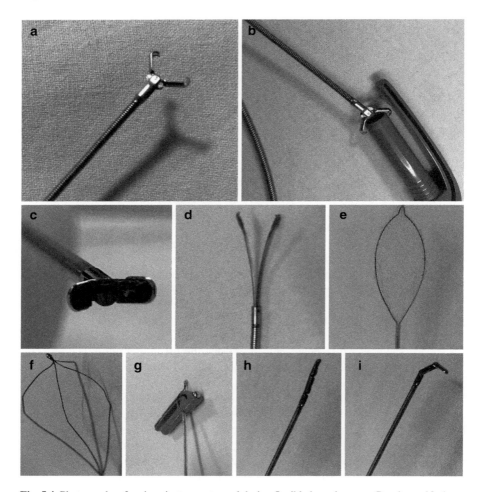

Fig. 5.4 Photographs of various instruments used during flexible bronchoscopy. Panel **a** and **b** demonstrating rat tooth forceps. Panel **c** demonstrating a rubber tip forceps that is used for removing soft foreign bodies and those with flat surface. Panel **d** demonstrating a V forceps used to grasp flat objects. Panel **e** demonstrating a fishnet. Panel **f** and **g** showing a Dormia basket with four wires attached to a lead point. Panel **h** and **i** demonstrating a curette used to mobilize foreign bodies from difficult areas

tooth alligator jaw grasping forceps (for soft and flat objects), three-nail grasping forceps, rubber tip grasping forceps (for sharp objects and smooth objects), shark tooth grasping forceps (for flat objects) and V-shaped forceps (for flat objects) [1–3]. The cupped forceps are generally not used for FB retrieval [1, 3]. The magnetic extractor is used to retrieve metallic foreign bodies such as broken cytology brush, pins or needles that are displaced in the distal airways and are not directly visible [39]. The magnetic extractor is advanced under fluoroscopic guidance to the FB. Once the FB is in contact with the magnetic extractor, it is withdrawn gently to bring the FB in more proximal airways. The magnetic extractor is then withdrawn and the FB is grasped with a grasping forceps and retrieved via oral route [39].

Snare   is used to extract large foreign bodies that cannot be grasped with the grasping forceps [40, 41]. The FB is entangled in the snare and secured. The snare with the FB is then withdrawn as a single unit [40]. The snare is helpful in retrieving large round foreign bodies with smooth margins that are difficult to grasp with routine forceps.

Baskets   are useful for retrieving foreign bodies that are large and slippery [42–45]. The Dormia baskets come in various sizes and require a minimum working channel of 2–2.8 mm depending on the size of the basket [46–48]. Baskets are usually made of three to eight wires that are attached to a lead point. The basket is passed distally to the FB and is opened just distal to the object. The basket is then withdrawn gently and manipulated to entangle the FB within the wires of the basket. Once the object is secured in the basket, the catheter is pulled to make it firmly hold the FB, which is then retrieved together with the basket and the bronchoscope as a single unit. The number of wires in the basket is determined by the size of the FB. Fewer wires are generally needed for a large FB, while more wires are required for smaller foreign bodies to prevent slippage. A fishnet basket has a mesh of thin wires that are attached to a wire snare [1, 3]. The fishnet is used like a basket by placing the net distal to the object. The net is manipulated gently to surround the FB that gets trapped in the fishnet.

Cryoprobe   The cryoprobes can also be used for retrieving airway foreign bodies. The rigid cryoprobes are larger in size but are not stable and there is a tendency for the objects to fall off. The flexible cryoprobes that are passed through the working channel of the flexible bronchoscope are more commonly used. The cryoprobe is generally suited best for organic foreign bodies with a large water content. Occasionally, inorganic foreign bodies can also be removed after instilling saline over the FB [49, 50]. After identifying the location of the FB, the cryoprobe is advanced and contact is made at the centre of the FB avoiding any contact with the surrounding bronchial tissue [35]. The cryoprobe is activated and after ensuring cryo-adherence, the cryoprobe, the FB and the bronchoscope are withdrawn before thawing occurs.

Practical tips Before attempting to remove airway FB, proper selection of the instruments must be done depending on the type of FB. For soft organic foreign bodies, the use of rubber tip forceps, cryoprobe or the Dormia basket should be used to avoid breakage of the FB. For inorganic foreign bodies, grasping forceps are preferred. For large mucus plugs and blood clots, a cryoprobe is the best method.

What Is the Role of Rigid Bronchoscopy in Removal of Airway FB?

Rigid bronchoscopy is an invasive technique for removal of airway FB [51]. It is performed by introducing rigid barrels of various sizes [51]. The advantage of the rigid bronchoscopy is that it secures the airways and enables ventilation during the procedure. It is usually performed in the operating room under general anaesthesia [32, 52]. A tracheobronchoscope of at least 11 mm internal diameter is used for retrieving tracheobronchial foreign bodies in adults, while 3.5–5.5 mm barrels are used in children. The use of a large-sized barrel enables the use of multiple instruments (optical telescope, forceps, suction catheters, Fogarty balloon and others). In children, generally an optical forceps is used to remove the FB. The rigid barrel is placed in the trachea, and a flexible bronchoscope is then introduced through the barrel of the rigid scope to perform complete examination of the tracheobronchial tree. Once the FB is localized, it can be removed either using the rigid forceps or with a flexible bronchoscope, as described above.

Rigid bronchoscopy is the preferred modality for removing airway foreign bodies in children. In adults, the use of rigid bronchoscopy is limited to large foreign bodies, foreign bodies with smooth margins and sharp foreign bodies and in situations where initial attempts to remove a FB using a flexible bronchoscope are unsuccessful [1, 7]. It is also the preferred method where the presentation is with respiratory failure.

The forceps used with the rigid scope are large and are enabled with the optics (Hopkins telescope). The optical forceps with alligator jaws has a force-limited handle and is used for grasping hard foreign bodies. The optical forceps with Killian bean jaws is used for grasping peanuts and soft foreign bodies. The optical forceps with 2 × 2 teeth is used for grasping coins and flat foreign bodies.

How Is a Metallic or an Inorganic FB Removed?

During flexible bronchoscopy, the sharp metallic foreign bodies including pins, nails or screws are first mobilized and are held from the pointed end. The types of forceps used include the grasping alligator forceps and the shark or the rat tooth forceps. Once the FB is held from its pointed end, it is held firmly with the forceps and is brought closer to the distal end of the bronchoscope in order to firmly secure the FB [53, 54]. It is important to hold the sharp FB by its pointed end; otherwise, it may injure the airways or embed itself in the mucosa during extraction [1, 7]. In case the FB is embedded in the bronchial mucosa, the object is held from its proximal end and is pushed down so that the sharp end becomes free, which is then held. In any situation where damage due to the airway is contemplated with a sharp FB, the procedure should be performed through an endotracheal tube or the rigid bronchoscope. Once the sharp tip of the FB is brought into the endotracheal tube/barrel of the rigid bronchoscope, the whole assembly can be removed *en bloc* as described earlier.

Pen caps and plastic whistle are removed using larger forceps such as the rat tooth or the shark tooth forceps [55–57]. Utmost care should be given while pulling the scope as the FB may get impacted in the subglottic region. A long-standing FB (a tooth or a denture) may result in stenosis or granulation tissue that may hinder mobilization of the FB. In such a situation, argon photocoagulation (APC) or laser may be used to remove the granulation tissue and the FB can be removed later [58, 59]. In case of bronchostenosis, a controlled radial expansion (CRE) balloon can be used to dilate the stenosed segment and the FB can be removed [60–62]. The stenosis can also be negotiated by using electrocautery enabled knife. Once the FB is visualized, a Fogarty balloon is passed distal to it and inflated. The balloon is then gently pulled to bring the FB across the granulation tissue or the stenosed segment. Once the FB is mobilized in the proximal airways, it is grasped with grasping forceps and extracted en bloc.

A large smooth FB such as a office magnet or a glass FB requires the use of a rigid bronchoscope. The FB is brought to the proximal airways and held with a large optical alligator forceps. The FB is brought into the barrel of the rigid scope and removed safely avoiding impaction of the large FB in the narrow subglottic region. Occasionally, a large magnet cannot be grasped in forceps even during rigid bronchoscopy. In such a scenario, the FB is first mobilized and brought to the proximal large airways, and a magnet placed externally over the chest wall can be used to mobilize the FB that can then be easily brought out [63].

Inorganic foreign bodies such as tablets and iron pills incite intense inflammatory response and may get dissolved over time [1, 3]. In such a situation, the airways should be examined thoroughly, and a short course of oral glucocorticoids instituted. Glucocorticoids resolve the inflammation and can enable removal of the FB remnants during a subsequent procedure.

How Is an Organic FB Removed?

The organic foreign bodies include seeds, peanuts, nuts and vegetable matter. The organic foreign bodies are more likely to cause inflammation and formation of granulation tissue. Also, the organic foreign bodies such as seeds, corn and others absorb moisture and swell, thus causing a more complete obstruction. In such a scenario, the foreign bodies are more difficult to mobilize. Soft and friable foreign bodies such as peanuts, nuts and vegetable matter disintegrate if excessive force is applied. Here, the FB should be held gently using a rubber tipped forceps that would avoid breakage of the FB. The friable foreign bodies can also be completely removed using a cryoprobe. A large organic FB such as a seed can also be easily removed with a cryoprobe due to high water content that enables cryo-adherence. In one such instance, we were unable to remove a large organic FB (*Terminalia chebula* seed) using the routine grasping forceps and the Dormia basket [35]. We then used the cryoprobe to extract the large FB successfully [35].

What Are the Recent Advances in the Management of Airway FB?

The main challenge in the management of foreign bodies is difficulty in locating the FB in the distal subsegmental bronchi that are not visualized with the current equipment. Thus, the advancement is likely to result from improvement in the broncho-scopes and the localization of the FB techniques. The thinner bronchoscopes with small external diameter (<3 mm) can reach up to the subsegmental bronchi and enable removal of the foreign bodies [64]. The only caveat is the smaller working channel that hinders the use of a larger forceps. However, once located, the FB can be removed using combination of instruments such as Fogarty balloon, magnetic extractor, fluoroscopic guidance and others [64]. Takenaka et al. described the use of virtual bronchoscopic navigation in successful localization and removal of a sur-gical gauge [65]. One report describes the use of electromagnetic navigation bron-choscopy to remove a distal FB that was not visible during routine bronchoscopy [66]. The use of electromagnetic navigation bronchoscopy not only enabled suc-cessful removal of the FB but also avoided surgery [66]. One of the authors has described the use of a ureteroscope for locating and removing the FB that was placed distally and could not be visualized using the conventional broncho-scope [67].

What Is the Efficacy of Flexible and Rigid Bronchoscopy for Managing Airway FB?

There is no head-to-head comparison of rigid versus flexible bronchoscopy in retrieving the airway FB. In a pooled analysis of studies describing the use of flex-ible bronchoscopy in the management of airway FB in adults, flexible bronchos-copy was successful in 90% of the cases [7]. The success of the procedure is highly dependent on the operator's experience and the availability of various instruments required for FB removal [1, 5]. In a retrospective study, rigid bronchoscopy had a significantly higher success rate in retrieving the airway FB compared to the flexible bronchoscopy (95% vs 40%). However, majority of their patients were <12 years [6]. In another study, rigid bronchoscopy was successful in 92% of the cases [5]. A yet another case series reported a success rate of 98% with rigid bronchoscopy including six instances where flexible bronchoscopy was unsuccessful [12]. We believe that flexible bronchoscopy should be the initial procedure of choice and rigid bronchoscopy should be performed when flexible bronchoscopy has failed to remove a FB.

How Is the Management of Foreign Body Aspiration Different in Children Compared to Adults?

The incidence of foreign body aspiration is higher in children compared to adults, especially in children less than 3 years old [68, 69]. The presentation of airway FB is more often acute and generally associated with hypoxemia due to smaller airway size [70]. The most common site for airway FB in children is in proximal bronchi followed by the trachea [6]. Unlike adults, rigid bronchoscopy is the preferred initial modality due to imminent risk of death and is more successful than flexible bronchoscopy [6]. Flexible bronchoscopy is generally reserved for children older than 12 years and in children where the history of FB aspiration is not clear. The commonly used flexible scope in children is that with an outer diameter of 4.2 mm, which has a working channel of 2 mm that allows only selective instruments. Even with rigid bronchoscopy, there can be practical issues. For example, due to small airways, only smaller-sized rigid scopes can be used. This not only restricts the instruments that can be introduced for foreign body removal but may also result in difficulty in ventilation during the procedure [71]. An important consideration during anaesthesia for foreign body in children is to maintain spontaneous ventilation, especially for those with tracheal FB. Theoretically, positive pressure ventilation may migrate a foreign body in the airway and potentially convert a partial obstruction to a complete obstruction.

Conclusion

In conclusion, airway FB is an important clinical problem that requires a high clinical suspicion for early diagnosis and requires skill set, experience and teamwork for successful management. In non-asphyxiating airway foreign bodies, flexible bronchoscopy is the initial preferred modality to confirm and retrieve the FB. The use of rigid bronchoscopy is limited to removal of foreign body in smaller children, in management of asphyxiating foreign bodies and in situations where initial attempts with flexible bronchoscopy have failed.

References

1. Rafanan AL, Mehta AC. Adult airway foreign body removal. What's new? Clin Chest Med. 2001;22(2):319–30.
2. Blanco Ramos M, Botana-Rial M, Garcia-Fontan E, Fernandez-Villar A, Gallas TM. Update in the extraction of airway foreign bodies in adults. J Thorac Dis. 2016;8(11):3452–6.
3. Dikensoy O, Usalan C, Filiz A. Foreign body aspiration: clinical utility of flexible bronchoscopy. Postgrad Med J. 2002;78(921):399–403.
4. Ali SR, Mehta AC. Alive in the airways: live endobronchial foreign bodies. Chest. 2017;151(2):481–91.
5. Baharloo F, Veyckemans F, Francis C, Biettlot MP, Rodenstein DO. Tracheobronchial foreign bodies: presentation and management in children and adults. Chest. 1999;115(5):1357–62.
6. Goyal R, Nayar S, Gogia P, Garg M. Extraction of tracheobronchial foreign bodies in children and adults with rigid and flexible bronchoscopy. J Bronchology Interv Pulmonol. 2012;19(1):35–43.
7. Sehgal IS, Dhooria S, Ram B, Singh N, Aggarwal AN, Gupta D, et al. Foreign body inhalation in the adult population: experience of 25,998 bronchoscopies and systematic review of the literature. Respir Care. 2015;60(10):1438–48.
8. Debeljak A, Sorli J, Music E, Kecelj P. Bronchoscopic removal of foreign bodies in adults: experience with 62 patients from 1974-1998. Eur Respir J. 1999;14(4):792–5.
9. Banerjee A, Rao KS, Khanna SK, Narayanan PS, Gupta BK, Sekar JC, et al. Laryngo-tracheobronchial foreign bodies in children. J Laryngol Otol. 1988;102(11):1029–32.
10. Johnson K, Linnaus M, Notrica D. Airway foreign bodies in pediatric patients: anatomic location of foreign body affects complications and outcomes. Pediatr Surg Int. 2017;33(1):59–64.
11. Adjeso T, Damah MC, Murphy JP, Anyomih TTK. Foreign body aspiration in northern Ghana: a review of pediatric patients. Int J Otolaryngol. 2017;2017:1478795.
12. Limper AH, Prakash UB. Tracheobronchial foreign bodies in adults. Ann Intern Med. 1990;112(8):604–9.
13. Friedman EM. Tracheobronchial foreign bodies. Otolaryngol Clin N Am. 2000;33(1):179–85.
14. Emir H, Tekant G, Besik C, Elicevik M, Senyuz OF, Buyukunal C, et al. Bronchoscopic removal of tracheobronchial foreign bodies: value of patient history and timing. Pediatr Surg Int. 2001;17(2-3):85–7.
15. Ali MS, Musani AI, Gaurav K. Pulmonary foreign body: an unusual cause of recurrent pneumonia. Arch Bronconeumol. 2018;54(1):39.
16. Dabu J, Lindner M, Azzam M, Al-Khateeb A, Kadri M, Bellary S, et al. A case of chronic cough and pneumonia secondary to a foreign body. Case Rep Med. 2017;2017:3092623.
17. Samprathi M, Acharya S, Biswal B, Panda SS, Das RR. An unusual foreign body masquerading as pneumonia. J Pediatr. 2016;178:300-.e1.
18. Adegboye VO, Osinowo O, Adebo OA. Bronchiectasis consequent upon prolonged foreign body retention. Cent Afr J Med. 2003;49(5-6):53–8.
19. Lin L, Lv L, Wang Y, Zha X, Tang F, Liu X. The clinical features of foreign body aspiration into the lower airway in geriatric patients. Clin Interv Aging. 2014;9:1613–8.
20. Mu LC, Sun DQ, He P. Radiological diagnosis of aspirated foreign bodies in children: review of 343 cases. J Laryngol Otol. 1990;104(10):778–82.
21. Zissin R, Shapiro-Feinberg M, Rozenman J, Apter S, Smorjik J, Hertz M. CT findings of the chest in adults with aspirated foreign bodies. Eur Radiol. 2001;11(4):606–11.
22. Kosucu P, Ahmetoglu A, Koramaz I, Orhan F, Ozdemir O, Dinc H, et al. Low-dose MDCT and virtual bronchoscopy in pediatric patients with foreign body aspiration. AJR Am J Roentgenol. 2004;183(6):1771–7.
23. Jackson CL. [Foreign bodies in the bronchi and esophagus in children and adults]. Ann Otolaryngol. 1955;72(2–3):179–82.

24. Killian G. Meeting of the Society of Physicians of Freiburg, Dec. 17, 1897. Munchen Med Wschr. 1898;45:378.
25. Jackson C. Diseases of the air and food passages of foreign body origin. Philadelphia: WB Saunders; 1936.
26. Ikeda S. Atlas of flexible bronchofiberoscopy. Baltimore: University Park Press; 1974. p. 220.
27. Zavala DC, Rhodes ML. Foreign body removal: a new role for the fiberoptic bronchoscope. Ann Otol Rhinol Laryngol. 1975;84(5 Pt 1):650–6.
28. Zavala DC, Rhodes ML. Experimental removal of foreign bodies by fiberoptic bronchoscopy. Am Rev Respir Dis. 1974;110(3):357–60.
29. Cunanan OS. The flexible fiberoptic bronchoscope in foreign body removal. Experience in 300 cases. Chest. 1978;73(5 Suppl):725–6.
30. Fieselmann JF, Zavala DC, Keim LW. Removal of foreign bodies (two teeth) by fiberoptic bronchoscopy. Chest. 1977;72(2):241–3.
31. Heinz GJ 3rd, Richardson RH, Zavala DC. Endobronchial foreign body removal using the bronchofiberscope. Ann Otol Rhinol Laryngol. 1978;87(1 Pt 1):50–2.
32. Farrell PT. Rigid bronchoscopy for foreign body removal: anaesthesia and ventilation. Paediatr Anaesth. 2004;14(1):84–9.
33. Helmers RA, Sanderson DR. Rigid bronchoscopy. The forgotten art. Clin Chest Med. 1995;16(3):393–9.
34. Gupta AA, Sehgal IS, Dhooria S, Singh N, Aggarwal AN, Gupta D, et al. Indications for performing flexible bronchoscopy: trends over 34 years at a tertiary care hospital. Lung India. 2015;32(3):211–5.
35. Sehgal IS, Dhooria S, Behera D, Agarwal R. Use of cryoprobe for removal of a large tracheo-bronchial foreign body during flexible bronchoscopy. Lung India. 2016;33(5):543–5.
36. Wankhede RG, Maitra G, Pal S, Ghoshal A, Mitra S. Successful removal of foreign body bronchus using C-arm-guided insertion of Fogarty catheter through plastic bead. Indian J Crit Care Med. 2017;21(2):96–8.
37. Elsharkawy H, Abd-Elsayed AA, Karroum R. Management challenges in the passing-through technique using a Fogarty catheter to remove an endobronchial foreign body from an infant. Ochsner J. 2015;15(1):110–3.
38. Banerjee A, Khanna SK, Narayanan PS. Use of Fogarty catheters for removal of tracheobronchial foreign bodies. Chest. 1984;85(3):452.
39. Saito H, Saka H, Sakai S, Shimokata K. Removal of broken fragment of biopsy forceps with magnetic extractor. Chest. 1989;95(3):700–1.
40. Ichimura H, Maeda M, Kikuchi S, Ozawa Y, Kanemoto K, Kurishima K, et al. Endobronchial dental prosthesis retrieval by a snare technique using a flexible bronchoscope and fluoroscopy: two case reports and technical tips. Respir Med Case Rep. 2016;19:187–9.
41. Tu CY, Chen HJ, Chen W, Liu YH, Chen CH. A feasible approach for extraction of dental prostheses from the airway by flexible bronchoscopy in concert with wire loop snares. Laryngoscope. 2007;117(7):1280–2.
42. Lando T, Cahill AM, Elden L. Distal airway foreign bodies: importance of a stepwise approach, knowledge of equipment and utilization of other services' expertise. Int J Pediatr Otorhinolaryngol. 2011;75(7):968–72.
43. Kim K, Lee HJ, Yang EA, Kim HS, Chun YH, Yoon JS, et al. Foreign body removal by flexible bronchoscopy using retrieval basket in children. Ann Thorac Med. 2018;13(2):82–5.
44. Hata A, Nakajima T, Ohashi K, Inage T, Tanaka K, Sakairi Y, et al. Mini grasping basket forceps for endobronchial foreign body removal in pediatric patients. Pediatr Int. 2017;59(11):1200–4.
45. Lax EA, Kiran SH, Lee MW. Bronchoscopic retrieval of a bullet using a Dormia basket: a case report. J Med Case Rep. 2014;8:358.
46. Moss R, Kanchanapoon V. Stone basket extraction of a bronchial foreign body. Arch Surg. 1986;121(8):975.
47. McCullough P. Wire basket removal of a large endobronchial foreign body. Chest. 1985;87(2):270–1.

48. Dajani AM. Bronchial foreign-body removed with a Dormia basket. Lancet. 1971;1(7708):1076–7.
49. Fruchter O, Kramer MR. Retrieval of various aspirated foreign bodies by flexible cryoprobe: in vitro feasibility study. Clin Respir J. 2015;9(2):176–9.
50. Srinivasan A, Sivaramakrishnan M, Vallandramam PR, Yadav P. Whistle lower-better late than never. Lung India. 2016;33(3):310–2.
51. Rigid bronchoscopy. Chest. 2003;123(5):1695–6.
52. Alraiyes AH, Machuzak MS. Rigid bronchoscopy. Semin Respir Crit Care Med. 2014;35(6):671–80.
53. Hamad AM, Elmistekawy EM, Ragab SM. Headscarf pin, a sharp foreign body aspiration with particular clinical characteristics. Eur Arch Otorhinolaryngol. 2010;267(12):1957–62.
54. Murthy PS, Ingle VS, George E, Ramakrishna S, Shah FA. Sharp foreign bodies in the tracheobronchial tree. Am J Otolaryngol. 2001;22(2):154–6.
55. Kumar J, Saini I, Yadav DK, Jana M, Kabra SK. Cap of pen aspiration causing multiple lung lesions. Indian J Pediatr. 2016;83(8):866–7.
56. Soong WJ, Tsao PC, Lee YS, Yang CF, Liao J, Jeng MJ. Retrieving difficult aspirated pen caps by balloon catheter with short working-length flexible endoscopy and noninvasive ventilation support in intensive care unit. Int J Pediatr Otorhinolaryngol. 2015;79(9):1484–9.
57. Chen M, Zhang J, Liu W, Zhao J, Liu B, Zhang Y. Clinical features and management of aspiration of plastic pen caps. Int J Pediatr Otorhinolaryngol. 2012;76(7):980–3.
58. Shu L, Hu Y, Wei R. Argon plasma coagulation combined with a flexible electronic bronchoscope for treating foreign body granulation tissues in children's deep bronchi: nine case reports. J Laparoendosc Adv Surg Tech A. 2016;26(12):1039–40.
59. Jabbardarjani H, Kiani A, Arab A, Masjedi M. Foreign body removal using bronchoscopy and argon plasma coagulation. Arch Iran Med. 2010;13(2):150–2.
60. Strychowsky JE, Roberson DW, Martin T, Smithers J, Herrington H. Proximal bronchial balloon dilation for embedded distal airway foreign bodies. Laryngoscope. 2016;126(7):1693–5.
61. Thornton CS, Yunker WK. Rigid bronchoscopy and balloon dilation for removal of aspirated thumbtacks: case series and literature review. Int J Pediatr Otorhinolaryngol. 2015;79(9):1541–3.
62. McAfee SJ, Vashisht R. Removal of an impacted distal airway foreign body using a guidewire and a balloon angioplasty catheter. Anaesth Intensive Care. 2011;39(2):303–4.
63. Hegde S, Bahadur U, Kanojia RP, Bawa M, Samujh R. Bronchoscopic airway foreign body extraction without using optical forceps. J Indian Assoc Pediatr Surg. 2018;23(2):87–9.
64. Hirai Y, Oura S, Yoshimasu T, Hirai I, Kokawa Y, Nakamura R, et al. Removal of an endobronchial foreign body using an ultrathin flexible bronchoscope and a novel suction system. J Bronchology Interv Pulmonol. 2013;20(4):363–4.
65. Takenaka T, Katsura M, Shikada Y, Furuya K, Takeo S. Intrapulmonary foreign body removal under virtual bronchoscopic navigation. J Bronchology Interv Pulmonol. 2012;19(2):159–61.
66. Karpman C, Midthun DE, Mullon JJ. A distal airway foreign body removed with electromagnetic navigation bronchoscopy. J Bronchology Interv Pulmonol. 2014;21(2):170–2.
67. Goyal R, Gogia P, Chachra V, Hibare K. Foreign body in the lung following dental procedure. Lung India. 2016;33(6):664–6.
68. Zhong B, Sun SL, Du JT, Deng D, Liu F, Liu YF, et al. Risk factors for lower respiratory tract infection in children with tracheobronchial foreign body aspiration. Medicine (Baltimore). 2019;98(10):e14655.
69. Tan GX, Boss EF, Rhee DS. Bronchoscopy for pediatric airway foreign body: thirty-day adverse outcomes in the ACS NSQIP-P. Otolaryngol Head Neck Surg. 2019;160(2):326–31.
70. Tenenbaum T, Kahler G, Janke C, Schroten H, Demirakca S. Management of foreign body removal in children by flexible bronchoscopy. J Bronchology Interv Pulmonol. 2017;24(1):21–8.
71. Woo SH, Park JJ, Kwon M, Ryu JS, Kim JP. Tracheobronchial foreign body removal in infants who had very small airways: a prospective clinical trial. Clin Respir J. 2018;12(2):738–45.

Chapter 6
Management of Bronchopleural Fistula

Normand R. Caron, Jeremy C. Johnson, and Satish Kalanjeri

Definition of Bronchopleural Fistula (BPF)

A bronchopleural fistula is a communication between a mainstem bronchus, a lobar bronchus, and a segmental bronchus with the pleural space. This is quite different from an alveolopleural fistula and its management is completely different. An alveolopleural fistula refers to a communication between the lung parenchyma at a level distal to a subsegmental bronchus and the pleural space.

Risk Factors Associated with the Bronchopleural Fistula

Bronchopleural fistulas can occur from multiple causes. Some such causes include underlying disease, lung abscesses, pneumonias with associated empyemas, and major chest trauma. However, bronchopleural fistulas most commonly occur after lung surgery. There is a 1–3% rate of developing a bronchopleural fistula after a lobectomy and up to a 12% rate of developing a bronchopleural fistula after a bilobectomy or a pneumonectomy. Empyemas after a pneumonectomy are associated with a bronchopleural fistula in 75–80% of the time [1]. Early bronchopleural fistulas that arise after surgery usually occur within 14 days and are often attributed to technical causes. Such causes include leaving a large diameter or long bronchial

N. R. Caron
Thoracic Surgery, Harry S. Truman Memorial Veterans Hospital, Columbia, MO, USA

J. C. Johnson · S. Kalanjeri (✉)
Pulmonary and Critical Care Medicine, Harry S. Truman Memorial Veterans Hospital and University of Missouri, Columbia, MO, USA
e-mail: kalanjeris@health.missouri.edu

© The Author(s), under exclusive license to Springer Nature Switzerland AG 2021
J. F. Turner, Jr. et al. (eds.), *From Thoracic Surgery to Interventional Pulmonology*, Respiratory Medicine,
https://doi.org/10.1007/978-3-030-80298-1_6

stump, performing an extensive dissection around the bronchial stump (lymph node dissection), or leaving residual tumor at the bronchial margin.

Other factors also increase the risk of developing a postoperative bronchopleural fistula and include older age at the time of surgery, previous ipsilateral chest surgery, right side surgery, neoadjuvant chemotherapy and radiation therapy, and the need for postoperative ventilatory support. In addition, patient-related causes include malnutrition (low albumin), diabetes, chronic steroid use, and COPD (low FEV_1, low DLCO). Also, complications from adjuvant chemotherapy or radiation therapy including ablative therapies can result in bronchopleural fistulas [2–4].

Benign causes include bacterial and fungal infections which can occasionally extend to the pleural space creating a bronchopleural fistula.

At the time of pneumonectomy, there are technical considerations to which the surgeon must strictly adhere. These include avoidance of bronchial stump devascularization, avoiding tension on the suture line, ensuring the bronchial stump is short, and obtaining clean margins if pneumonectomy is performed for a malignant etiology [4]. Most surgeons usually cover the bronchial stump with viable tissue. This includes surrounding tissue such as the pericardium, prepericardial fat, pleura, and right azygos vein for right pneumonectomies. Also, mobilization of an intercostal muscle or a pedicle of the diaphragm can be mobilized to cover the bronchial stump. It is unknown whether bronchial stump coverage after pneumonectomy is beneficial. The bronchial stump is usually covered with viable tissue in high-risk patients [2, 5]. Postoperatively after pneumonectomy, ventilatory support is best avoided. If this is needed, then the endotracheal tube should be guided into the nonoperative mainstem bronchus to avoid barotrauma to the bronchial stump.

Clinical Presentation

Patients who develop postoperative bronchopleural fistulas can present with sudden, acute symptoms or with more gradual, subacute symptoms.

Acute symptoms of bronchopleural fistula can occur at any time but are usually seen in the early postoperative period. The patient usually has a sudden onset of severe dyspnea often with chest pain and hemodynamic instability. They may also develop subcutaneous emphysema since the incision is still fresh. Should the bronchopleural fistula develop in the immediate postoperative period while the chest tube is still present, the symptoms may be less severe with a large increase in the chest tube air leak and the patient having some malaise.

Patients in whom bronchopleural fistulas occur later in the postoperative period have usually been discharged from the hospital often present with fever, malaise, and very productive cough that usually contains purulent material. They can present in extreme distress if the nonoperated lung develops an aspiration pneumonia. This is especially true if the operation was a pneumonectomy. Additionally, if a post-pneumonectomy patient presents with hemodynamic instability from a tension pneumothorax, then a bronchopleural fistula is almost always the cause.

Diagnostic Studies

The diagnosis of a bronchopleural fistula requires astute clinical skills with a reliable history, imaging studies, and bronchoscopic evaluation.

Clinical decision-making requires noting the appearance of the patient, the amount of distress he/she is having, the appearance of the incision and the surrounding skin, the symmetry of the chest during respiration, and any changes in voice or diaphoresis. On examination, the patient often will have some fever, tachypnea, tachycardia, and perhaps hypotension. There may be some subcutaneous emphysema along the chest wall or around the base of the neck. On auscultation, the breath sounds are often reduced on the affected side and crackles may be heard on the nonoperated side.

Definitive diagnosis includes lab work especially a CBC with differential and a chest radiograph (Fig. 6.1). The chest radiograph is especially useful in a postoperative patient if compared to a previous postoperative chest x-ray. If the patient had a pneumonectomy and the postoperative chest x-ray showed a pleural cavity that was completely opacified with pleural fluid but now has an air fluid level, then the formation of a bronchopleural fistula is most likely the cause. The nonoperative lung can also be assessed for possible contamination from the bronchopleural fistula (Fig. 6.1). Sometimes pneumomediastinum and subcutaneous emphysema can be visualized on a posteroanterior and lateral chest x-ray. A better imaging study is a computerized tomography scan (CT scan) of the chest (Fig. 6.2). This imaging study is often performed with coronal and sagittal reformatting and can detect any shift of the mediastinum and any subcutaneous and

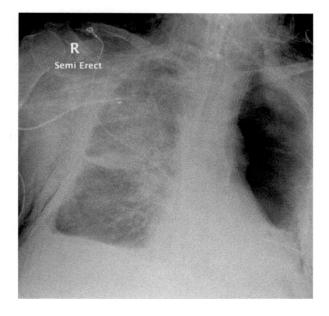

Fig. 6.1 Portable chest x-ray showing contamination of the right lung in a 72-year-old postpneumonectomy patient who developed a left bronchopleural fistula that has just been drained by tube thoracostomy

Fig. 6.2 CT scan of the
chest after right upper
lobectomy demonstrating a
bronchopleural fistula
involving the right upper
lobe bronchus in a
63-year-old cancer patient

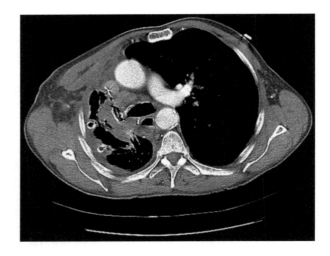

mediastinal emphysema. It can also localize the site of the bronchopleural fistula where there is communication between the pleural space and the main airway (Fig. 6.2). It may also demonstrate bubbles within the pleural fluid indicating an infection within the pleural cavity.

Once a postoperative empyema that contains a bronchopleural fistula is confirmed, then the next immediate steps are beginning intravenous broad-spectrum antibiotics, laying the patient onto the operative side to protect the contralateral lung, placement of a chest tube into the empyema for immediate drainage, and obtaining cultures. This is especially crucial in a postpneumonectomy with bronchopleural fistula. The next steps in management depend on the time since the surgery and the development of the empyema. Also, the size of the bronchopleural fistula and the clinical status of the patient will impact what follows next.

If the patient is stable enough, fiber-optic bronchoscopy should be performed on any patient suspected of having a bronchopleural fistula. This is most important in assessing the site of the fistula as well as its size. It can also assess the noninvolved lung for possible contamination. Cultures can also be obtained during bronchoscopy. If there is a long bronchial stump, its length can be estimated. Sometimes, the fistula is small and difficult to detect. Other times, the opening of the bronchopleural fistula cannot be detected upon direct visualization of the surgical site. It may be detected by instillation of normal saline and observing for bubbling. If the patient has a chest tube in the pleural space, sequential balloon occlusion may show stoppage of the air leak seen in the collection system's bubble chamber. This can help locate the site of the bronchopleural fistula. If the bronchopleural fistula can be seen on bronchoscopy, then an assessment can be made as to whether the patient will require surgical exploration and repair or whether it can be treated nonoperatively or by interventional bronchoscopy.

Initial Management of Bronchopleural Fistulas

The initial approach to the management of a patient with a bronchopleural fistula depends a lot on the experience of the thoracic surgical team and the interventional pulmonary team. Usually, a multidisciplinary team approach offers the best chance for success in treating this morbid and often fatal condition. Most patients require surgical closure of the bronchopleural fistula while at the same time undergoing chest debridement and covering the repaired bronchus with viable tissue. This is often the case if the patient has had recent surgery within the past 2 weeks. The viable tissue usually consists of intercostal muscle, but extrathoracic muscle such as the serratus anterior or the latissimus dorsi [6]. Also, a pedicle of the diaphragm can be used as well as omentum when other chest wall muscles are not usable. These patients need to be hemodynamically stable and able to tolerate a reoperation.

Patients who present with a bronchopleural fistula and are not candidates for immediate surgical repair because of hemodynamic instability, sepsis, and shock or they require ventilatory support need to be temporized until their condition is improved enough to tolerate reoperation. This is usually done in an ICU setting where a chest tube is placed in the empyema to drain it, cultures are obtained, and broad-spectrum antibiotics are started. Inotropic and ventilator support are also started if needed. If the patient has had a pneumonectomy and requires intubation, the endotracheal tube should be guided into the remaining mainstem bronchus to avoid ventilating the mainstem bronchus with the bronchopleural fistula. Once the cultures are known, the antibiotics can be tailored to the causative bacteria.

Patients who are not well enough to go directly to the operating room for debridement of the pleural cavity and bronchial stump revision with viable tissue coverage and chest closure will require a staged procedure with an open window thoracostomy.

Surgical Repair of Bronchopleural Fistulas

If the patient recovers well enough to tolerate surgery, then he should be taken to the operating room for debridement of the pleural cavity, suture closure of the bronchopleural fistula, and covering the stump with omentum or viable muscle. Instead of closing the chest, the patient will require either packing the chest with dilute povidone-iodine or 1/4 strength Dakin's soaked gauze packing through an open window thoracostomy (Clagett procedure) or placing a wound VAC within the pleural space [4, 7–9].

The surgical repair usually involves a redo thoracotomy or a VATS procedure. Usually, a thoracotomy is preferred for thoroughly debriding the pleural space. Also, suture repair of the bronchopleural fistula can be difficult. It requires dissecting the bronchus for repair while at the same time avoiding any injury to the nearby main pulmonary artery. This is especially true for postpneumonectomy broncho-pleural fistulas. Also, if viable tissue is to be used to reinforce the repair site, then muscle or omentum needs to be mobilized and placed within the pleural cavity.

After the pleural cavity is well debrided and the bronchopleural fistula is repaired and covered with viable tissue, the pleural cavity is packed with either antibiotic or antimicrobial gauze through an open window thoracostomy or wound VAC sponges are placed within the chest cavity and the chest wall remains partially open while the wound VAC is placed to 125 mmHg suction. The antimicrobial packing or the VAC sponges are usually left for 3 days while attempts are made to extubate the patient. The affected pleural cavity is usually well stabilized by the packed dress-ings or the wound VAC until the next dressing change. This is usually preplanned for the third postoperative day. The patient is returned to the operating room and the dressings or wound VAC sponges are removed with care not to dislodge or damage the viable tissue covering the bronchial stump. Our group no longer favors the use of antibiotic or antimicrobial chest packings with a Clagett window unless there is a large air leak that prevents the use of a wound VAC. Instead, we prefer using a wound VAC and the reason for this is because the wound VAC promotes granulation tissue formation, contracts the size of the pleural space, requires a lesser number of operative debridement, usually shortens the hospital stay, and allows the patient to be discharged with the wound VAC. The patient can return twice a week for wound VAC changes. These can even be performed in a procedure room once the patient has had several wound VAC changes and less extensive pleural debridements are required [9].

Once the pleural cavity exhibits good granulation tissue throughout, a decision is made to close the chest wall. The antibiotic solution used to fill the pleural space when closing the chest after removal of the wound VAC sponges is the solution derived from the Clagett procedure. It is an antibiotic solution composed of 500 mg of neomycin, 100 mg of polymyxin B sulfate, and 80 mg of gentamicin in 1 liter of normal saline.

After filling the entire pleural cavity with the antibiotic solution, the chest wall closure needs to be watertight to prevent any loss of the antibiotic solution from the pleural cavity [7].

Other methods of obliterating the pleural space include transposition of extratho-racic muscle into the pleural space, mobilization of omentum into the pleural cavity, or performing a thoracoplasty. Thoracic surgeons are usually adept at mobilizing intercostal muscles or the serratus anterior muscle and using it to cover the bron-chial stump. It also helps to fill in the residual space if there is remaining lung within the pleural cavity. When it comes to obliterating the entire pleural space after a pneumonectomy, it is wise to have the assistance of a plastic surgeon to mobilize large muscle flaps that have a narrow pedicle and excellent blood supply [9]. This allows placement of large muscles within the pleural cavity.

The transposition of omentum from the abdomen into the chest also brings a large amount of viable tissue into the pleural space. However, it requires a separate laparotomy to mobilize the omentum and with this comes the inherent risk of con-taminating the abdominal cavity with the empyema.

Thoracoplasty is still a viable option, whereby large portions of ribs are removed, and the overlying soft tissues of the chest wall are allowed to fill in the residual space in the chest. This was more common in the days when tuberculosis was more prevalent and when there was no effective antibiotics to treat the disease. However, thoracoplasty has fallen out of favor and most younger surgeons have never seen or performed a thoracoplasty [10, 11].

Nonsurgical Treatment of Bronchopleural Fistulas

For smaller bronchopleural fistulas, usually less than 8 mm, nonsurgical therapies can be tried to close the bronchopleural fistula. If the bronchopleural fistula is small and well drained with not much soilage of the pleural space, then the fistula could heal on its own. However, most specialists prefer using bronchoscopic therapies to try to close the fistula or at least reduce the air leak and pleural soilage with occlusive materials such as fibrin glue. Sometimes, this can be done to allow the patient to recover from the sepsis and to be liberated from the ventilator and allow the patient to become an operative candidate. Larger bronchopleural fistulas greater than 8 mm can also be treated by interventional bronchoscopy with covered airway stents, spigots, fibrin glue, blood patch, Amplatzer device, or endobronchial valves [12, 13].

Endobronchial Valves

The most widely used bronchoscopic modality in managing BPF is the use of endobronchial valves (EBV). Two types of valves are currently approved by the US Food and Drug Administration (FDA) for bronchoscopic lung volume reduction. These are the umbrella-shaped Spiration valve (Olympus, USA) and the duckbill-shaped Zephyr valve (Pulmonx Corporation, USA). However, as of writing of this book, only the Spiration valve has been approved by the FDA for management of prolonged air leak under a Humanitarian Use Device (HUD) exemption. The FDA-approved indication for use of this device is to control prolonged air leaks of the lung, or significant air leaks that are likely to become prolonged air leaks, following lobectomy, segmentectomy, or lung volume reduction surgery (LVRS). An air leak present on postoperative day 7 is considered prolonged unless present only during forced exhalation or cough. An air leak present on day 5 should be considered for treatment if it is (1) continuous, (2) present during normal inhalation phase of inspiration, or (3) present upon normal expiration and accompanied by subcutaneous emphysema or respiratory compromise. The Spiration valve system use is limited to 6 weeks per prolonged air leak.

The Spiration valve is an umbrella-shaped device which is designed to prevent air from flowing through the airway within which the valve is placed. The design allows for air and secretions to be relieved from the segment of the lung beyond the valve. The procedure involves use of a balloon such as Fogarty catheter to occlude lobar bronchi of the affected lung until the air leak diminishes or stops (Figs. 6.3 and 6.4). This is typically easy in the case of a BPF as the target lobe is usually identifiable on a CT scan as opposed to persistent air leak after spontaneous pneumothorax. Upon identifying the target lobe, segmental airways are occluded to identify if a particular segmental or subsegmental bronchus is responsible for the air leak. Once a target airway is identified, the sizing catheter is used to measure airway diameter and choose an appropriately sized valve. The valves come in various sizes (5 mm, 6 mm, 7 mm, 9 mm). In our experience, the 9 mm valve is the most often used because of its ability to occlude a segmental bronchus which obviates the need to use multiple valves in subsegmental bronchi. The valve is deployed using a dedicated deployment catheter (Figs. 6.5 and 6.6). Early data suggested use of four to six valves per patient, but this number is lower with the availability of the 9 mm valve. Complications include granulation tissue, pneumonia, empyema, and bleeding upon removal of the valve(s). Although ipsilateral pneumothorax is a common complication with EBV after bronchoscopic lung volume reduction, the presence of pre-procedural pneumothorax and chest tube in patients with BPF makes it challenging to determine if this occurs in these patients.

Fig. 6.3 Fogarty balloon catheter positioned within a segmental bronchus

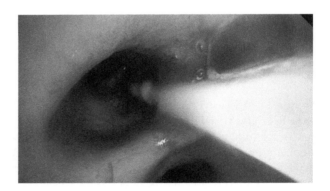

Fig. 6.4 Fogarty balloon inflated to occlude segmental bronchus to isolate the location of air leak

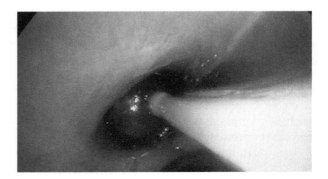

Fig. 6.5 Valve deployment catheter positioned in a segmental bronchus just before valve insertion

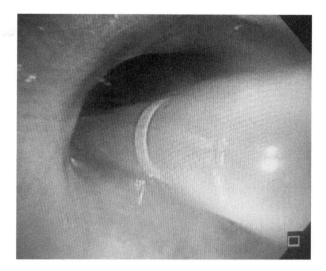

Fig. 6.6 Endobronchial valve position immediately after deployment

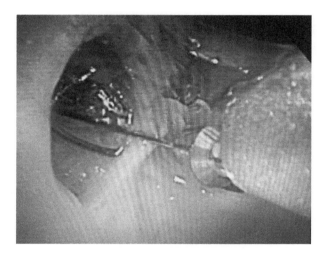

In a multicenter experience with cases sourced from eight centers, Gilbert et al. [14] studied the efficacy of EBV in 75 patients. Twenty-five percent of the cases were post-surgery. One hundred percent success in resolution in air leak was noted in patients with persistent air leak after surgery and 58% success in patients with other causes. The median time to resolution of air leak in BPF after surgery was 10 days, and 15 days after secondary spontaneous pneumothorax. Two patients suffered complications related to EBV use – empyema and contralateral pneumothorax. It is anticipated that both Spiration and Zephyr valves will receive full FDA approval for persistent air leak management in the foreseeable future.

Refractory Patients

There are some patients who are not candidates for surgery, are in an unstable condition, and have had previous unsuccessful attempts at treating their bronchopleural fistula or in whom the bronchopleural fistula cannot be closed or eliminated. Their air leak will continue for many months. These patients can be treated on a long-term basis with an open window thoracostomy. This can be either an Eloesser flap or a Clagett window with daily packing of the chest cavity. A wound VAC will not work if the bronchopleural fistula is not closed.

Eloesser Flap

An Eloesser flap is a surgical procedure that allows chronic drainage of the pleural cavity by creating an opening in the chest wall that will remain open. It usually involves making a U-shaped incision down to the chest wall to create a tongue flap, partial resection of two ribs, folding the tongue flap into the pleural cavity, and sewing it to the parietal pleura to create a permanent open window. This open window can be used to irrigate the pleural cavity or to pack it. If the window is small and the space still has some remaining lung, then it can heal spontaneously with granulomatous tissue. However, these spaces are often too large to heal spontaneously and usually require the transposition of a myocutaneous flap to fill in the space and close the defect. The benefit of an Eloesser flap is that the communication between the pleural space and the chest wall will remain open permanently. This allows control of the infected space for long periods of time [15].

Clagett Window

A Clagett window (Figs. 6.7 and 6.8) is also an opening in the chest wall with partial resection of a posterolateral lower rib but is intended to be temporary and allows irrigation and packing of the pleural space until the pleural cavity is sufficiently debrided. Antimicrobial packings are performed daily. This mechanical action debrides the pleural space. At some point, the packings can be changed to normal saline wet-to-dry gauze. When the pleural space demonstrates good granulation tissue throughout the pleural cavity, closure of the chest wall can be attempted by instillation of an antibiotic solution. For this, we use the original Clagett solution mentioned above [7]. This has an approximately 80% success rate. If it should fail, one may consider mobilizing extrathoracic muscle to place within the chest cavity [6].

Fig. 6.7 Malnourished
64-year-old man with a
MAC complex and fungal
ball within the pleural
cavity

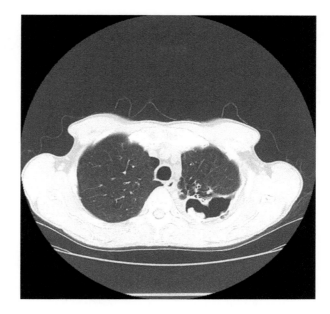

Fig. 6.8 After resection of
right upper lobe MAC
complex. Clagett window
with packing was required
to sterilize the pleural
space that had a persistent
air leak

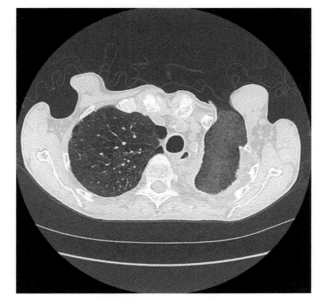

Prognosis

Overall, a significant amount of morbidity and mortality is associated with bronchopleural fistulas. According to Bribriesco and Patterson [4], pneumonectomy by
itself carries a morbidity of greater than 50% and a mortality of 5–7%. They also

state that in the setting of postpneumonectomy empyema, bronchopleural fistulas are present in 60–80% of patients, and the mortality rates range from 21% to 71%.

Summary

Operative management remains the gold standard definitive management of BPF. However, with the advent of bronchoscopic interventions particularly EBV, minimally invasive procedures offer an attractive alternative when surgery is not possible or deemed high risk.

References

1. Varker KA, Ng T. Management of empyema cavity with the vacuum-assisted closure device. Ann Thorac Surg. 2006;81:723–5.
2. Okuda M, Go T, Yokomise H. Risk factor of bronchopleural fistula after general thoracic surgery: review article. Gen Thorac Cardiovasc Surg. 2017;65:679–85.
3. Farkas EA, Detterbeck FC. Airway complications after pulmonary resection. Thorac Surg Clin. 2006;16:243–50.
4. Bribriesco A, Patterson GA. Management of postpneumonectomy bronchopleural fistula: from thoracoplasty to transternal closure. Thorac Surg Clin. 2018;28:323–35.
5. Di Maio M, Perrone F, Deschamps C, Rocco G. A metaanalysis of the impact of bronchial stump coverage on the risk of bronchopleural fistula after pneumonectomy. Eur J Cardiothorac Surg. 2015;48:196–200.
6. Deschamps C, Pairolero PC, Allen MS, et al. Management of postpneumonectomy empyema and bronchopleural fistula. Chest Surg Clin N Am. 1996;6:519–27.
7. Clagett OT, Geraci JE. A procedure for the management of postpneumonectomy empyema. J Thorac Cardiovasc Surg. 1963;45:141–5.
8. Weissberg D. Empyema and bronchopleural fistula: experience with open window thoracostomy. Chest. 1982;82:447–50.
9. Palmen M, Nathalie H, van Breugel AM, Geskes GG, van Belle A, Swennen JMH, Drijkoningen AHM, van der Hulst RR, Maessen JG. Open window thoracostomy treatment of empyema is accelerated by vacuum-assisted closure. Ann Thorac Surg. 2009;88:1131–7.
10. Hysi I, Rousse N, Claret A, Bellier J, Pincon C, Wallet F, Akkad R, Porte H. Open window thoracostomy and thoracoplasty to manage 90 postpneumonectomy empyemas. Ann Thorac Surg. 2011;92:1833–9.
11. Deslauriers J, Jaques LF, Gregoire J. Role of eloesser flap and thoracoplasty in the third millennium. Chest Surg Clin N Am. 2002;12:605–23.
12. Watanabe S-i, Shimokawa S, Yotsuimoto G, Sakasegawa K-i. The use of a dumon stent for the treatment of a bronchopleural fistula. Ann Thorac Surg. 2001;72:276–8.
13. Passera E, Guanella G, Meroni A, Chiesa G, Rizzi A, Roccco G. Amplatzer device and vacuum-assisted closure therapy to treat a thoracic empyema with bronchopleural fistula. Ann Thorac Surg. 2011;92:e23–5.
14. Gilbert CR, Casal RF, Lee HJ, Feller-Kopman D, Frimpong B, Dincer HE, Podgaetz E, et al. Use of one-way intrabronchial valves in air leak management after tube thoracostomy drainage. Ann Thorac Surg. 2016;101(5):1891–6.
15. Eloesser L. An operation for tuberculous empyema. Surg Gynecol Obstet. 1935;60:1096–7.

Chapter 7
Management of Acquired Tracheoesophageal Fistula in Adults

Danai Khemasuwan and David Griffin

Introduction

Tracheoesophageal fistula (TEF) is defined as a pathologic connection between the airway and the esophagus, leading to a spillover of oral and gastric secretions into the respiratory tract [1]. TEF is classified into two main categories: congenital and acquired. Congenital TEF is frequently associated with esophageal atresia (EA), which was first described by Thomas Gibson in 1697 [2]. Since then, the diagnosis and surgical repair techniques for correction of a congenital TEF have been well-established, resulting in a significant improvement in its outcomes. Meanwhile, acquired TEF is further divided into malignant and benign categories. Approximately half of acquired TEF are caused by malignancies [1]. The most common cancer associated with malignant TEF is esophageal cancer, with more than 10% of patients developing the condition during the clinical course [1, 3]. The most common presentations of a TEF are respiratory distress, dysphagia, and recurrent lung infections, with the magnitude of symptoms largely dependent on the size and location of TEF. The management of TEF requires a prompt multidisciplinary approach including interventional pulmonology (IP), gastroenterology, and thoracic surgery [4]. Surgical correction can be considered in certain instances, particularly with benign fistulas, but less invasive management strategies are often pursued. This often involves placement of stents but alternative approaches with new devices and technologies have emerged in the past years. This chapter describes the available

D. Khemasuwan (✉)
Virginia Commonwealth University Medical Center, Richmond, VA, USA
e-mail: danai.khemasuwan@vcuhealth.org

D. Griffin
Intermountain Medical Center, Murray, UT, USA
e-mail: david.griffin@imail.org

© The Author(s), under exclusive license to Springer Nature Switzerland AG 2021
J. F. Turner, Jr. et al. (eds.), *From Thoracic Surgery to Interventional Pulmonology*, Respiratory Medicine,
https://doi.org/10.1007/978-3-030-80298-1_7

117

data on risk factors, clinical manifestations, diagnostic approaches, management algorithm, traditional and novel management methods, and prognosis of acquired TEF.

Etiology and Risk Factors

Benign TEF occurs in tracheobronchial injury from blunt trauma to the chest or the neck, traumatic airway injury, prolonged intubation, traumatic intubation, injury from tracheostomy tubes, granulomatous mediastinal infections, stent-related injuries, and ingestions of foreign body or corrosives [5]. In the past, the most common cause of acquired benign TEF was from granulomatous mediastinal infections such as tuberculosis. However, more recently, the most common etiology is iatrogenic from cuff-related injury from prolonged intubation and injury from a tracheostomy tube [4]. As the mechanism of injury stems from pressure necrosis from the cuff, tracheostomies do not reduce the incidence of acquired TEF when compared to endotracheal tubes, given the similar mechanism of injury. Predisposing conditions such as diabetes, prior airway infections, use of steroids, and the presence of nasogastric tubes also increase the risk of TEF formation [6].

On the other hand, malignant TEFs are found in a setting of cancers arising from the esophagus, trachea, lungs, larynx, and thyroid. In one of the largest case series of malignant TEF involving 207 patients, 77% was attributed to primary esophageal cancer and only 16% to primary lung cancer [7]. Given the anatomic proximity of the upper and middle esophagus to the posterior wall of the trachea and the left mainstem bronchus, tumors originating from the esophagus can readily invade into the nearby airways. In malignant TEF, the size will grow over time due to the combination of recurrent aspiration injuries, corrosive injuries from gastric acid, pooling of respiratory and gastric secretions, and poor tissue healing particularly from concurrent steroid use or cancer treatment with radiation or chemotherapy. One of the clinical challenges in the management of a TEF is that the fistula can form due to both cancer progression and cancer treatment. When the tumor cells bridging the structures necrose, usually because of treatment with chemotherapy or radiation therapy, then the void of the tumor cells creates a communication, a fistula, between the aerodigestive tracts. A "clean-edge" airway wall defect can be observed in this setting, and the biopsies are often negative for any malignancies. Choi et al. reported that out of 52 patients with TEF and esophageal cancer, 28.8% of cases were thought to be related to the treatment of cancer rather than the progression of cancer [9]. Furthermore, Balazs et al. found that the latency from the initial radiation therapy to the detection of TEF was approximately 4.4 months (range, 1–13; SD, 2.98; CI, 3.5–5.4) [8]. This highlights the need for close monitoring for patients undergoing cancer treatment, especially 3–6 months after the initial cancer treatment. Endoscopic examination is warranted if patients become symptomatic or if clinicians have high suspicion based on radiographic findings. Similarly, stents have been associated with TEF formation. The incidence of esophageal stent-related TEF is estimated to be 4% with a median latency of 5 months (range 0.4–53 months) after the placement of the stent [10].

Clinical Manifestations

Patients with TEF can have varying clinical presentations, depending on such factors as the rate of its formation, size, location, patient comorbidities, and nutritional status. In a case series involving over 200 patients by Burt et al., symptoms and signs were cough (56%), aspiration (37%), fever (25%), dysphagia (19%), pneumonia (5%), hemoptysis (5%), and chest pain (5%) [7]. Ono's sign (worsening cough with swallowing solid/liquid) was present in 81% of patients with known TEF, though it is neither sensitive nor specific [11]. The average time for malignant TEF from onset of symptoms to detection is approximately 7.3 months (range 1–58 months; SD 4.25; CI 6.5–8.1). The onset of symptoms from benign cases is more variable, ranging from 5 to 15 days for traumatic causes to 21–30 days for iatrogenic cuff-related injuries [8] (Table 7.1).

In sedated and ventilated patients, TEF should be suspected if a continuous air leak in the ventilator circuit is detected despite a well-inflated cuff. Other signs such as abdominal distension, bloating, loss of ventilator tidal volume, worsening oxygenation, recurrent pulmonary sepsis, and repeated failures to wean can be observed. As TEF is unlikely to spontaneously heal and will eventually lead to respiratory complications and death, a prompt risk stratification and diagnostic efforts should be made.

Diagnostic Evaluation

The diagnosis of TEF is made by a combination of thoracic imaging studies and endoscopy – both flexible bronchoscopy and upper endoscopy if possible. An initial investigation of respiratory symptoms with a chest radiograph is a reasonable approach. Depending on the duration of symptoms, early findings of bibasilar infiltrates to more defined basilar consolidative changes can be seen. In addition to aspiration-related changes, the etiology of TEF may be apparent on initial radiographic evaluation such as a lung mass or an over-inflated cuff of endotracheal/

Table 7.1 Time course of symptoms of acquired benign TEF

Causes	Time (days)
Surgical	1–5
Ischemic/traumatic	5–15
Local infection	15–21
Tracheal cuff-related injury	21–30

tracheostomy tube. Although there are no formal guidelines, most experts agree that esophagogram and endoscopy are necessary to diagnose the disease and to perform preoperative planning. Esophagogram is performed preferentially with barium, given its favorable physiologic profile compared to gastrografin. The latter has been associated with pulmonary edema and death due to its hypertonic nature [12]. In the presence of TEF, the oral contrast will traverse through the fistula and will be visualized in the airways at the time of esophagogram (Fig. 7.1). The contrast-enhanced esophagogram demonstrates the defect in approximately 70% of patients with TEF [13]. The study is not ideal for patients who are not able to swallow the contrast such as those who are sedated and/or ventilated. In these patients, computed tomography (CT) scan of the chest can be performed to evaluate for signs of fistula, aerodigestive tract anatomy, and mediastinal pathology. There are no available data assessing the sensitivity, specificity, negative predictive value, and positive predictive value of CT scans in settings of known TEF.

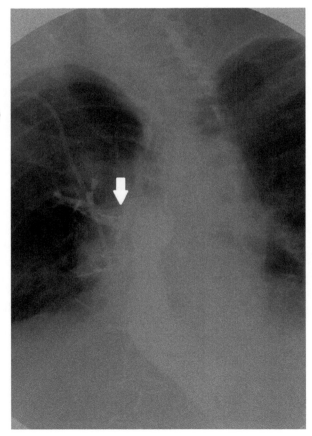

Fig. 7.1 Esophagogram showing the contrast leak in right upper lobe airways (arrowhead). (Reproduced with permission of the © ERS 2021: *European Respiratory Review* 29 (158) 200094; DOI: https://doi.org/ 10.1183/16000617.0094-2020 Published 5 November 2020)

Once the thoracic imaging confirms the presence of TEF, the next step in evaluation is to assess the anatomy further via upper endoscopy and bronchoscopy. Endoscopic visualization allows for better localization, characterization, and potentially treatment of the TEF (Figs. 7.2, 7.3, and 7.4) and can be performed with moderate sedation or general anesthesia. Direct visualization can be difficult in the setting of a mucosal inflammation, edema, and gastric debris, which can obscure a small TEF. Gentle maneuvers with the tip of the endoscope with judicious suctioning can dislodge debris, froth, or gastric content, leading to an improved visualization of the obscured TEF. Similarly, a flexible or a rigid bronchoscope can be used to express purulent material or dislodge spilled gastric contents in the airways to improve the visualization in the respiratory tract. For patients with poorly visualized fistula due to its size, location, or mucosal debris, an administration of methylene blue via oral route or feeding tube at the time of an endoscopic evaluation can be

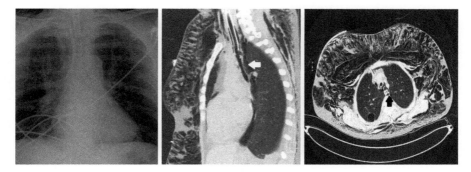

Fig. 7.2 Massive pneumomediastinum and subcutaneous emphysema from tracheoesophageal fistula. (Courtesy of Harpreet Singh Grewal MD. Reproduced with permission of the © CHEST 2021: *Chest* 2019 Mar;155(3):595–604. doi: https://doi.org/10.1016/j.chest.2018.07.018. Epub 2018 Jul 27)

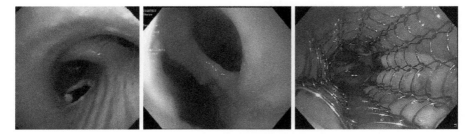

Fig. 7.3 (Left) Bronchoscopic view of the TEF at the posterior wall of proximal right bronchus intermedius; (Middle) esophageal endoscopic view of the same TEF showing the fistula and mucosal abnormalities; (Right) TEF closure utilizing Alloderm (*) and self-expanding metallic stent in the trachea. (Reproduced with permission of the © ERS 2021: *European Respiratory Review* 29 (158) 200094; DOI: https://doi.org/10.1183/16000617.0094-2020 Published 5 November 2020)

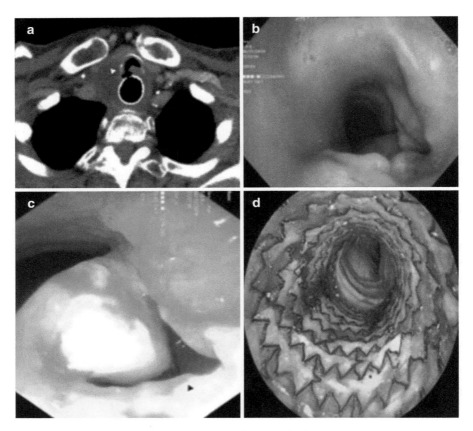

Fig. 7.4 A case of malignant tracheoesophageal fistula (TEF) from metastatic esophageal cancer after radiation treatment followed by esophageal self-expandable metallic stent placement: (**a**) computed tomography scan of the chest showing TEF (arrowhead) at the level of proximal end of the esophageal stent, (**b**) bronchoscopic view showing mucosal abnormality obscuring the view of the fistula at the posterior wall of the trachea. (**c**) A close-up bronchoscopic view of TOF; the esophageal sent can be seen at the bottom of TEF (arrowhead). (**d**) A case of iatrogenic TOF: closure with Alloderm (*) and covered, self-expandable metallic stent in the trachea. (Reproduced with permission of the © ERS 2021: *European Respiratory Review* 29 (158) 200094; DOI: https://doi.org/10.1183/16000617.0094-2020. Published 5 November 2020)

helpful in the identification of TEF [14]. There is a small risk of serotonin syndrome with methylene blue in patients on certain medications, particularly serotonin reuptake inhibitors (SSRIs), like fluoxetine, paroxetine. If the patient is intubated with an endotracheal tube for the procedure, maneuvering the tip of the ETT should be carried out to allow for a complete visualization of the airway during the bronchoscopic exam. Endoscopic and/or bronchoscopic biopsies of the lesions should be considered to investigate the underlying etiology of TEF. The information obtained may be helpful for further management and/or palliative care discussion.

Location of TEF

The location of TEF depends on the etiology and the nature of the inciting injury. For iatrogenic TEFs from cuff-related injuries, the defect will occur in mid- to distal trachea corresponding to the location of the cuff. Most traumatic TEFs are the results of motor vehicle accidents and occur mostly at the level of the carina where the chest wall suffers a forceful crushing injury while striking the steering wheel. The location of TEFs caused by inhalation injuries, aspiration of toxic chemicals, and mediastinal infections are less well defined.

The location of malignant TEF largely depends on the location of the primary tumor. From a study by Burt and colleagues [7] investigating patients with malignant TEFs that were mostly due to esophageal cancer (77%), the airway location of the fistula was the trachea in 110 (53%), left main bronchus in 46 (22%), right main bronchus in 33 (16%), multiple sites in 5 (2%), and bronchopleural fistula (BPF) in 13 (6%). Another study by Balazs and colleagues [8] who looked at patients with esophageal cancer with concurrent TEF showed similar trend with the fistula in the trachea/carina in 120 (46%), right main bronchus in 118 (45%), left main bronchus in 22 (8%), and distal airways in 4 (2%) of patients. The difference in these two studies is likely related to patient population and proportion of patients with esophageal cancer, but the two studies highlight the consistent relationship between esophageal cancer and fistula development in the trachea.

Management

Preoperative Management

The management strategy for TEF should consider multiple aspects of the disease, which includes identifying the underlying etiology, patient comorbidities, nutrition status, and goals of care. Prior to undertaking therapeutic interventions, it is crucial to determine and treat the underlying condition implicated in TEF formation. The general principle of preoperative management is to treat complications arising from the anatomic deformity while addressing modifiable risk factors of fistula formation. The most worrisome complication is soiling of the respiratory tract, leading to pneumonitis and ultimately respiratory sepsis. Patients should be made NPO, and gastric acid-suppressive therapy should be used to decrease the acidity and the volume of gastric acid. Patient positioning with the head of the bed elevated to 45° or greater, strict limitation of oral intake, and frequent oral suctioning are used in conjunction with the pharmacologic therapy. For ventilated patients, the endotracheal tube can be advanced to position the cuff distal to the fistula to prevent soiling of the respiratory tract. Nasogastric and orogastric tubes should be removed to prevent propagation of the pressure necrosis around the fistula, especially in intubated patients. Placement of gastrostomy tubes for evacuation of residual gastric contents and jejunostomy tubes for enteric feeding can also be considered in appropriate clinical circumstances.

Intraoperative Management

The key principles of intraoperative management parallel the key concepts of pre-operative management. It is crucial to consider the aerodigestive tract anatomy and the location of TEF to formulate strategies to minimize spillover of gastric contents into the respiratory tract. As the fistula must be visualized for the bronchoscopic treatment of TEF, the tip of endotracheal tube is positioned proximally to the TEF, thus potentially exposing the respiratory tract to gastric contents. Aggressive suctioning via flexible bronchoscope or a suction catheter through the rigid broncho-scope is usually sufficient to clear the gastric spillover in the airways and can result in improved visualization.

During endoscopy, care must be taken to overdistension of the stomach via positive pressure ventilation causing gastric spillover, and with esophagoscopy, a potentially unique respiratory complication can also occur. Depending on the size and the location of the fistula, the insufflated air from the endoscope can traverse into the airway, leading to increased airway pressures, ineffective ventilation, and parenchymal barotrauma. Prompt communication between the endoscopist and the anesthesiologist is of the utmost importance in minimizing complications during the procedure.

Stenting Strategy in TEF

There are two clinical circumstances that stents can be utilized: bridging benign TEF to definitive surgical therapy and palliating symptoms of a malignant TEF such as aspiration, dysphagia, worsening respiratory status, and improving poor nutritional status. In general, benign TEF is more amenable for a definitive surgical intervention due to the nature of the injury and better nutritional status. However, cardiopulmonary instability may prohibit definite surgical intervention, and may require medical optimization, and in extreme circumstances, extracorporeal device therapy can be used to stabilize pulmonary function and hemodynamics. In contrast, patients with malignant TEF are frequently malnourished and usually are undergoing treatment with chemotherapy and/or radiation, making them poor surgical candidates. Minimally invasive endoscopic procedures including stenting are typically preferred in these cases to improve nutritional status while preventing further complication from pneumonia and sepsis.

The main endoscopic technique to manage a TEF is esophageal and/or airway stenting with the goal to seal the fistula and prevent the spillover to the respiratory tract [15]. Most of the stents are cylindrical in shape, which allow them to exert

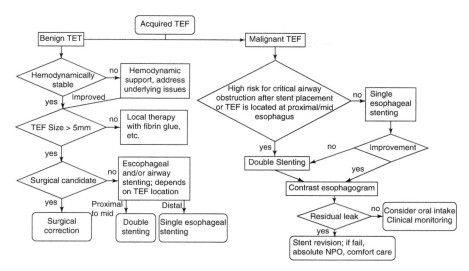

Fig. 7.5 Management algorithm for acquired tracheoesophageal fistula (TEF). (Reproduced with permission of the © ERS 2021: European Respiratory Review 29 (158) 200094; DOI: https://doi.org/10.1183/16000617.0094-2020 Published 5 November 2020)

radial force in the lumen when fully deployed. Thus, oversized stents can stretch the lumen with their expansile radial forces, resulting in an enlargement of the fistula, thus decreasing the possibility of healing. Therefore, stent placement is generally considered a palliative measure that may increase the quality of life, but it may not promote healing of a fistula [15]. In patients with a malignant TEF, stent placement is considered the treatment of choice based on poor prognosis with a mean survival expectancy between 1 and 6 weeks [16]. The management algorithm of TEF is showed in Fig. 7.5. The type of the stent, quantity of stent, and location of stent are very important decisions that clinicians must make, and the strategy will be reviewed here.

Single Esophageal Stenting

Esophageal stenting is a good option to seal the fistula in the middle-to-lower section of esophagus, especially in patients without known airway stenosis. This rationale is due to the potential of the esophageal stent to cause an airway obstruction via extrinsic compression and/or fistula formation. In addition, the esophageal wall is quite pliable which allows the wall to conform to the cylindrical shape of stent. The choice of esophageal stent for malignant cases is generally self-expandable metallic stents (SEMSs) over other available stents such as self-expandable plastic stents or biodegradable stents. This is due to overall durability, availability, and well-established efficacy in a wide variety of malignant esophageal diseases. When comparing covered SEMSs with uncovered SEMSs, the covered stents showed increased resistance to tumor ingrowth but had higher migration rates [17, 18]. For benign cases, self-expandable plastic stents are generally used given their ease of retrieval – as stenting for benign TEF cases is used as a bridge to definitive surgery [19]. For sizing, an endoscopic balloon dilator in the esophagus can be used to approximate the appropriate diameter to aid in the stent selection. Known complications from esophageal stenting are extrinsic airway compression, bleeding, esophageal perforation, and, paradoxically, the formation of new TEF [20]. For patients at high risk for airway obstruction from the extrinsic compression by the esophageal stent placement, concomitant airway and esophageal "double" stenting should be considered under selected circumstances.

Single Airway Stenting

There are two main types of airway stents that are available in the United States: silicone and metallic stents. In patients with TEF, the use of self-expandable metallic stents (SEMSs) is generally preferred, owing largely to their ease of deployment, robust radial expansile forces, and the ability to achieve better apposition to the airway mucosa. They can be placed both with a flexible or rigid bronchoscope using a guidewire/fluoroscopy and under a direct visualization and can be deployed in technically difficult locations compared to silicone stents. One of the advantages of SEMSs over silicone stents is the ease of rapid revision immediately after the deployment, though this can depend significantly on the experience and technical skills of the bronchoscopist. As mal-positioned stents can obstruct the airways and cause further damage to the fistula or nearby structures, the ability to revise the stent placement is crucial. In addition, SEMSs achieve better apposition with the airway wall, which may lower the incidences of migration [21]. However, SEMSs have less durability by design which can lead to metal fatigue and stent fracture. This durability is less of a concern in malignant TEF, as these patients rarely outlive the stent and develop this complication. Overall, SEMSs are more favorable profiles in malignant TEF, evidenced by a study by Wang et al. demonstrating a 71% complete closure rate in patients with malignant TEF [22].

In contrast, silicone stents are available in different configurations: straight and Y-stents. Silicone stents have studs on external surfaces which are designed to prevent migration and reduce mucosal ischemia [23]. However, these studs may prevent a complete apposition to the airway wall, thus making it difficult to obtain a seal overlying the TEF. In the management of benign TEFs, silicone stents may be favored due to better durability compared to SEMSs. Due to the C-shaped airway anatomy and dynamic motion during the respiratory cycle, airways do not conform to the "one size fits all" principle, and the choice to use a particular stent should be individualized. The comparison between SEMSs and silicone stent is showed in Table 7.2.

The ideal indication of single airway stenting is for TEF in the proximal trachea where the esophageal stent placement can be technically challenging. This can be

Table 7.2 A comparison of airway stents used for TEF management

Self-expandable metallic stent	Silicone stent
Advantages	*Advantages*
Easy to deploy	Durability
Less stent migration	Customizable
Better apposition/sealing with airway wall	Easy to revise and remove
Disadvantages	*Disadvantages*
Complications include membrane damage or dislocation, metal fatigue, and granulation tissue formation	Outer studs may affect the sealing effect
Less durability due to risk of stent fracture	More difficult to insert (need rigid scope)
Fistula size may increase after stent deployment	Fistula size may increase after stent deployment

related to the location of TEF (usually very proximal fistulas) or an occlusion of the esophageal lumen from a stenosis or a bulky tumor, making dilation or stenting challenging. The airway stent must be positioned so that the fistula is completely covered, ideally with a covered safety or "landing" zone of 20 mm at both ends [24]. Theoretically, this approach provides reassurance against the vertical expansion of the fistula following the stent deployment. However, the 20 mm safety margin may not be achieved due to the location of the fistula.

Double Airway and Esophageal Stenting

Double stenting may be considered a first-line intervention in the management of malignant TEF cases involving mid- to distal trachea [25–28], although this practice is controversial especially in the patients with low risk of airway compromise after proper sizing and deployment of esophageal stent. Double stenting approach provides protective strategy against airway compression by the esophageal stents and their migration into the airways. To further prevent airway compromise, the airway stents are always placed first, followed by esophageal stents. An additional strategy to ameliorate esophageal stent migration is placing the proximal end of the esophageal stent higher than the airway stent's upper margin, although the efficacy of this technique is unclear. Endoscopic clips can also be used to provide a point of fixation. After the deployment of esophageal stent, it is important to confirm the position of airway stent with either bronchoscopic or radiographic examination. One of the main issues of double stenting is the risk of fistula enlargement from a friction point or pressure necrosis between airway and esophageal stenting especially in metal on metal contact of both luminal stents.

Although these strategies for placement of both single and double stents have been accepted based on anecdotal success and smaller case series, there has not been a head-to-head trial assessing the efficacy of the two approaches. The only available prospective data that studied the efficacy of double stenting versus single stenting comes from Herth and colleagues [16]. Involving 112 patients, 65 (58%) received single airway stent, 37 (33%) received single esophageal stent, and 10

Table 7.3 Single versus double stents

Authors	Method	Etiology	Location/ fistula size	Sample size	Outcomes
Ke M, et al. (2015)	Retrospective case series	Undefined	Undefined	61 (26 tracheal, 35 double)	Better resolution of TEF contrast-enhanced imaging and clinical symptoms for double stents
Herth F, et al. (2010)	Prospective case series	Malignant	Trachea, mainstem bronchi, size not reported	112 (65 tracheal, 37 esophageal, 10 double)	Increased mean survival time (182d tracheal vs 249d esophageal vs 245d double)
Freitag L, et al. (1996)	Retrospective case series	Malignant	Trachea, 1–4 cm	30 (12 tracheal, 18 double)	Increased mean survival time (24d vs 110d) for double stents

(9%) received double stents. The unadjusted median survival time was 182, 249, and 245 days, respectively. There are other smaller retrospective case series that are summarized in Table 7.3.

Assessing the Efficacy of Airway Stent

There are several methods to assess the efficacy of stenting in adequately sealing a TEF. Using a naso-/orogastric tube, methylene blue can be utilized to confirm the proper approximation of stenting and successful closure of the fistula. The dye is instilled into the esophagus and the bronchoscope is used to assess for any leakage of the dye into the airways. If no soilage is noted on bronchoscopy, this suggests successful closure of the fistula. Another method of assessment is using barium swallow test to identify any leakage into the airway.

For most patients, stent placement helps to prevent pulmonary complications including aspiration pneumonia. Occasionally, oral intake can be resumed with a complete coverage of the fistula in selected patients. However, most patients will require nutritional support via gastrostomy, jejunostomy, nasojejunal tube, or parenteral nutrition.

Other Therapeutic Modalities

Several alternative therapeutic modalities have been described. But majority of these modalities are less well-studied, with only case reports to support their use. These modalities are fibrin glue injections, atrial closure devices, and other surgical tools. Fibrin glue injections have been used to treat small fistulas (<5 mm). This method has high failure rates in larger fistulas (>8 mm) due to the rapid dissolution of coagulative effect, leading to a recanalization of the fistula [29–31]. The atrial closure device (Amplatzer), which was originally designed for transcatheter closure of cardiac defects, has been used to successfully close TEFs and bronchio-esophageal fistulas related to nonmalignant etiologies [32–35]. However, significant airway complications have been reported with Amplatzer device use, ranging from airway obstruction from mucostasis and granulation tissue formation to a new TEF from erosive changes relating to the device itself. In addition, unlike airway stents, the Amplatzer decreases the airway cross-sectional area. Thus, this device is generally not used in the management of TEF [32]. ACell® matrix is a decellularized porcine urinary bladder matrix used to facilitate the natural healing process. There was an off-label use of this device to promote the healing process in patients with benign TEF with a complete closure at 10 days [36]. However, these methods are less often used due to anecdotal nature and lack of proven efficacy in larger cohorts. Other investigational and alternative therapeutic methods are summarized in Table 7.4.

There are a few endoscopic repair techniques that have been described on esophageal side. Several techniques have been described, for example, (1) a knot pusher which is an extracorporeal suturing device [37], (2) a Cor-Knot device [38], and (3) trans-tracheostomy repair [39]. In the report by Mozer et al. [38], the benign TEF was closed by suturing the fistula via a rigid esophageal tube, and securing with a Cor-Knot device. They observed a full post-procedural closure of the fistula on the esophagogram, and the patient was able to resume full oral intake at 6-month follow-up. Endoluminal vacuum-assisted closure (EVAC) therapy can potentially be used in the repair of TEF. EVAC creates a negative pressure while placing a sponge in the lumen of the fistula. The sponge is connected via a nasogastric tube that continuously removes secretions. This process induces the granulation tissue formation and closure of the fistula [40].

Outcomes

TEF is a condition that is found in many different conditions – benign, as well as malignant. Thus, it is very difficult to establish concrete outcomes in TEF due to its heterogeneity on affected population. Benign TEFs have more favorable clinical outcomes due to several factors including better nutritional status, less comorbidities, and feasibility of definitive surgical intervention. In two of the largest recent case series in surgical literatures, perioperative mortality ranged from 0% to 2.8% and morbidity ranged from 32% to 56% (pneumonias, respiratory failures, and fistula recurrences). In a series by Marulli and colleagues, all 25 patients who underwent surgical intervention for benign TEF survived with a median of 41 months of follow-up [41].

For malignant TEF, the available data suggests drastically worse outcomes. Although there was less than 0.5% procedure-related mortality, the mean survival of

Table 7.4 Alternative bronchoscopic approaches to stent placement – summary of anecdotal approaches

Authors	Method	Etiology	Location/ fistula size	Improvement	Complications
Scappaticci et al. (2004)	Fibrin glue – Tissucol	Benign – Post-intubation	Trachea, <5 mm	Near-complete closure in <24 hr	None
Miller PE, et al. (2014)	Atrial septal occluders – Amplatzer® (AGA Medical; Golden Valley, Minnesota, USA)	Benign – prolonged stenting	Trachea, not reported	Complete closure	Dislodged, airway obstruction, infection at 3 months after placement
Traina M, et al. (2018)	Atrial septal occluders – Amplatzer® (AGA Medical; Golden Valley, Minnesota, USA)	Benign – post-tracheostomy	Trachea, not reported	Complete closure	None
Mahajan AK, et al. (2018)	ACell® decellularized porcine urinary bladder matrix; Y-stent	Benign – Inflammation	RMS, 2 cm	Complete closure after 10 days	None
Traina M, et al. (2010)	Over the scope clipping (Ovesco Endoscopy GmbH)	Benign – post-tracheostomy	Trachea, 4 cm below VC – 1 cm	Complete closure/ resume diet	None
Mozer AB, et al. (2019)	Endobronchial suture (Cor-Knot device)	Benign – iatrogenic surgery	Trachea, 12 mm	Complete closure	None
Wong, An-Kwok et al. (2019)	Fibrin sealant (Ethicon Evicel)/ silicone-covered stent (Bonastent)	Benign – broncholith	RMS, 2 cm	Complete closure/ resume diet	None
Lee HJ, et al. (2015)	Endoscopic vacuum-assisted closure (EVAC)	Esophageal cancer, post-esophagectomy	N/A	Complete closure after 10 days	None

patients with malignant TEF was only 2.8 months from the time of TEF diagnosis from a large case series by Balazs and colleagues [8]. The patients who underwent esophageal stenting had mean survival of 3.4 months in this study suggesting potential survival benefits [8]. The clinical efficacy of double stenting was seen in a retrospective study by Freitag and colleagues who found increased survival time in double stenting compared to single tracheal stenting (110 days vs 24 days). This was supported by a larger prospective study by Herth and colleagues, with a median survival of 245 days in double stent population and 182 days in single tracheal stent population [16]. Patients who underwent stenting reported a significant improvement in dyspnea and dysphagia scores, and quality of life measured by the European Organization for Research and Treatment of Cancer quality of life questionnaire (EORTC QLQ-C30) supporting its role in palliative therapy [16, 41].

Conclusions

Due to heterogeneity in inciting factors and underlying conditions, the diagnosis of TEF is often significantly delayed or undiagnosed. The first step in prompt diagnosis is understanding the pathophysiology of fistula formation between the airways and the esophagus, and being cognizant of associated conditions. Clinical signs and symptoms can be often helpful but are often nonspecific, requiring careful review of symptoms, ventilatory variables (i.e., loss of tidal volume), frequency of respiratory infections, and evolution of chest radiographs. The next step in diagnosis is visualizing the fistula via contrast esophagogram or endoscopy/bronchoscopy, which provides crucial pre-procedural planning in addition to the diagnosis. The choice between definitive surgery, palliative stenting, use of investigational methods, and conservative approach will depend on combination of patient's condition, underlying etiology of TEF, goals of care, and availability of expertise.

Currently, endoscopic stenting is the most viable and well-studied intervention for patients with malignant TEF requiring palliative intervention or patients with a benign TEF who require stenting as a bridge to a definitive surgery. In this case, stenting has been shown to improve quality of life in patients with TEF and lessen symptoms of dyspnea and dysphagia. The choice of silicone stent versus metal stent is largely up to the comfort and the experience of the bronchoscopist, as there are advantages and disadvantages to both stents. Single esophageal stenting is preferred for TEF in distal esophagus without known airway compromise. Single tracheal stenting is ideal in very proximal TEF where esophageal stenting is technically challenging. Otherwise, double stenting may be favored as it provides structural support from both sides of the fistula while creating a seal to prevent spillovers but may lead to pressure necrosis. Close monitoring of the symptoms and signs of procedural complication is warranted in these highly complex patients to sustain desired clinical outcomes.

Acknowledgments Harpreet Singh Grewal, MD, for sharing his figures in this chapter.

References

1. Davydov M, Stilidi I, Bokhyan V, et al. Surgical treatment of esophageal carcinoma complicated by fistulas. Eur J Cardiothorac Surg. 2001;20(2):405–8.
2. Gibson T. The anatomy of humane bodies epitomized. 5th ed. T. W. for Awnsham and John Churchill; 1647.

3. Reed MF, Douglas JM. Tracheoesophageal fistula. Chest Surg Clin N Am. 2003;13(2):271–89.
4. Diddee R, Shaw IH. Acquired tracheo-oesophageal fistula in adults. Contin Educ Anaesth Crit Care Pain. 6(3):105–8.
5. Santosham R. Management of acquired benign tracheoesophageal fistulae. Thorac Surg Clin. 2018;28(3):385–92.
6. Macchiarini P, Verhoye JP, Chapelier A, et al. Evaluation and outcome of different surgical techniques for postintubation tracheoesophageal fistulas. J Thorac Cardiovasc Surg. 2000;119(2):268–76.
7. Burt M, Diehl W, Martini N, et al. Malignant esophagorespiratory fistula: management options and survival. Ann Thorac Surg. 1991;52(6):1222–8.
8. Balazs A, Kupcsulik PK, Galambos Z. Esophagorespiratory fistulas of tumorous origin. Non-operative management of 264 cases in a 20-year period. Eur J Cardiothorac Surg. 2008;34(5):1103–7.
9. Choi MK, Park YH, Im YH, et al. Clinical implications of esophagorespiratory fistulae in patients with esophageal squamous cell carcinoma. Med Oncol. 2010;27:1234–8.
10. Bick LB, Song LMWK, Buttar NS, et al. Stent-associated esophagorespiratory fistulas: incidence and risk factors. Gastrointest Endosc. 2013;77:181–9.
11. Gerzić Z, Rakić S, Randjelović T. Acquired benign esophagorespiratory fistula: report of 16 consecutive cases. Ann Thorac Surg. 1990;50(5):724–7.
12. Gore R, Levine M. Textbook of gastrointestinal radiology. 3rd ed. Philadelphia: W. B. Saunders Company; 2007.
13. Couraud L, Ballester MJ, Delaisement C. Acquired tracheoesophageal fistula and its management. Semin Thorac Cardiovasc Surg. 1996;8(4):392–9.
14. Mathisen DJ, Grillo HC, Wain JC, et al. Management of acquired nonmalignant tracheoesophageal fistula. Ann Thorac Surg. 1991;52(4):759–65.
15. Freitag L, Tekolf E, Steveling H, et al. Management of malignant esophagotracheal fistulas with airway stenting and double stenting. Chest. 1996;110:1155–60.
16. Herth FJ, Peter S, Baty F, et al. Combined airway and oesophageal stenting in malignant airway oesophageal fistulas: a prospective study. Eur Respir J. 2010;36:1370–4.
17. Sarper A, Oz N, Cihangir C, et al. The efficacy of self-expanding metal stents for palliation of malignant esophageal strictures and fistulas. Eur J Cardiothorac Surg. 2003;23(5):794–8.
18. Sharma P, Kozarek R. Practice Parameters Committee of American College of Gastroenterology. Role of esophageal stents in benign and malignant diseases. Am J Gastroenterol. 2010;105(2):258.
19. Verschuur E, et al. New design esophageal stents for the palliation of dysphagia from esophageal or gastric cardia cancer: a randomized trial. Am J Gastroenterol. 2008;103(2):304–12. Epub 2007 Sep 25.
20. Sze D, et al. Delayed complications after esophageal stent placement for treatment of malignant esophageal obstructions and esophagorespiratory fistulas. J Vasc Interv Radiol. 2001;12(4):465–74.
21. Avasarala SK, Freitag L, Mehta AC. Metallic endobronchial stents: a contemporary resurrection. Chest. 2019;155(6):1246–59.
22. Wang H, Tao M, Zhang N, et al. Airway covered metallic stent based on different fistula location and size in malignant tracheoesophageal fistula. Am J Med Sci. 2015;350(5):364–8.
23. Flannery A, Daneshvar C, Dutau H, Breen D. The art of rigid bronchoscopy and airway stenting. Clin Chest Med. 2018;39(1):149–67.
24. Hurtgen M, Herber SC. Treatment of malignant tracheoesophageal fistula. Thorac Surg Clin. 2014;24(1):117–27.
25. Matsumoto K, Yamasaki N, Tsuchiya T, et al. Double stenting with silicone and metallic stents for malignant airway stenosis. Surg Today. 2017;47(8):1027–35.
26. Machuzak MS, Santacruz JF, Jaber W, et al. Malignant tracheal-mediastinal-parenchymal-pleural fistula after chemoradiation plus bevacizumab: management with a Y-silicone stent inside a metallic covered stent. J Bronchology Interv Pulmonol. 2015;22(1):85–9.

27. Zhou C, Hu Y, Xiao Y, Yin W. Current treatment of tracheoesophageal fistula. Ther Adv Respir Dis. 2017;11(4):173–80.
28. Nomori H, Horio H, Imazu Y, Suemasu K. Double stenting for esophageal and tracheobronchial stenoses. Ann Thorac Surg. 2000;70(6):1803–7.
29. Scappaticci E, Ardissone F, Baldi S, et al. Closure of an iatrogenic tracheo-esophageal fistula with bronchoscopic gluing in a mechanically ventilated adult patient. Ann Thorac Surg. 2004;77:328–9.
30. Sharma M, Somani P, Sunkara T, et al. Trans-tracheal cyanoacrylate glue injection for the management of malignant tracheoesophageal fistula. Am J Gastroenterol. 2018;113(6):800.
31. Wong AI, et al. Patch-and-Glue: Novel Technique in Bronchoesophageal Fistula Repair and Broncholith Removal With Stent and Fibrin Glue. J Bronchology Interv Pulmonol. 2021;28(3):e45–e49.
32. Miller PE, Arias S, Lee H, et al. Complications associated with the use of the amplatzer device for the management of tracheoesophageal fistula. Ann Am Thorac Soc. 2014;11(9):1507–9.
33. Marwah V, Rajput AK, Madan H, et al. Closure of chronic bronchopleural fistula using atrial septal occluder device. J Bronchology Interv Pulmonol. 2014;21:82–4.
34. Traina M, Amata M, De Monte L, et al. Chronic tracheoesophageal fistula successfully treated using Amplatzer septal occluder. Endoscopy. 2018;50(12):1236–7.
35. Fruchter O, Kramer MR, Dagan T, et al. Endobronchial closure of bronchopleural fistulae using amplatzer devices: our experience and literature review. Chest. 2011;139:682–7.
36. Mahajan AK, et al. Successful endobronchial treatment of a non-healing tracheoesophageal fistula from a previous histoplasmosis capsulatum infection using decellularized porcine urinary bladder matrix†. J Surg Case Rep. 2018(8):rjy187.
37. Galluccio G. Endoscopic treatment of tracheo-oesophageal fistulae: an innovative procedure. Multimed Man Cardiothorac Surg. 2016;201:mmw015.
38. Mozer AB, Michel E, Gillespie C, et al. Bronchoendoscopic repair of tracheoesophageal fistula. Am J Respir Crit Care Med. 2019;200:774–5.
39. Caronia FP, Reginelli A, Santini M, et al. Trans-tracheostomy repair of tracheo-esophageal fistula under endoscopic view in a 75-year-old woman. J Thorac Dis. 2017;9:E176–9.
40. Lee HJ, Lee H. Endoscopic vacuum-assisted closure with sponge for esophagotracheal fistula after esophagectomy. Surg Laparosc Endosc Percutan Tech. 2015;25:e76–7.
41. Marulli G, et al. Early and late outcome after surgical treatment of acquired non-malignant tracheo-esophageal fistulae. Eur J Cardiothorac Surg. 2013;43:e155–61.

Chapter 8
Lung Volume Reduction: Surgical Versus Endobronchial

Pallav L. Shah and Samuel V. Kemp

Introduction

Chronic obstructive pulmonary disease is a heterogeneous disease predominantly caused by cigarette smoking, and in some developing economies by the indoor use of biomass fuels for cooking in poorly ventilated homes [1]. The condition consists of chronic bronchitis, airflow obstruction and alveolar destruction. This latter component is known as emphysema, and was first alluded to in 1679 by Bonet [2] where he described 'voluminous lungs', with the first case series of 19 patients [3] published in 1769 by Morgagni, where he described lungs that were 'turgid with air'. It was Laënnec who made the first detailed description of the pathology of emphysema [4]. He reported on some post-mortem observations where he found that the lungs were hyperinflated and frequently obstructed by mucus and did not empty well. Emphysema is defined as the abnormal, permanent enlargement of airspaces distal to the terminal bronchioles, accompanied by the destruction of their walls and without obvious fibrosis. Patients with advanced emphysema are breathless despite the use of anticholinergic drugs, beta-2 agonists, long-acting bronchodilators, inhaled steroids and oral steroids, and whilst oxygen has some role in palliation, it barely alters the disability and breathlessness experienced by these patients. Lung

P. L. Shah (✉)
Royal Brompton Hospital, London, UK

National Heart & Lung Institute, Imperial College, London, UK

Chelsea and Westminster Hospital NHS Foundation Trust, London, UK
e-mail: pallav.shah@imperial.ac.uk

S. V. Kemp
National Heart & Lung Institute, Imperial College, London, UK

Nottingham City Hospital, Nottingham, UK

J. F. Turner, Jr. et al. (eds.), *From Thoracic Surgery to Interventional Pulmonology*, Respiratory Medicine,
https://doi.org/10.1007/978-3-030-80298-1_8

transplantation and lung volume reduction remain the only realistic options for significant improvements in lung function, exercise tolerance and quality of life in these patients.

Pathophysiology of Emphysema

The destruction of the elastic tissue of the lung leads to the enlargement of airspaces, small airway collapse and progressive hyperinflation. This shifts the compliance curve of the lung towards the right. Consequently, greater pressure changes are required for any given tidal volume. Hence, greater effort is required for breathing. The destructive process of emphysema also reduces the degree of tethering leading to early collapse of the airways in expiration, with prolonged expiratory air flow and air trapping. This effect is exacerbated during exercise or any significant effort as an increase in the respiratory rate further reduces the time allowed for expiration. Hence, patients with emphysema exhibit both static and dynamic hyperinflation. The hyperinflation further increases the effort of breathing as the inspiratory muscles are at a mechanical disadvantage owing to changes in the length-tension relationship [5].

Besides the changes in lung mechanics already discussed, dynamic hyperinflation also leads to a number of other deleterious consequences: significant V/Q mismatching, increased dead space and the generation of high intrinsic positive end-expiratory pressure (PEEP). The latter compresses pulmonary vessels giving rise to pulmonary hypertension during exercise, impairing venous return to the heart and therefore reducing cardiac output. The air trapping per se also leads to hypercapnia and hypoxia during exercise.

There are three main subtypes of emphysema described: centrilobular, panlobular or panacinar and paraseptal. Centrilobular emphysema refers to abnormal enlargement of the airspaces centred on the respiratory bronchiole. It tends to have an upper lobe preponderance and is the most common pathological form in smokers. The computed tomographic (CT) features are foci of low attenuation at the centre of the secondary pulmonary lobule. With advancing disease, these centrilobular low attenuation areas may coalesce to form bullae of increasing size. Panlobular emphysema involves the whole secondary pulmonary lobule and is classically associated with alpha-1 antitrypsin deficiency where it typically occurs in the lower lobes. There is diffuse destruction of the alveolar and respiratory bronchiolar walls, giving rise to widespread low attenuation of the affected areas on CT. Paraseptal emphysema arises at the distal portion of the secondary pulmonary lobule and typically affects areas of the lung adjacent to the pleura. This type of emphysema may give rise to 'vanishing lung syndrome' or giant bullous emphysema. It has an upper lobe predominance and is associated with an increased risk of pneumothorax.

Lung Transplantation

Lung transplantation is the only potential cure for emphysema. However, this treatment option is limited by an inadequate supply of donor organs, although recent advances in organ harvesting and preservation (such as ex vivo lung perfusion) [6] have helped to increase availability. Strict eligibility criteria are applied in most countries, and lung transplantation is a realistic option for only a few patients. Even in those transplanted, there is a significant mortality and morbidity; 90-day mortality is 13%, with 22% dead at 1 year [7]. The trend towards double lung transplantation rather than single lung transplantation in emphysema has further reduced the number of patients that can be treated with the available organs but has improved the longer-term outlook (66.7% vs. 44.9% 5-year survival) [8]. Whilst transplantation is a surgical treatment for emphysema, this chapter mainly concerns itself with techniques for lung volume reduction.

Lung Volume Reduction Surgery

Surgical procedures for the palliation of symptoms in emphysema have been attempted over many years, with widely varying approaches, including artificial pneumoperitoneum, phrenic nerve dissection, thoracoplasty, costochondrectomy and procedures to improve pulmonary blood flow. All were soon abandoned following universally disappointing or disastrous outcomes. However, lung volume reduction by removing a portion of diseased lung appeared to have some merit and was first reported by Brantigan in 1957 [9]. The concept was simply that reducing the volume of the overinflated lung would enable improved function of both the diaphragm and the respiratory muscles. His group published a series of 33 patients and suggested symptomatic improvements in 75% of survivors. However, they presented no objective measurements of improvement, and concerns regarding operative morbidity and mortality (18%) lead to the procedure being abandoned.

A series published by Delarue and colleagues [10] in 1977 resulted in a 21% post-operative mortality, but they also demonstrated functional benefits in some survivors, suggesting that LVRS had something to offer the carefully selected patient. Surgical lung volume reduction only gained credibility in the 1990s after improvements in surgical techniques by Joel Cooper. Cooper and colleagues [11] resected 20–30% of the most emphysematous lung using a stapling technique performed through a median sternotomy. At a mean follow-up of 6 months, they reported significant improvements in lung function with an 82% improvement in FEV1 and 27% improvement in FVC. Symptom scores also improved substantially but there was no change in walking distance. Whilst prolonged air leaks occurred in over half of the patients, there were no deaths during the follow-up period. These striking results led to a resurgence in interest in LVRS. A larger series of 150 consecutive patients published the following year demonstrated sustained benefits to 2 years and a relatively low overall mortality of 4% at 90 days [12].

The evidence base for LVRS was supported by several small, short-term, randomised controlled studies. One study in 37 patients who were randomised to either LVRS or pulmonary rehabilitation demonstrated that surgical intervention improved pulmonary function parameters at 3 months [13]. A study performed at the Royal Brompton Hospital in the UK compared LVRS to medical treatment [14]. Potentially eligible patients were given intensive medical treatment, and completed a smoking cessation program and a 6-week outpatient rehabilitation program before randomisation. Forty-eight patients were randomised to either surgery or continued medical treatment. At 6 months, there was no significant difference in the rates of death between the two groups, but there were statistically significant improvements in the forced expiratory volume in 1 second (FEV1; $p = 0.02$) and shuttle walking distance ($p = 0.02$) in the surgical group over the medical group. However, in the surgical arm, 5 of the 19 surviving patients derived no measurable benefit from the treatment. Medium-term follow-up (median 25 months) demonstrated that the immediate increase in FEV1 was not sustained, although beneficial changes in the forced vital capacity and a reduction in hyperinflation remained. There was also a gradual and sustained increase in transfer factor accompanied by improved oxygen saturations [15].

The Canadian Lung Volume Reduction (CLVR) study and the Overholt-Blue Cross Emphysema Surgery Trial (OBEST) were two similar, independently conceived and conducted, multicentre, randomised clinical trials of LVRS, but their results were published as a single (meta-) analysis [16]. Patients were required to have severe airflow obstruction, hyperinflation and measurable dyspnoea. Optimal medical therapy included pulmonary rehabilitation in both arms of both studies. The CLVR study randomised 58 patients and the OBEST 35 patients (a total of 93 patients), with 54 patients randomised to undergo surgery, and 39 randomised to receive medical treatment. Six-month results were similar to the Brompton trial, with no difference between arms in mortality, and significant beneficial changes in spirometry, hyperinflation and exercise capacity. Two further small clinical studies also reported improvements in pulmonary function and quality of life measures, but in the latter study, there was a higher surgical mortality (12%) [17, 18].

These encouraging reports led to a dramatic uptake in LVRS, but the Centers for Medicare & Medicaid Services (CMS) published data in 1998 showing mortality rates of 14.4% at 3 months and 23% at 12 months from claims submitted between October 1995 and January 1996, together with a high rate of rehospitalisation, and subsequently stopped reimbursements for the procedure [19]. This led to the development of a multicentre, prospective, randomised trial between LVRS and medical care (National Emphysema Treatment Trial (NETT)) [20]. Funded by the CMS and the National Heart, Lung, and Blood Institute (NHLBI), it aimed to answer two fundamental questions – could a sustained survival benefit from surgery be demonstrated, and would LVRS improve measures of lung function, exercise capacity and quality of life? Seventeen designated centres in the USA recruited patients with severe airflow obstruction together with bilateral emphysema and hyperinflation on chest radiograph and randomised them to best medical care or best medical care plus lung volume reduction surgery. One thousand two hundred eighteen patients were randomised.

Results at 24 months showed a higher early mortality in the surgical arm than the medical arm (2.2% vs. 0.2% at 30 days; 5.1% vs. 1.5% at 90 days), but no overall difference in mortality at 24 months [21]. A greater proportion of patients in the surgical arm had an increase in exercise capacity at each time point (24% vs. 4% at 6 months; 22% vs. 5% at 12 months; 15% vs. 3% at 24 months), and there was a greater chance of improvements in FEV1, health-related quality of life and dyspnoea scores in the surgical arm. There was also a reduction in exacerbation frequency and an increase in time to first exacerbation [22].

The safety monitoring board identified a group of patients that appeared to have a greater mortality [23]. By six months, 35% of patients with FEV1 <20% and either a TLco <20% predicted or emphysema that was homogeneously distributed had died. Enrolment of patients with these characteristics was stopped in May 2001, by which time 140 had been recruited, 70 in each arm of the trial. Of these, all had an FEV1 <20% predicted, 94% had homogeneous disease, and 87% had a TLCO <20% predicted. Forty one patients met all three criteria. Mortality in those who underwent surgery was 0.43 per person year, compared to 0.11 per person year in those treated medically. Thirty-day mortality was 16% in this high-risk surgical group and 0% in the medical group, with poor outcomes persisting to 2 years [21].

Short-term safety analysis identified that the only two statistically significant independent pre-operative factors that predicted mortality in the surgical arm were the presence or absence of upper lobe predominant disease on CT scanning and baseline exercise tolerance (cut-off for low exercise capacity that determined risk of death was the 40th centile, 25 Watts in females and 45 Watts in males). When divided into four patient groups on the basis of these two parameters at 24 months, a clear stratification of benefit between groups could be seen, summarised in Table 8.1. Subject monitoring continued beyond the 24-month trial period, with 70% of survivors participating in extended follow-up. Overall, a significant survival advantage in the LVRS group emerged at 5 years (0.11 deaths per patient year in the surgical arm vs. 0.13 deaths per patient year in the medical arm; 283 vs. 324 deaths, respectively), with improvements in exercise capacity out to 3 years, and quality of life out to 5 years [24]. In the survivors, there were small but significant improvements in FEV1, exercise capacity and walking distance, but no improvement in

Table 8.1 NETT outcomes stratified by disease distribution and baseline exercise capacity

	Upper lobe predominant disease	Non-upper lobe predominant disease
Low baseline exercise capacity	Survival ↑ Quality of life ↑ Exercise capacity ↑	Survival ↔ Quality of life ↑ Exercise capacity ↔
High baseline exercise capacity	Survival ↔ Quality of life ↑ Exercise capacity ↑	Survival ↓ Quality of life ↔ Exercise capacity ↔

quality of life. High-risk patients continued to demonstrate excessive mortality without functional benefit, whilst those in the upper lobe predominant, low exercise capacity group were consistently shown to benefit the most from surgery. This improvement came at considerable financial cost, however, with an estimated $190,000 per quality adjusted life year (QALY) in all-comers, and $98,000 in those with upper lobe disease and low exercise tolerance [25].

The NETT study demonstrated significant benefits in survival, exercise capacity and quality of life in carefully selected patient groups, and also identified a clear higher responder group; patients with upper lobe predominant emphysema with low baseline exercise capacity. However, instead of signalling a resurgence in the numbers operated on, the high short-term mortality, significant morbidity and short-term costs have meant that very few operations are currently undertaken. Since the publication of the NETT study, there have been significant developments in surgical techniques. Greater use of video-assisted thoracoscopic approach and unilateral treatment and development of non-resectional lung volume reduction surgery. The latter involves using adapted staples which effectively separate two regions of the lung without cutting through and leaving the emphysematous parts of the lobe collapsed and folded in situ. Lung volume reduction surgery is now centralised in higher volume centres, and 90-day mortality in some groups has been reported as <1% over the past 5 years [26].

However, the challenges already discussed, invasive nature of surgery and unpredictable lengths of hospital stay have fuelled the development of non-surgical methods of lung volume reduction. Several different bronchoscopic techniques and devices have now been developed, employing a variety of ingenious strategies to achieve their desired effect. These can be grouped into airway blockers, sclerosants, coils and airway bypass techniques, each category being discussed separately below.

Endobronchial Valves

Endobronchial valves function as one-way valves which allow gas out during expiration, but prevent further inspired air reaching the treated area. They are only effective at inducing lung volume reduction when several valves are used together to completely occlude a lobe in the absence of significant collateral ventilation. Endobronchial valves are the most extensively evaluated bronchoscopic lung volume reduction technique. Clinical studies have yielded critical information on patient selection, treatment strategies and complications, and the strategies pursued by the different manufactures have had a major impact on the success or otherwise of those devices.

Two valve systems are currently commercially available. The earliest valves for human use were developed by Emphasys Medical (Redwood City, CA), which were subsequently acquired by Pulmonx Corporation (Redwood City, CA). Similar in shape to a spigot, they consisted of a framework of nitinol (a super-elastic memory shape alloy) surrounding a silicone duck-billed valve in a stainless steel cylinder

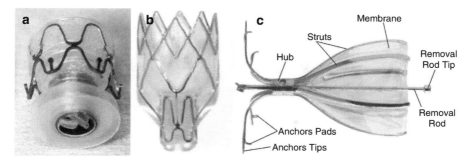

Fig. 8.1 Endobronchial valves. (**a**) First-generation Emphasys valve (**b**) Zephyr valve. (**c**) Spiration intrabronchial valve

(Fig. 8.1a). A more elegant second-generation valve (the Zephyr valve) was subsequently developed in order to reduce granulation tissue formation, with a framework of self-expanding nitinol and a latex one-way valve (Fig. 8.1b). This is available in three sizes, a 4.0 mm valve for airways of 4–7 mm diameter, a further of a framework 4.0 mm valve designed with a shorter length (4LP) and a 5.5 mm valve for airways from 5.5 to 8 mm diameter. The other commercially available valve is the Intrabronchial Valve© (IBV) developed by Spiration Incorporated (now acquired by Olympus Medical). The IBV consists of a nitinol frame covered by a latex membrane as shown in Fig. 8.1c. This 'umbrella valve' has five distal anchors which penetrate approximately 1 mm into the airway mucosa and six proximal struts. These struts are flexible, conform to the shape of the airway during both inhalation and exhalation and hold the latex membrane against the mucosa to prevent inspiratory airflow whilst allowing air and secretions to pass from distal to proximal. These are available in 5 mm, 6 mm, 7 mm and 9 mm diameter sizes. One significant advantage of such devices over surgery, and indeed other bronchoscopic interventions, is the reversibility of the procedure, with valves removable via a flexible bronchoscope.

The first clinical study performed at the Royal Brompton Hospital confirmed the feasibility and safety of endobronchial valve placement, and a number of early studies reported improvements in lung function parameters, quality of life and exercise capacity [27–29]. A retrospective collection of the early experience at several centres demonstrated encouraging results with mean changes in FEV1 of +10.7% ($p = 0.007$), FVC +9.0% ($p = 0.024$), RV −4.9% ($p = 0.025$) and 6MWD +23.0% ($p = 0.001$) [30]. In this series of 98 patients, the clinical practice was varied, with a combination of unilateral and bilateral treatments, some with complete lobar occlusion and some with only segmental occlusions. Those in whom lobar occlusion was attempted (70.4% of subjects) demonstrated the greatest response to treatment, and interestingly those treated unilaterally (65.3%) had greater improvements in measured parameters than those treated bilaterally (34.7%).

The Valves for Emphysema palliatioN Trial (VENT) [31] was designed as a multicentre, prospective, randomised controlled trial in severe heterogeneous emphysema (FEV1 <45% predicted, TLC >100% predicted, RV >150% predicted). Patients were randomised 2:1 procedure to control, with the aim of assessing the safety and efficacy of unilateral complete lobar occlusion. A co-primary end point of mean per cent change in FEV1 and 6-minute walking distance (6MWD) at 180 days were used.

Three hundred twenty-one patients were enrolled and randomised to endobronchial valve treatment (220 subjects) or standard medical care (101 subjects) in the US arm of the trial [32]. Statistically significant improvements in the treatment group were seen at 6 months when compared to changes in the control group with respect to both primary end points – FEV1 $p = 0.005$; 6MWD $p = 0.04$. There were also statistically significant improvements in the SGRQ and dyspnoea scores. However, whilst statistically significant, most clinicians considered these changes as modest and not meeting minimum clinically important differences. Subsequent analysis revealed subject characteristics that were associated with better outcomes. Quantitative density analysis of subject scanning bet was used to derive a heterogeneity score from the difference in the percentage of pixels below −910HU between the target lobe and the adjacent ipsilateral non-target lobe, demonstrating significant changes in both FEV1 ($p = 0.003$) and 6MWD ($p = 0.009$) in subjects with a heterogeneity score of 25%. The more important finding, however, was that in subjects with complete lobar occlusion (evaluated on post-treatment CT scans) and anatomically isolated upper lobes (also determined by CT analysis of fissural integrity), FEV1 was increased by 16.2% relative to the control arm ($p < 0.001$), a benefit that persisted out to 1 year of follow-up (17.9%; $p < 0.001$).

A parallel study using an identical protocol was conducted in Europe, recruiting 171 patients randomised to either endobronchial valve treatment ($n = 111$) or medical management ($n = 60$) [33]. The results again demonstrated statistically significant improvements, but below those considered clinically meaningful, in FEV1 (valves vs. medical care, $7 \pm 20\%$ vs. $0.5 \pm 19\%$; $p = 0.067$), cycle ergometry (2 ± 14 W vs. -3 ± 10 W; $p = 0.04$) and St George's Respiratory Questionnaire (SGRQ; -5 ± 14 points vs. 0.3 ± 13 points; $p = 0.047$), with improvements maintained out to 1 year of follow-up. Rates for complications did not differ significantly between the groups. Once again, those with a complete fissure(s) adjacent to the treatment lobe and a correctly performed procedure (i.e. lobar occlusion) had a mean lobar volume reduction of 80%, and greater than half met minimal clinically important difference thresholds.

The Intrabronchial Valve (Spiration/Olympus) was initially used to treat patients by implanting valves into the airways of both upper lobes. A report on the first 30 patients demonstrated a clinically significant improvement in the SGRQ (>4 point reduction, although >8 points was taken to be significant in the NETT) in greater than 50% of participants. However, there were no significant changes in any measured lung function parameters or in exercise tolerance [34]. This open-label study was subsequently expanded to several centres worldwide and recruited 98 patients, and initial reports suggested reductions in the volume of the treated lobes with improvements in quality of life [35]. Atelectasis was documented in nine subjects (9.2%) at 2 weeks, and five of these experienced a pneumothorax (one fatal).

Three pneumothoraces occurred in those without atelectasis, and six pneumothoraces occurred in patients who had the lingula segments treated ($n = 18$) leading to the discontinuation of lingular treatments after enrolment of subject 65.

Unfortunately, the high incidence of pneumothoraces in patients who developed atelectasis (55.6%) influenced the subsequent randomised trial [36], which employed a treatment strategy of bilateral incomplete occlusions of both upper lobes in a single procedure. This European multicentre trial (73 patients in 7 centres) in heterogeneous emphysema demonstrated shifts in lobar volume compared with control subjects at 3 months, with a significant decrease in upper lobe lung volumes ($-7.3 \pm 9.0\%$), but a similar and significant corresponding increase in non-treated lobe volumes ($-6.8 \pm 6.9\%$). Six-month CT analysis showed a slight reduction in the amount of volume loss in the upper lobes to -5.3 ± 7.8. There was no change in volumes in the control group. A responder analysis was conducted, with a responder being a subject with a 7.5% decrease in treated lobar volumes and a ≥ 4 point fall in the SGRQ at 3 months. The treatment group had a 24% responder rate, against 0% in the control group. This result was used by the authors to suggest a beneficial treatment effect of bilateral incomplete lobar occlusions with the IBV. However, there was no overall difference in the change in SGRQ between groups and no difference in SGRQ 'responders', and changes in SGRQ did not correlate with volume shifts. The changes in SGRQ were randomly distributed across both groups, and were independent of any treatment effects. Furthermore, there were no differences in changes in lung function parameters, breathlessness or 6MWD between the two groups.

What was not fully appreciated during the enrolment phase of the VENT trial was the critical role that collateral ventilation plays in the success or failure of endobronchial valve therapy. Collateral ventilation is the ventilation of alveolar structures through passages or channels that bypass the normal airways [37]. These high resistance channels become increasingly important with increasing airflow obstruction, as airway resistance in the airways approaches that of the collateral channels, and alveolar destruction causes coalescence of airspaces. The likelihood is that collateral ventilation between lobes is largely secondary to incomplete fissures, and these can be a feature of normal health [venuta respiration ref] [38], or secondary to the proteolytic damage to pulmonary tissue that occurs in emphysema. Correct technical placement of the valves is also essential, and in the VENT studies, 46.9% of procedures (US arm 85/194 and European arm 58/111) did not achieve complete lobar exclusion due to inadequate valve placement [32, 33]. A direct comparison of the two strategies was performed by Eberhardt and colleagues [39], who randomised 22 patients to receive either a bilateral incomplete occlusions or a unilateral complete occlusion. Beneficial changes were seen in the complete but not incomplete occlusion group. The changes seen in this subgroup do seem to indicate clinically as well as statistically meaningful changes with correct patient selection, and indeed long-term survival data has been published showing a survival benefit in patients in whom lobar collapse was achieved [40–42].

A system for predicting the presence of collateral ventilation has subsequently been developed, comprising of a balloon catheter incorporated with a pressure and flow sensor [43]. The balloon catheter is manoeuvred into the target lobe and the balloon inflated to fully occlude the lobe, with the pressure and flow pattern measured via a central channel in the catheter. Where there is no collateral ventilation, there should be a steady reduction in the flow over several minutes whilst maintaining the inspiratory pressure changes. In contrast, where there is collateral ventilation, there is sustained flow beyond 5 minutes with the emptying of several litres of air. This method has an accuracy of 75% in predicting whether or not significant treated lobe atelectasis (≥350 mls volume loss) will occur, and those predicted to respond have been shown to have greater improvements in FEV1 and greater volume loss [44]. Subsequent Zephyr valve trials utilised the Chartis system to determine collateral ventilation status prior to valve placement.

The Brompton randomised, double blind, sham controlled study of endobronchial valves (BeLieVer-HiFI study) [45] selected patients with major lobar fissures that were assessed as being >90% intact on CT imaging. The Chartis procedure was also performed, but the patients were randomised to treatment or sham irrespective of the Chartis-assessed collateral ventilation status. Fifty patients were randomised to endobronchial valve insertion with usual medical care ($n = 25$) or a sham procedure and usual medical care ($n = 25$). The patient group had severe disease with a mean FEV1 of 31.7% predicted and severe hyperinflation with residual volumes (RV) of 232% predicted. FEV1 was improved by a mean of 24.8% (median change 8.8%) in the intervention group compared to 3.9% (median change 2.9%) in the sham group. However, in this study, four patients in the treatment group had collateral ventilation present on the Chartis assessment, and a further four subjects had an indeterminate assessment. Excluding the patients with collateral ventilation improves the responder rate for a number of parameters. There were 23 episodes described as exacerbations in 16 patients in the treatment group and 22 events in 20 patients in the sham group. There were two episodes of pneumonia, two pneumothoraces and two deaths in the treatment group.

The STELVIO trial [46] was a single centre randomised but un-blinded trial which also selected patients with severe emphysema with intact lobar fissures on CT. The Chartis procedure was also performed, and in the STELVIO trial, only patients that were considered collateral ventilation negative after the Chartis assessment were included. Furthermore, patients in whom complete occlusion was not possible for technical or anatomical reasons were excluded. Sixty-eight patients were randomised, 34 to treatment with endobronchial valves and 34 to usual medical care. Patients had severe disease with a baseline FEV1 of 29% predicted, RV of 218% predicted, 6MWT of 337 metres and total SGRQ score of 59.2. The intention to treat analysis demonstrated a 20.9% (95% CI 11.1 to 30.7) improvement in FEV1 in the intervention group compared to a 3.1% (CI −0.4 to 6.6) in the control group. There were clinically meaningful improvements in 6MWT (increase by 92 m, CI 64 to 120) and SGRQ scores (−17.4, CI-24.75 to −10.0) in the treatment group that completed the study ($n = 23$). The main adverse events observed in the study were exacerbations of COPD and pneumothoraces. In total, there were six pneumothoraces (18%), three of which settled within 14 days, and three which required removal of a valve. About 35% of the patients required a further bronchoscopy for valve removal or repositioning.

The LIBERATE [47] and TRANSFORM [48] trials were two very similar randomised controlled studies (2:1 in favour of intervention), the former predominantly undertaken in the USA and the latter in Europe. In both studies, patients were selected on the basis of severe emphysema, hyperinflation, intact fissures on CT scans and heterogeneous distribution of disease. Both studies only recruited patients who were confirmed as collateral ventilation negative on Chartis assessment. TRANSFORM 6-month data demonstrated statistically and clinically meaningful benefits in multiple parameters over standard of care, including FEV1 (+29.3%), RV (−0.67 L), 6MWD (78.9 m), SGRQ (−6.9 points) and BODE index (−1.75 points), confirming the improvements seen in earlier trials. The LIBERATE trial extended the control data collection period out to 1 year, showing a durable response to EBV therapy, with improvements again seen in FEV1 (+18.0%), RV (−0.52 L), 6MWD (39.3 m), SGRQ (−7.1 points) and BODE index (−1.2 points). These trials expanded the evidence base sufficiently to allow approval for routine clinical use of the Zephyr valve in the USA, Europe and several other territories.

Although a majority of the evidence for +EBVs has been collected in heterogeneous emphysema, their benefit in homogeneous disease has also been demonstrated in a dedicated [49]. Ninety-three patients were randomised to endobronchial valves ($n = 43$) or standard of care ($n = 50$). The difference in change in FEV1 between groups was 13.5%, 6MWT 22.6 m and SGRQ −8.63 points. COPD exacerbations and pneumothoraces were the commonest adverse events.

The main adverse event observed has been the higher incidence of pneumothorax [50]. The latest results and current clinical practice suggest a pneumothorax rate around 15–25%. Hence, it is crucial that treating centres have experience in the management of often complex pneumothoraces. The sharing of experiences and data should allow for the development of robust treatment algorithms, and a recent expert statement has been published to provide guidance in this often tricky area [51]. The evidence base demonstrates that endobronchial valves are a genuine alternative to lung volume reduction surgery, with a similar magnitude of benefit but with a less invasive procedure and potentially lower morbidity. Furthermore, the improved safety profile of EBVs has enabled treatment in patients with homogeneous destruction and alpha-1-antitrypsin deficiency.

Endobronchial Lung Volume Reduction Coils

Endobronchial coils comprise a pre-shaped nitinol wire which is introduced into the segmental airway under fluoroscopy, and once released reverts to its original shape (Fig. 8.2) [52]. After a number of coils are placed in a target lobe, tension is created between them, which is thought to promote small airway splinting and improved lung emptying on expiration. The effect is to reduce lung compliance and reduce

Fig. 8.2 A lung volume
reduction coil

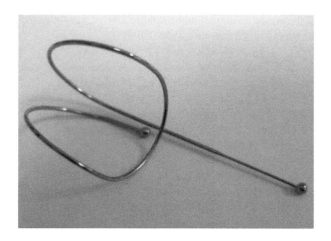

Fig. 8.2 A lung volume
reduction coil

hyperinflation. In patients where there is significant parenchymal compression with
some coil-associated pulmonary consolidation, the effects appear to be greater.

A first in man study [53] with 11 patients and 21 procedures under general anaesthetic demonstrated the safety of the procedure, with no severe adverse events. A
subsequent prospective, non-randomised, efficacy study in 16 patients with heterogeneous emphysema [54] demonstrated statistically significant benefits in SGRQ
(-14.9 points), FEV_1 ($+14.9\%$) and 6MWD ($+84.4$ m). A median of ten coils were
implanted per lung, with 12 patients having both lungs treated in sequential procedures. One pneumothorax occurred in the first month after treatment, with the predominant adverse event being COPD exacerbation, particularly in the immediate
post-procedure period. Outcomes were better with ten than five coils per lobe, and
this has now become the treatment strategy of choice.

Outcomes of two trials, one recruiting only heterogeneous patients [52] and the
other only homogeneous patients [55], appear comparable. Mean improvements in
FVC of 13.4% and 17.5%, reductions in RV of 11.4% and 11.9% and improvements
in 6MWD of 84.4 m and 61 m, respectively, were seen. Quality of life as measured
by the SGRQ was very significantly improved in both studies, with mean falls of
14.9 points and 15 points. Interestingly, different treatment strategies for homogeneous disease patients have been implemented in different centres, without any
obvious difference in outcomes. One strategy is to place a coil in each bronchopulmonary segment of the whole lung [56], and the other to treat only the upper lobes
as one would for heterogeneous upper lobe disease [55].

The first randomised controlled study with the RePneu Lung Volume Reduction
Coils (LVRC) in comparison to Standard of Care for the Treatment of Emphysema
(RESET) study [56] recruited 47 patients. Patients were randomised in a 1:1 ratio to
either treatment with endobronchial coils (23 subjects) or usual care (24 subjects).
After randomisation, treatment arm patients underwent treatment of one lung, with
the contralateral lung treated about 1 month later. End points were assessed at
3 months after the last treatment. The results showed substantial between-group

differences in mean changes from baseline in the SGRQ (-8.4 points; $p = 0.04$), 6MWD ($+63.55$ m; $p < 0.001$) and FEV1 ($+10.6\%$; $p = 0.03$). The RESET study reported six serious adverse events (SAEs) in the treatment group within the first 30 days, and three events between 30 and 90 days. The control group experienced one and three SAEs, respectively, with all SAEs in both groups beyond 30 days related to infection or exacerbation. There were no late pneumothoraces, and no deaths occurred within the follow-up period.

A second randomised study was performed in ten centres in France and randomised 100 patients to either endobronchial coil treatment or regular care (control) [57]. Forty-seven of the 50 patients randomised to endobronchial coils underwent bilateral treatment. Eighteen patients (36%) had an improvement in their 6MWT by ≥ 54 metres compared to only nine patients (18%) in the control group ($p = 0.03$). Hence, the trial achieved its primary end point, but the 6MWT in the treated patients was improved by a mean of only 18 metres at 6 months, and had declined to 2 metres at 12 months. However, when compared to the control group, there was a persistent mean difference of 21 metres at both 6 and 12 months. At 1 year, the mean difference in FEV1 was 11% ($p = 0.002$), and the mean difference in SGRQ was -10.6 ($p < 0.001$), both in favour of the active treatment group. At 1 year, there were four deaths in the treatment group compared to three in the control group. Four pneumothoraces occurred in the treatment group compared to one in the controls. The occurrence of COPD exacerbations did not differ between the two groups, but in the endobronchial coil group, significantly more pneumonias were observed (11 vs. 2). Some of these patients did not have any features of infection, and now are considered to have developed coil-associated inflammatory opacities rather than bacterial pneumonia.

The most recent randomised study, the RENEW trial [58], conducted in 21 centres in the USA and 5 centres in Europe randomised 157 patients to best medical therapy and 158 patients to bilateral endobronchial coil treatment. Median change in the 6MWT at 12 months was only 10.3 metres versus a decrease of 7.6 metres in the standard of care group. The mean in-group difference is 14.6 m ($p = 0.02$), although 40% of patients did improve by a clinically meaningful amount. There were greater improvements in quality of life scores with a mean 8.1 point reduction in SGRQ. There was a greater rate of adverse events in the treated patients (34.8%) compared to the control group (19.1%), with key adverse events such as pneumothorax (9.7% vs. 0.6%) and pneumonia (20% vs. 4.5%) also more frequent in coil-treated patients. The overall results of the RENEW trial are modest and appear to have been influenced by a change in inclusion criteria allowing patients with a residual volume between 175% and 225% predicted to be enrolled. This group appeared to have significant comorbidity which adversely affected the primary end point of 6MWT.

Hartman and colleagues [59] have been reporting data on 38 patients recruited to several earlier trials at one study site, and Zoumot [60] reported on the 2-year data in patients treated in the original RESET study. Clinical benefit appears to gradually decline over time, but even at 3 years post-treatment, approximately 50% of patients maintained improvement in 6MWD, SGRQ and mMRC. Early theoretical concerns with endobronchial coils had been the development of bacterial or fungal colonisation, migration of coils over time and tearing of lung parenchyma, but no microbiological or imaging evidence of any of these was seen throughout the follow-up period.

Endobronchial coils may be considered in patients with emphysema and severe hyperinflation. Patients both homogeneously and heterogeneously distributed can be considered, but patients with paraseptal disease, gross bullous destruction and giant bullae should be avoided. There are still a number of procedural uncertainties that need resolving, such as the precise location of coil placements during treatment, size of coils and number of coils that should be deployed.

Sealants

Sealants reduce lung volumes by tissue remodelling, through the induction of an inflammatory response and then fibrotic scarring. The first such technique was developed by Aeris Therapeutics, Inc. (Woburn, MA), which designed a fibrinogen biopharmaceutical suspension and thrombin solution that polymerised in situ to form a hydrogel (so-called BioLVR) for deployment via a standard bronchoscope. Early results indicated benefits could be seen in both heterogeneous upper lobe emphysema [61] and advanced homogeneous emphysema [62]. Two treatment regimens were followed, with a high-dose (HD) and a low-dose (LD) group. In heterogeneous subjects, there were statistically significant improvements in hyperinflation at 12 weeks and in spirometric values at 6 months in both LD and HD cohorts, although changes were greater with high-dose treatment. Homogeneous subjects also exhibited a better response to HD than LD therapy, with a significant reduction in gas trapping at 3 months in HD subjects.

The sealant was subsequently refined to create a more stable hydrogel foam using a solution containing aminated polyvinyl alcohol and glutaraldehyde. As the air contained within the hydrogel foam diffuses out, it collapses leading to approximation of the tissues to which the surface of the hydrogel foam has attached. A pilot study conducted across several sites in Germany enrolled 25 patients with heterogeneous emphysema, treating two to four subsegments initially with the potential to repeat therapy in two additional sites if deemed necessary by the treating physician [63]. Quality of life scores and 6-minute walking distance were improved in subjects with both severe (GOLD III; $n = 14$) and very severe (GOLD IV; $n = 7$) airflow obstruction (SGRQ -9.9 ± 15.3 points and -6.7 ± 7.0 points; 6MWD $+28.7 \pm 59.6$ m and $+28.3 \pm 58.4$ m). Meaningful improvements in RV/TLC ($-7.4\% \pm 10.3\%$), FEV1 ($+15.9\% \pm 22.6\%$) and diffusing capacity ($+19.3 \pm 34.8\%$) were observed in GOLD III but not in GOLD IV subjects.

The second study evaluated the effects in ten patients with upper lobe disease and ten with homogeneous disease [64]. Subjects received treatment to four subsegments, two in each upper lobe. Upper lobe lung volumes assessed by quantitative CT scan analysis were decreased by nearly 1 litre (-895 ± 484 mL, $p < 0.001$) with improvements in lung function-derived measures of hyperinflation (RV/TLC 7.2% ± 12.7% and 10.9% ± 14.0%). There were corresponding improvements in FEV_1 (31.2% ± 36.6% and 25.0% ± 33.4%) and quality of life (SGRQ 8.0 ± 17.2 points and 7.0 ± 15.8 points) at both 6 and 12 months of follow-up. Improvements relative to baseline in spirometry (FEV1 + 14.3% ± 33.1%; FVC + 5.8% ± 23.2%) and diffusing capacity (+10.6% ± 20.6%) continued to be seen at 2 years of follow-up [65].

Despite these encouraging early results, development of the product was hampered by the presence of a severe inflammatory response in some subjects. A pivotal randomised controlled trial was initiated (95 out of planned 300 patients recruited) but was not completed owing to funding shortfalls [66]. Nonetheless, at 3 months, there were significant improvements in lung function, dyspnoea and quality of life from baseline in the treatment group ($n = 34$) compared to the control group ($n = 23$). However, there were two deaths in the treated cohort, and 44% of treated patients experienced an adverse event requiring hospitalisation. The technology has now been acquired by Pulmonx, which is currently focussed on improving the safety profile of the product.

Vapour Therapy

Vapour treatment utilises the effects of thermal energy to induce a localised fibrotic response and subsequent lung volume reduction. This bronchoscopic thermal vapour ablation (BTVA) technology uses steam delivered via the central channel of a simple endobronchial balloon catheter to induce tissue remodelling and scarring, resulting in volume loss in the target area. Animal studies demonstrated a dose-dependent reduction in volumes of treated lobes [67], and whilst this was not demonstrated in a first-in-human trial [68], there were clinically significant improvements in the SGRQ (−15.3 points) and a reduction in the MRC dyspnoea score of 0.5 points, together with a 16% improvement in gas transfer. This trial demonstrated the feasibility and safety of the technology, and a subsequent larger clinical trial in 44 subjects with upper lobe predominant disease [69] demonstrated significant changes from baseline in FEV_1 (+141 ml), RV (−406 ml), 6MWD (+46.5 m), SGRQ (−14.0 points) and mMRC dyspnoea score (−0.9 points) at 6 months of follow-up. Some benefit persisted out to 1 year, with sustained meaningful improvements in the SGRQ, and statistically but not necessarily clinically significant changes in spirometry, lung volumes and exercise capacity [70]. The main limitation was the incidence of a more severe inflammatory response.

The STEP-UP study [71] was a randomised multicentre study which enrolled subjects with upper lobe predominant emphysema to staged therapy with vapour. The study was designed to exclude patients with too much lung destruction and focussed more on patients with upper lobe predominant disease with a difference in emphysema destruction scores of at least 15% between ipsilateral lobes. The treatment algorithm was calculated for each individual patient based on the tissue-to-air ratio at a segmental level on CT scanning. The most destroyed segments were identified, and the dose of vapour energy to be delivered at the treatment site was calculated. The intention was that only one segment was treated at the first treatment and up to two segments were treated during the second treatment (about 3 months later). Forty-six patients were randomised to vapour therapy and 24 to standard of care. The mean change in FEV1 in the treatment group was 11.0% (SD +/− 16.2) at 6 months compared to a change of −3.7% (+/−11.1) in the SOC group ($p < 0.0001$). The mean change in SGRQ-C was −9.7 (+/−14.4) points at 6 months, compared to 0 (+/−9.8) points in the control group ($p = 0.0021$). At 6 months, there was an absolute difference between the two arms in the 6MWT of 30·5 (+/−32) metres, but the difference was not statistically significant. There was a greater incidence of adverse events in the vapour treatment group: exacerbations (24%), pneumonitis (18%) and one death (2%).

The 12-month data [72] demonstrated significant improvements in FEV1 (between-group difference 12.8%) and SGRQ (between group difference − 12.1 points) in patients treated with vapour. However, in this study, there were no significant improvements in 6MWT at 12 months. As expected, there was an excess of adverse events in the peri-procedure period with significantly more events in the vapour group in the first 90 days post-treatment. However, there were no differences in adverse event rates in the subsequent period (days 90–360) between the groups.

Accessory Airway Formation

In spite of the apparent successes of the techniques so far discussed, not all attempts at minimally invasive lung volume reduction have lasted the course, and accessory airway formation has been the conspicuous loser in this regard. The concept of using extra-anatomical passages for the venting of trapped gas in severe emphysema was first proposed by Peter Macklem in 1978 [73]. This idea has been developed in two different approaches, one venting air into the larger non-collapsible airways (Broncus Technologies, Inc., Mountain View, CA) and the other taking the more extreme option of venting directly through the chest wall (Portaero, Inc., Cupertino, CA).

Macklem's basic concept was adapted by Joel Cooper and his group at Washington University who developed a technique of creating bronchial fenestrations held open by transbronchial stents to connect the diseased parenchyma with the large airways. Whilst targeting the most severely affected areas of emphysema, the procedure, unlike with endobronchial valves, also relied on the *presence* of collateral ventilation to reduce the residual volume of the whole lung, and was shown to improve the mechanical properties of explanted lungs [74, 75]. Experiments in canine models indicated that the patency of plain stents was short-lived (all stents occluded at 1 week), but that excellent stent patency rates could be achieved with the regular application of mitomycin C [76]. Owing to the impracticality of topical mitomycin C applications in patients, the anti-proliferative drug paclitaxel was used to coat the stents (Fig. 8.3a). Safety of the procedure was demonstrated in feasibility studies in patients undergoing lobectomies for cancer or lung transplantation [77], with significant improvements in lung function, dyspnoea, exercise capacity and quality of life at 1 month, with the improvements in lung function and dyspnoea remaining significant at 6 months.

Following on from these early results, the multicentre, randomised, double blind, sham controlled Exhale Airway Stents for Emphysema (EASE) trial [78] investigated the use of transbronchial airway stents in subjects with severe homogeneous emphysema, creating connections between the coalesced airspaces of the emphysematous lung and the (sub)segmental bronchi. Under bronchoscopic control, a needle was used to puncture the airway, the tract was dilated with a balloon, and a 5 mm stent was placed across the airway wall (Fig. 8.3b). Subjects in the sham arm of the trial had a bronchoscopy under general anaesthesia, with a scripted running commentary delivered by the operator(s) to minimise the risk of unblinding owing to partial anaesthesia. The bronchoscope was left in the trachea for a total of 1 hour during these sham procedures. The primary end point combined a $\geq 12\%$ change in FVC *and* a 1 point or greater fall in mMRC, and a subject had to meet both criteria to be considered a 'responder'.

Although early improvements in lung function and breathlessness were apparent, these were not sustained beyond 1 month, and a significant difference in the primary end point responder rate existed only at day 1 post-procedure. The lack of response appeared to be a result of an ongoing process of stent occlusion as the airway wall attempted to repair itself, overcoming the anti-proliferative effects of paclitaxel. Further work is needed to determine the exact nature of the airway reaction to stent placement, and to identify better anti-proliferative drugs with which to coat the stents (e.g. sirolimus, which is used to good effect in coronary artery stents), although the cost of repeating such a large trial is likely to be prohibitive.

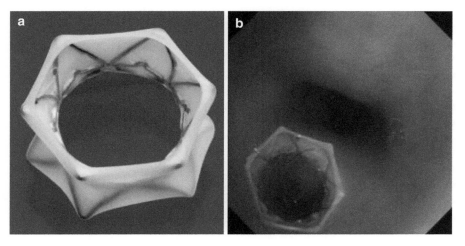

Fig. 8.3 Airway bypass stent (**a**) ex vivo and (**b**) placed across the wall in a segmental airway

The second method involved the surgical creation of a transthoracic pneumono-stoma (meaning that this technique can be considered to be only 'less invasive' rather than 'minimally invasive'), through which a small plastic tube was inserted to maintain patency and vent air. A pilot study reported changes in lung function mea-sures, although not in exercise capacity or quality of life [79], and a larger multicen-tre trial was initiated but never completed, and no results have ever been published. Maintenance of tract patency was a particular issue, in much the same way as with the airway bypass stents in the EASE trial [78], and some of the pilot study patients subsequently required multiple tract dilatations.

Whilst the theory of accessory airways appears sound, the practical aspects of implementing that theory have been more challenging than anticipated. These investigations have not, however, been futile. The principle has been established, in particular with the early EASE trial follow-up results, and the technique for airway bypass has recently been adopted for use in the investigation of pulmonary nodules, allowing direct access to parenchyma not otherwise accessible via the broncho-scope [80].

Treatment of Giant Bullae

A bulla is defined as an airspace in the lung measuring more than 1 cm in diameter in the distended state. Bullae are termed 'giant' when they occupy one third of the volume of the hemithorax, and can cause significant compression of the surround-ing lung parenchyma [81]. Known as vanishing lung syndrome, or idiopathic giant bullous emphysema, it is typically a consequence of cigarette smoking, although increasingly the smoking of marijuana and other drugs is recognised as a causative factor [82], possibly owing to the inhalation of hot gas through 'bongs' and associ-ated breath holding.

Although the aetiology may be subtly different, giant bullous disease could be seen as heterogeneous disease taken to its extreme, and surgery for giant bullous disease, unlike traditional LVRS, has been practiced for several decades [83, 84]. However, there are no universally accepted criteria for intervention, and the litera-ture is in very large part restricted to case series of surgical treatments with surpris-ingly little prospective long-term data available, and no comparison of different techniques for achieving decompression or excision. The received wisdom is that surgical treatment of giant bullae gives universally excellent results, but what evi-dence there is does not necessarily support this view even in stable patients. Nonetheless, results following surgical bullectomy can be spectacular and genu-inely life-changing in individual patients, with evidence to show persistence of ben-efit out to at least 5 years [85]. Palla and colleagues recruited 41 patients undergoing either thoracotomy or video-assisted thoracoscopy for the removal of giant bullae. After surgery, there was a fall in dyspnoea scores, and a mean increase in FEV_1 at the second year of follow-up of 489 mls, with a mean annual decrease thereafter of

46mls. The mean intrathoracic gas volume decreased significantly and remained constant throughout the entire follow-up period.

A less invasive method for surgically treating giant bullae is the use of intracavity drainage, with a chest tube inserted into the bullous space via a minithoracotomy, with localised pleurodesis [86], also known as the Brompton technique. Suction can be applied to the drain to assist with the evacuation of air [87].

As with the surgical literature, there is a much smaller body of evidence for bronchoscopic interventions for giant bullous disease. The first published technique, a single case report, involved the direct aspiration of air from a bulla using a transbronchial aspiration needle followed by 5 mls of autologous blood in a similar fashion to blood pleurodesis [88]. The FEV_1 was seen to rise from 0.68 L to 1.20 L, and there was an unquantified improvement in exercise capacity.

Two publications from Japan have reported significant reductions in static lung volumes and dyspnoea in the treatment of a giant bulla [89] and bullous disease associated with lymphangioleiomyomatosis [90] using the infusion of a blood and thrombin mixture into the damaged lung via a flexible bronchoscope. This is similar to the initial concept behind the forerunner to the emphysema lung sealant system [61] which used a fibrinogen and thrombin mixture to induce volume loss. One unanswered question with this technique, however, was how much of its action could be attributed to the blood component of the mixture and how much to the thrombin solution.

A pilot study of the use of 240 mls of autologous blood delivered via an extended working channel under fluoroscopic guidance into the bullae of five patients [91] has demonstrated dramatic clinical improvements, with large reductions in RV (mean − 0.73 L), increases in FEV1 (mean + 17.3%), reductions in the SGRQ (mean − 11.1 points) and increases in the 6MWD (mean + 88 m), all exceeding minimal clinically important differences. Three patients had noticeable reductions in the size of the bullae on CT scanning at 3 months, and these patients had considerable and almost universal improvements across all outcome measures. Kanoh and colleague [89] had already demonstrated a similar response, but crucially Zoumot and colleagues did not use any additional clotting products in their procedures. Success potentially provides the benefits of bullectomy without the surgical risk, and failure would not hinder any subsequent surgical intervention. The slow reduction in the size of the bulla mitigates against the risk of pneumothorax from rapid decompression, or any problems associated with rapid re-expansion of the compressed lung. The exact mechanism of action, however, has yet to be determined for intrabullous blood injection, but is probably a combination of inflammatory reaction, obliteration of small ventilatory channels and other as yet undefined processes. Although blood can cause the pleural surfaces to adhere and sclerose together, the volume of blood injected into these non-decompressed bullae was not sufficient to fill the bullae and for that mechanism of action to explain the bullous collapse/reabsorption seen. A larger multicentre study is ongoing to further characterise the potential benefits of this procedure.

Summary

There has traditionally been a rather nihilistic attitude towards emphysema and COPD, but with recent advances in the understanding of aetiological, pathophysiological and prognostic mechanisms, and the increase in treatment options, this approach is no longer appropriate. The reported morbidity and mortality with surgical approaches have driven the development of bronchoscopic lung volume reduction, but recent data showing zero mortality across 81 unilateral LVRS procedures (bilateral procedures were performed in the NETT [21]) suggests that with appropriate patient selection and in the right hands, the risks of surgery can be minimised [26]. However, safety concerns about mortality and morbidity, in particular prolonged air leaks, persist.

Ironically, this interest in non-surgical treatments has actually resulted in a resurgence in surgical lung volume reduction, as multidisciplinary team meetings have been developed and more patients with severe emphysema are being reviewed and discussed. This increase in activity is likely to produce data supporting the role of LVRS in special circumstances for new patient subgroups, but this is one area where BLVR has the potential to increase the availability of treatment to those with severe emphysema. The potential avoidance in risk directly associated with surgery (and the replacement of general anaesthetic with conscious sedation in some circumstances) allows for those with other medical co-morbidities to be treated.

There is undoubtedly still a need for surgical lung volume reduction (e.g. in predominantly paraseptal disease), but the range of bronchoscopic treatments currently under assessment should help to provide a wide range of patients with a number of treatment options, and even combined treatments using different techniques to achieve individualised treatment plans for best outcomes. However, one current problem with the entire field of BLVR is the lack of robust control data. The open-label nature of studies in which a number of efficacy parameters are subjective means that one cannot exclude a significant placebo effect. The importance of this in bronchoscopic intervention trials was well illustrated in the randomised, double blind, sham controlled trial of bronchial thermoplasty in patients with asthma [92], which demonstrated a large and significant increase in the asthma-related quality of life in the placebo arm.

It may be that it is not the actual method of volume reduction per se that counts, rather the choice of device based on patient characteristics. Results of recent BLVR trials demonstrate very similar outcomes, with largely similar entry criteria. Some techniques claim better results with certain outcome measures, and whether this simply represents statistical variation is unclear. However, if these results hold true in larger controlled studies, then they may allow further tailoring of products to individuals depending on the severity of impairment of various parameters at the time of treatment.

Pivotal trial data is certainly needed to establish BLVR as a routine treatment option in most healthcare systems, and ultimately what is needed are large randomised trials of the various BLVR techniques against each other, and including

LVRS in those with upper lobe heterogeneous emphysema. These, however, are unlikely ever to be performed owing to the huge investment (both of time and money) that would be required to demonstrate differences between methods with similar results.

One factor that could restrict access to BLVR is pricing. Publicly funded healthcare systems (and indeed insurance companies) may not be able to afford to offer some or any of these technologies, and whilst there may be good reasons for using BLVR over LVRS, such as disease distribution or co-morbidities, it is unappealing to funding bodies to pay large sums of money (e.g. endobronchial coils cost around €1000 per coil, and a complete bilateral procedure involves the insertion of 20 or more coils) for a procedure with less substantial evidence of benefit than LVRS. Companies now need to provide robust safety and cost-effectiveness analyses, and this is one of the major challenges faced by the field. Nonetheless, BLVR represents one of the few interventions shown to benefit those with emphysema, and when used alongside surgical treatment options, provides a suite of interventions for patients with severe emphysema in whom traditional medical management is not sufficient.

References

1. Kemp SV, Polkey MI, Shah PL. The epidemiology, etiology, clinical features and natural history of emphysema. In: Choong C, Fergusuon M, editors. Thoracic surgical clinics: update on surgical and endoscopic management of emphysema, vol. 2. Pennsylvania: WB Saunders; 2009. p. 149–58. ISBN 978-1-4377-0552-2.
2. Bonet T. Geneva: 1679. Sepulchretum sive anatonia pructica ex Cadaveribus Morbo denatis, proponens Histoa's Observations omnium pené humani corporis affectuum, ipsarcomoue Causas recorditas revelans.
3. Morgagni GB. The seats and causes of disease. In: Alexander B, Miller A, Caldwell T, translators. Investigated by anatomy; in five books, containing a great variety of dissections, with remarks. London: Johnson and Payne; 1769.
4. Laennec RTH. A treatise on the diseases of the chest and on mediate auscultation. Translated by J. Forbes. Fourth London edition. Philadelphia: Thomas and Co.; 1835.
5. Gauthier AP, Verbanck S, Estenne M, et al. Three-dimensional reconstruction of the in vivo human diaphragm shape at different lung volumes. J Appl Physiol. 1994;76:495–506.
6. Cypel M, Yeung JC, Liu M, et al. Normothermic ex vivo lung perfusion in clinical lung transplantation. N Engl J Med. 2011;364:1431–40.
7. Trulock EP, Christie JD, Edwards LB, et al. Registry of the International Society for Heart and Lung Transplantation: twenty-fourth official lung and heart-lung transplantation report – 2007. J Heart Lung Transplant. 2007;26:782–95.
8. Cassivi SD, Meyers BF, Battafarano RJ, et al. Thirteen-year experience in lung transplantation for emphysema. Ann Thorac Surg. 2002;74:1663–70.
9. Brantigan OC, Mueller E. Surgical treatment of pulmonary emphysema. Am Surg. 1957;23:789–804.
10. Delarue NC, Woolf CR, Sanders DE, et al. Surgical treatment for pulmonary emphysema. Can J Surg. 1977;20:222–31.
11. Cooper JD, Trulock EP, Triantafillou AN, et al. Bilateral pneumonectomy (volume reduction) for chronic obstructive pulmonary disease. J Thorac Cardiovasc Surg. 1995;109:106–16.

12. Cooper JD, Patterson GA, Sundaresan RS, et al. Results of 150 consecutive bilateral lung volume reduction procedures in patients with severe emphysema. J Thorac Cardiovasc Surg. 1996;112:1319–29.
13. Criner GJ, Cordova FC, Furukawa S, et al. Prospective randomized trial comparing bilateral lung volume reduction surgery to pulmonary rehabilitation in severe chronic obstructive pulmonary disease. Am J Respir Crit Care Med. 1999;160(6):2018–27.
14. Geddes D, Davies M, Koyama H, et al. Effect of lung-volume-reduction surgery in patients with severe emphysema. N Engl J Med. 2000;343:239–45.
15. Lim E, Ali A, Cartwright N, Sousa I, et al. Effect and duration of lung volume reduction surgery: mid-term results of the Brompton trial. Thorac Cardiovasc Surg. 2006;54:188–92.
16. Miller JD, Berger RL, Malthaner RA, et al. Lung volume reduction surgery vs medical treatment: for patients with advanced emphysema. Chest. 2005;127:1166–77.
17. Bingisser R, Zollinger A, Hauser M, et al. Bilateral volume reduction surgery for diffuse pulmonary emphysema by video-assisted thoracoscopy. J Thorac Cardiovasc Surg. 1996;112(4):875–82.
18. Daniel TM, Chan BB, Bhaskar V, et al. Lung volume reduction surgery. Case selection, operative technique, and clinical results. Ann Surg. 1996;223(5):526–31.
19. Health Care Financing Administration. Report to congress. Lung volume reduction surgery and Medicare coverage policy: implications of recently published evidence. Baltimore: Health Care Financing Administration; 1998.
20. National Emphysema Treatment Trial Research Group. Rationale and design of the National Emphysema Treatment Trial (NETT): a prospective randomized trial of lung volume reduction surgery. Chest. 1999;116(6):1750–61.
21. Fishman A, Martinez F, Naunheim K, et al. National Emphysema Treatment Trial Research Group. A randomized trial comparing lung-volume-reduction surgery with medical therapy for severe emphysema. N Engl J Med. 2003;348:2059–73.
22. Washko GR, Fan VS, Ramsey SD, et al. The effect of lung volume reduction surgery on chronic obstructive pulmonary disease exacerbations. Am J Respir Crit Care Med. 2008;177(2):164–9.
23. National Emphysema Treatment Trial Research Group. Patients at high risk of death after lung-volume-reduction surgery. N Engl J Med. 2001;345(15):1075–83.
24. Naunheim KS, Wood DE, Mohsenifah S, et al. Long term follow-up of patients receiving lung- volume-reduction surgery versus medical therapy for severe emphysema by the National Emphysema Treatment Trial Research Group. Ann Thorac Surg. 2006;82:431–43.
25. Ramsey SD, Sullivan SD, Kaplan RM. Cost-effectiveness of lung volume reduction surgery. Proc Am Thorac Soc. 2008;5(4):406–11.
26. Clark SJ, Zoumot Z, Bamsey O, Polkey MI, Dusmet M, Lim E, Jordan S, Hopkinson NS, et al. Surgical approaches for lung volume reduction in emphysema. Clin Med (Lond). 2014;14(2):122–7.
27. Toma TP, Hopkinson NS, Hillier J, et al. Bronchoscopic volume reduction with valve implants in patients with severe emphysema. Lancet. 2003;361:931–3.
28. Snell GI, Holsworth L, Borrill ZL, et al. The potential for bronchoscopic lung volume reduction using bronchial prostheses: a pilot study. Chest. 2003;124(3):1073–80.
29. Yim AP, Hwong TM, Lee TW, et al. Early results of endoscopic lung volume reduction for emphysema. J Thorac Cardiovasc Surg. 2004;127(6):1564–73.
30. Wan IY, Toma TP, Geddes DM, et al. Bronchoscopic lung volume reduction for end-stage emphysema: report on the first 98 patients. Chest. 2006;129(3):518–26.
31. Strange C, Herth FJ, Kovitz KL, et al. VENT Study Group. Design of the endobronchial valve for emphysema palliation trial (VENT): a non-surgical method of lung volume reduction. BMC Pulm Med. 2007;7:10.
32. Sciurba FC, Ernst A, Herth FJ, et al.; VENT Study Research Group.A randomized study of endobronchial valves for advanced emphysema. N Engl J Med. 2010;363:1233–44.
33. Herth FJF, Noppen M, Valipour A, Leroy S, Vergnon J-M, Ficker JH, et al. Efficacy predictors of lung volume reduction with Zephyr valves in a European cohort. Eur Respir J. 2012;39:1334–42.

34. Wood DE, McKenna RJ Jr, Yusen RD, et al. A multicenter trial of an intrabronchial valve for treatment of severe emphysema. J Thorac Cardiovasc Surg. 2007;133(1):65–73.
35. Springmeyer SC, Bolliger CT, Waddell TK, et al. Treatment of heterogeneous emphysema using the spiration IBV valves. Thorac Surg Clin. 2009;19(2):247–53, ix–x.
36. Ninane V, Geltner C, Bezzi M, et al. Multicentre European study for the treatment of advanced emphysema with bronchial valves. Eur Respir J. 2012;39:1319–25.
37. Van Allen CM, Lindskog GE, Richter HG. Collateral respiration. Transfer of air collaterally between pulmonary lobules. J Clin Invest. 1931;10:559–90.
38. Diso D, Anile M, Carillo C, et al. Correlation between collateral ventilation and interlobar lung fissures. Respiration. 2014;88(4):315–9.
39. Eberhardt R, Gompelmann D, Schuhmann M, et al. Complete unilateral versus partial bilateral endoscopic lung volume reduction in patients with bilateral lung emphysema. Chest. 2012;142(4):900–8.
40. Hopkinson NS, Kemp SV, Toma TP, et al. Atelectasis and survival after bronchoscopic lung volume reduction for COPD. Eur Respir J. 2011;37(6):1346–51.
41. Venuta F, Anile M, Diso D, Carillo C, De Giacomo T, D'Andrilli A, Fraioli F, Rendina EA, Coloni GF. Long-term follow-up after bronchoscopic lung volume reduction in patients with emphysema. Eur Respir J. 2012;39(5):1084–9.
42. Garner J, Kemp SV, Toma TP, et al. Survival after endobronchial valve placement for emphysema: a 10-year follow-up study. Am J Respir Crit Care Med. 2016;194(4):519–21.
43. Aljuri N, Freitag L. Validation and pilot clinical study of a new bronchoscopic method to measure collateral ventilation before endobronchial lung volume reduction. J Appl Physiol. 2009;106(3):774–83.
44. Herth FJ, Eberhardt R, Gompelmann D, Ficker JH, Wagner M, Ek L, Schmidt B, Slebos DJ. Radiological and clinical outcomes of using Chartis™ to plan endobronchial valve treatment. Eur Respir J. 2013;41(2):302–8.
45. Davey C, Zoumot Z, Jordan S, et al. Bronchoscopic lung volume reduction with endobronchial valves for patients with heterogeneous emphysema and intact interlobar fissures (the BeLieVeR-HIFi study): a randomised controlled trial. Lancet. 2015;386(9998):1066–73.
46. Klooster K, ten Hacken NH, Hartman JE, et al. Endobronchial valves for emphysema without interlobar collateral ventilation. N Engl J Med. 2015;373(24):2325–35.
47. Criner GJ, Sue R, Wright S, et al.; LIBERATE Study Group.A multicenter randomized controlled trial of Zephyr endobronchial valve treatment in heterogeneous emphysema (LIBERATE). Am J Respir Crit Care Med. 2018;198(9):1151–64.
48. Kemp SV, Slebos DJ, Kirk A, et al.; TRANSFORM Study Team.A multicenter randomized controlled trial of Zephyr endobronchial valve treatment in heterogeneous emphysema (TRANSFORM). Am J Respir Crit Care Med. 2017;196(12):1535–43.
49. Valipour A, Slebos DJ, Herth F, et al. IMPACT study team. Endobronchial valve therapy in patients with homogeneous emphysema. Results from the IMPACT study. Am J Respir Crit Care Med. 2016;194(9):1073–82.
50. Kemp SV, Zoumot Z, Mahadeva R, et al. Pneumothorax after endobronchial valve treatment: no drain, no gain? Respiration. 2014;87(6):452–5.
51. Valipour A, Slebos DJ, de Oliveira HG, Eberhardt R, Freitag L, Criner GJ, Herth FJ. Expert statement: pneumothorax associated with endoscopic valve therapy for emphysema--potential mechanisms, treatment algorithm, and case examples. Respiration. 2014;87(6):513–21.
52. Klooster K, Ten Hacken NH, Slebos DJ. The lung volume reduction coil for the treatment of emphysema: a new therapy in development. Expert Rev Med Devices. 2014;11:481–9.
53. Herth FJ, Eberhard R, Gompelmann D, Slebos DJ, Ernst A. Bronchoscopic lung volume reduction with a dedicated coil: a clinical pilot study. Ther Adv Respir Dis. 2010;4:225–31.
54. Slebos DJ, Klooster K, Ernst A, Herth FJ, Kerstjens HA. Bronchoscopic lung volume reduction coil treatment of patients with severe heterogeneous emphysema. Chest. 2012;142:574–82.
55. Klooster K, Ten Hacken NH, Franz I, Kerstjens HA, van Rikxoort EM, Slebos DJ. Lung volume reduction coil treatment in chronic obstructive pulmonary disease patients with homogeneous emphysema: a prospective feasibility trial. Respiration. 2014;88:116–25.

56. Shah PL, Zoumot Z, Singh S, Bicknell SR, Ross ET, Quiring J, Hopkinson NS, Kemp SV; RESET trial Study Group.Endobronchial coils for the treatment of severe emphysema with hyperinflation (RESET): a randomised controlled trial. Lancet Respir Med. 2013;1:233–40.
57. Deslée G, Mal H, Dutau H, et al.; REVOLENS Study Group.Lung volume reduction coil treatment vs usual care in patients with severe emphysema: the REVOLENS randomized clinical trial. JAMA. 2016;315(2):175–84.
58. Sciurba FC, Criner GJ, Strange C, et al.; RENEW Study Research Group.Effect of endobronchial coils vs usual care on exercise tolerance in patients with severe emphysema: the RENEW randomized clinical trial. JAMA. 2016;315(20):2178–89.
59. Hartman JE, Klooster K, Gortzak K, Ten Hacken NH, Slebos D. Long-term follow-up after bronchoscopic lung volume reduction treatment with coils in patients with severe emphysema. Respirology. 2015;20(2):319–26.
60. Zoumot Z, Kemp SV, Singh S, et al. Endobronchial coils for severe emphysema are effective up to 12 months following treatment: medium term and cross-over results from a randomised controlled trial. PLoS One. 2015;10(4):e0122656.
61. Criner GJ, Pinto-Plata V, Strange C, et al. Biologic lung volume reduction in advanced upper lobe emphysema: phase 2 results. Am J Respir Crit Care Med. 2009;179(9):791–8.
62. Refaely Y, Dransfield M, Kramer MR, et al. Biologic lung volume reduction therapy for advanced homogeneous emphysema. Eur Respir J. 2010;36:20–7.
63. Herth FJ, Gompelmann D, Stanzel F, Bonnet R, Behr J, Schmidt B, Magnussen H, Ernst A, Eberhardt R. Treatment of advanced emphysema with emphysematous lung sealant (AeriSeal®). Respiration. 2011;82(1):36–45.
64. Kramer MR, Refaely Y, Maimon N, Rosengarten D, Fruchter O. Bilateral endoscopic sealant lung volume reduction therapy for advanced emphysema. Chest. 2012;142(5):1111–7.
65. Kramer MR, Refaely Y, Maimon N, Rosengarten D, Fruchter O. Two-year follow-up in patients treated with emphysematous lung sealant for advanced emphysema. Chest. 2013;144(5):1677–80.
66. Come CE, Kramer MR, Dransfield, et al. A randomised trial of lung sealant versus medical therapy for advanced emphysema. Eur Respir J. 2015;46(3):651–62.
67. Emery MJ, Eveland L, Eveland K, et al. Lung volume reduction by bronchoscopic administration of steam. Am J Resp Crit Care Med. 2010;182:1282–91.
68. Snell GI, Hopkins P, Westall G, Holsworth L, Carle A, Williams TJ. A feasibility and safety study of bronchoscopic thermal vapor ablation: a novel emphysema therapy. Ann Thorac Surg. 2009;88(6):1993–8.
69. Snell G, Herth FJ, Hopkins P, Baker KM, Witt C, Gotfried MH, Valipour A, Wagner M, Stanzel F, Egan JJ, Kesten S, Ernst A. Bronchoscopic thermal vapour ablation therapy in the management of heterogeneous emphysema. Eur Respir J. 2012;39(6):1326–33.
70. Herth FJ, Ernst A, Baker KM, Egan JJ, Gotfried MH, Hopkins P, Stanzel F, Valipour A, Wagner M, Witt C, Kesten S, Snell G. Characterization of outcomes 1 year after endoscopic thermal vapor ablation for patients with heterogeneous emphysema. Int J Chron Obstruct Pulmon Dis. 2012;7:397–405.
71. Herth FJ, Valipour A, Shah PL, et al. Segmental volume reduction using thermal vapour ablation in patients with severe emphysema: 6-month results of the multicentre, parallel-group, open-label, randomised controlled STEP-UP trial. Lancet Respir Med. 2016;4(3):185–93.
72. Shah PL, Gompelmann D, Valipour A, et al. Thermal vapour ablation to reduce segmental volume in patients with severe emphysema: STEP-UP 12 month results. Lancet Respir Med. 2016;4(9):e44–5.
73. Macklem PT. Collateral ventilation. N Engl J Med. 1978;298:49–50.
74. Lausberg HF, Chino K, Patterson GA, et al. Bronchial fenestration improves expiratory flow in emphysematous human lungs. Ann Thorac Surg. 2003;75:393–8.
75. Choong CK, Macklem PT, Pierce JA, et al. Airway bypass improves the mechanical properties of explanted emphysematous lungs. Am J Respir Crit Care Med. 2008;178:902–5.

76. Choong CK, Haddard FJ, Gee EY, et al. Feasibility and safety of airway bypass stent placement and influence of topical mitomycin C on stent patency. J Thorac Cardiovasc Surg. 2005;129:632–8.
77. Rendina EA, De Giacomo T, Venuta F, et al. Feasibility and safety of the airway bypass procedure for patients with emphysema. J Thorac Cardiovasc Surg. 2003;125:1294–9.
78. Shah PL, Slebos DJ, Cardoso PF, Cetti E, Voelker K, Levine B, Russell ME, Goldin J, Brown M, Cooper JD, Sybrecht GW; EASE trial study group.Bronchoscopic lung-volume reduction with exhale airway stents for emphysema (EASE trial): randomised, sham-controlled, multicentre trial. Lancet. 2011;378(9795):997–1005.
79. Moore AJ, Cetti E, Haj-Yahia S, Carby M, Björling G, Karlsson S, Shah P, Goldstraw P, Moxham J, Jordan S, Polkey MI. Unilateral extrapulmonary airway bypass in advanced emphysema. Ann Thorac Surg. 2010;89(3):899–906, 906.e1-2
80. Herth FJ, Eberhardt R, Sterman D, et al. Bronchoscopic transparenchymal nodule access (BTPNA): first in human trial of a novel procedure for sampling solitary pulmonary nodules. Thorax. 2015;70(4):326–32.
81. Roberts L, Putman CE, Chen JT, et al. Vanishing lung syndrome: upper lobe bullous pneumopathy. Rev Interam Radiol. 1987;12:249–55.
82. Johnson MK, Smith RP, Morrison D, et al. Large lung bullae in marijuana smokers. Thorax. 2000;55:340.
83. Ray JF 3rd, Lawton BR, Smullen WA, Myers WO, Sautter RD. Effective surgical palliation of giant compressive bullous emphysema (vanishing lung syndrome): long-term follow-up. Am Surg. 1976;42:181–5.
84. Laros CD, Gelissen HJ, Bergstein PG, Van den Bosch JM, Vanderschueren RG, Westermann CJ, Knaepen PJ. Bullectomy for giant bullae in emphysema. J Thorac Cardiovasc Surg. 1986;91:63–70.
85. Palla A, Desideri M, Rossi G, Bardi G, Mazzantini D, Mussi A, Giuntini C. Elective surgery for giant bullous emphysema: a 5-year clinical and functional follow-up. Chest. 2005;128(4):2043–50.
86. Goldstraw P, Petrou M. The surgical treatment of emphysema. The Brompton approach. Chest Surg Clin N Am. 1995;5:777–96.
87. Wang H, Xu Z, Gao W. A modified Brompton technique for the treatment of giant bulla in patients with diffuse emphysema. Thorac Cardiovasc Surg. 2012;60:161–3.
88. Bhattacharyya P, Sarkar D, Nag S, Ghosh S, Roychoudhury S. Transbronchial decompression of emphysematous bullae: a new therapeutic approach. Eur Respir J. 2007;2:1003–6.
89. Kanoh S, Kobayashi H, Motoyoshi K. Bronchoscopic blood injection reducing lung volume in lymphangioleiomyomatosis. Ann Thorac Surg. 2009;87(4):1266–8.
90. Kanoh S, Kobayashi H, Motoyoshi K. Intrabullous blood injection for lung volume reduction. Thorax. 2008;63(6):564–5.
91. Zoumot Z, Kemp SV, Caneja C, Singh S, Shah PL. Bronchoscopic intrabullous autologous blood instillation: a novel approach for the treatment of giant bullae. Ann Thorac Surg. 2013;96(4):1488–91.
92. Castro M, Rubin AS, Laviolette M, Fiterman J, De Andrade LM, et al. Effectiveness and safety of bronchial thermoplasty in the treatment of severe asthma. A multicentre, randomized, double blind, sham controlled clinical trial. Am J Respir Crit Care Med. 2010;181:116–24.

Chapter 9
Surgical Versus Medical Management of Anastomotic Dehiscence

Amit K. Mahajan, Bethany Hampole, Priya P. Patel, and Wickii T. Vigneswaran

Anastomotic dehiscence is one of the most serious airway complications following lung transplantation. Development of airway dehiscence in the modern age of lung transplantation is rare. While anastomotic dehiscence is estimated to occur in less than 2 percent of transplantations, it is often associated with high morbidity and mortality [1–3]. The development of anastomotic dehiscence can occur from a number of etiologies, but the most common cause is thought to result from extreme mucosal necrosis [4, 5]. The diagnosis and treatment of anastomotic dehiscence following lung transplantation requires close collaboration between interventional pulmonologists and thoracic surgeons. Although management approaches may vary between the two specialties, the end goal is the same: salvage of the allograft. Expeditious treatment of anastomotic dehiscence is essential to ensure viability of the allograft and survival of the transplant recipient.

Anastomotic dehiscence following lung transplantation is characterized by necrosis leading to full-thickness anastomotic separation of the bronchial wall. Multiple grading systems have been proposed to describe airway complication following lung transplantation. Courad et al. published an early schema in 1992 based on bronchoscopic appearance of anastomosis on day 15 [6]. This system is graded

---

** Each author has contributed equally to this manuscript
*** This manuscript has not been submitted for publication in any other journals

---

A. K. Mahajan (✉) · P. P. Patel
Department of Surgery, Inova Schar Cancer Institute, Inova Fairfax Hospital, Falls Church, VA, USA
e-mail: Amit.Mahajan@inova.org

B. Hampole · W. T. Vigneswaran
Department of Thoracic and Cardiovascular Surgery, Loyola University Health System, Maywood, IL, USA

© The Author(s), under exclusive license to Springer Nature Switzerland AG 2021
J. F. Turner, Jr. et al. (eds.), *From Thoracic Surgery to Interventional Pulmonology*, Respiratory Medicine,
https://doi.org/10.1007/978-3-030-80298-1_9

as grade 1, complete primary mucosal healing; grade 2a, complete primary healing without necrosis, partial primary mucosal healing; grade 2b, complete primary healing without necrosis, no primary mucosal healing; grade 3a, limited focal necrosis (extending less than 5 mm from the anastomotic line); and grade 3b, extensive necrosis. However, this system does not address anastomotic stenosis, granulation tissue formation, or other potential findings with airway complications. Santacruz and Mehta have categorized airway complications following lung transplantation into six groups: stenosis, necrosis and dehiscence, exophytic granulation tissue, malacia, fistulae, and infections [7]. This system, however, does not differentiate anastomotic dehiscence from necrosis. The French Language Pulmonary Society (FLPS) has also proposed a system based on the macroscopic appearance, diameter, and suture (MDS) in 2013 [8]. The MDS system, however, lacks terminology for the severity of ischemia or necrosis. The International Society for Heart and Lung Transplantation (ISHLT) also offers a grade of dehiscence by location (cartilaginous, membranous, both) and extent (0–25%, >25–50%, >50% to 75%, >75% of circumference) [9].

While some of the major risk factors associated with anastomotic dehiscence include surgical technique, perioperative steroids, acute rejection, infection, inadequate organ preservation, and immunosuppression, the primary cause is thought to be anastomotic ischemia [10, 11]. Following transplantation, the bronchial arteries are not typically revascularized, and thus the donor tracheobronchial blood supply initially derives from retrograde perfusion from the pulmonary arteries. Ultimate formation of collateral blood supplies to the donor lung and the anastomosis may take up to 6 weeks. Additionally, infections including *Aspergillus* along with the use medications, such as sirolimus, in the early postoperative period have also been strongly correlated with anastomotic dehiscence [12].

Common clinical signs and symptoms of anastomotic dehiscence include shortness of breath, sudden subcutaneous emphysema, pneumomediastinum, pleural effusion on the affected side, or a pneumothorax on chest radiograph [11]. Placement of a chest tube into the affected pleural space may result in a persistent air leak or infected pleural fluid. Unfortunately, the development of dehiscence may quickly result in infection of the allograft with potential for respiratory failure, septic shock, and even death.

Interventional Pulmonologist Approach to Anastomotic Dehiscence

Bronchoscopic inspection is essential in diagnosing and assessing an anastomotic dehiscence. While radiographic imaging in the form of a computer tomographic (CT) scan of the chest is sensitive for detecting anastomotic breakdown, endobronchial assessment confirms the diagnosis and helps determine if a bronchoscopic intervention is feasible. If definitive bronchoscopic treatment is not feasible, temporizing interventions may be possible until surgical correction is performed.

The severity of anastomotic dehiscence determines if bronchoscopic treatments will be successful. Partial anastomotic dehiscence can often be treated conservatively with close surveillance and antibiotic therapy, in both intravenous and inhaled forms [1]. Conversely, full-thickness dehiscence without complete anastomotic breakdown can initially be managed with endobronchial stent placement. Utilization of an airway stent as the means for treatment must be closely monitored in the weeks and months following placement to ensure that the dehiscence is improving. Additional endoscopic treatments for severe anastomotic dehiscence include cyanoacrylate glue, growth factors, and autologous platelet-derived wound healing factor [13]. If no significant improvement is noted after initial bronchoscopic treatment, surgical treatment should be performed.

The use of self-expanding metallic stents (SEMS) is the cornerstone of the bronchoscopic treatment of severe anastomotic dehiscence without complete anastomotic breakdown. The ability to capitalize on scarring properties of uncovered SEMS allows for airway remodeling. The SEMS serves as a lattice for granulation tissue to form and reestablish a durable airway. The feasibility of treating severe anastomotic dehiscence bronchoscopically depends on the ability to stent across the defect. Uncovered SEMS are preferred to avoid bacterial colonization of the stent coating and to allow drainage of mediastinal and bronchial secretions while still allowing for ventilation of the involved lobes [11]. Typically, SEMS are left in place for 4 to 6 weeks to allow for adequate granulation formation to cover the defect. If sufficient scarring is not present after 4 to 6 weeks, regular surveillance bronchoscopies should be performed to determine when the defect is closed. When the defect is closed, the stent should be removed. Extreme caution must be exercised when removing the stent to avoid recreating the defect or making the dehiscence worse.

While the bronchoscopic interventions are the most desirable management option for anastomotic dehiscence, the potential for treatment failure exists. Stent migration, infection, and invasion into neighboring vascular structures are potential risks to consider. In circumstances when healing is not achieved or the risk of complication outweighs the benefits, surgical intervention should be seriously considered.

Surgical Approach to Anastomotic Dehiscence

Surgical Prevention of Anastomotic Dehiscence

Various surgical techniques have been developed and refined to reduce the incidence of anastomotic dehiscence and airway complications. Earlier anastomotic techniques involved a telescoping approach; however, this has been abandoned due to overall increased rates of anastomotic stenoses and infections [10, 11]. Some success has been achieved using a continuous running polydioxanone suture along the membranous portion and interrupted simple or figure-of-eight suture along the cartilaginous portion versus an interrupted simple suturing technique all around [4, 10, 14].

Care must also be taken to ensure adequate, but not excessive, length of the donor bronchus. The donor bronchus should be cut obliquely, within one to two rings of the upper lobe bronchus origin in order to minimize length of tissue at risk for perioperative ischemia [4, 9, 10], The use of autologous tissue flaps using the omentum, pericardium, or intercostal tissue have been tried during the primary procedure; however, randomized controlled trials have not demonstrated a significant difference in airway complication and routine use of anastomotic wrapping has fallen out of favor [15]. Bronchial artery revascularization (BAR) has also been used in an attempt to decrease airway complications. Although there is postoperative angiographic evidence of bronchial perfusion with BAR, this technique adds additional technical complexity, increases graft ischemic time, and often requires cardiopulmonary bypass [9, 16].

Surgical Treatment of Anastomotic Dehiscence

Regardless of classification schemes, most cases of anastomotic dehiscence are incomplete. The occurrence of partial dehiscence may respond to management with close bronchoscopic monitoring, aggressive treatment of associated infection with culture targeted antibiotic and antifungal medication, and endobronchial therapy [10, 11, 17, 18]. There are no published guidelines on absolute indicators for failure of conservative management as an indication for operative intervention for anastomotic dehiscence. Principles of surgical management of anastomotic dehiscence involve management of the ongoing air leak with chest tube drainage, debridement of devitalized tissue, and local and systemic control of infection. Most cases of anastomotic dehiscence requiring surgery necessitate more than local debridement of devitalized tissue and primary closure with pericardial buttress, pleural flap, or other autologous tissue pledget or reinforcement [19–23]. Thus, the major surgical approach for operative management of anastomotic dehiscence requires resection and reanastomosis of the airway or consideration of allograft pneumonectomy with or without re-transplantation.

Airway reanastomosis in these circumstances is challenging due to the re-operative nature of the field, the poor tissue quality, relative ischemia, and, in many cases, the presence of infection [9, 11, 24]. Preoperative planning should also consider the likelihood for need of extracorporeal membrane oxygenation (ECMO) assistance during and after the operation, if not before [19, 20]. Preoperative bronchoscopy can delineate the location and extent of the necrosis. Isolated necrosis from a donor main bronchus may demonstrate a clear technical cause for dehiscence. This pattern of dehiscence lends itself to resection with re-anastomosis. Much of our experience dealing with anastomotic complication is from treating post-lung resection bronchial complication or tracheobronchial strictures and fistula unrelated to transplantation [15, 21–23, 25]. Consideration ought to be given that in the post-transplant period, the bronchus is relatively ischemic due to the lack of bronchial blood supply. This emphasizes the need to reinforce most of the surgical re-intervention with vascularized tissue. The reanastomosis should be performed in a standardized fashion without undue telescoping and should be buttressed with autologous vascularized tissue. Autologous tissue options include pedicled mammary, omentum brought through a small central tendon incision, intercostal muscle flap, pericardial flap, pleural flap, and intra-thoracic transfer of serratus anterior muscle or latissimus dorsi on its vascular pedicle [10, 23–28].

Extensive necrosis at the site of dehiscence may require a significant amount of debridement, causing tissue loss and the shortening of distance between the donor and recipient bronchus. This places the patient at further risk of bleeding complications and need for tissue coverage. Aortic homograft may provide an option to bridge the gap between donor and recipient bronchi. The homograft may also be buttressed further with vascularized autologous tissue flap [19, 20]. In these circumstances, a serratus anterior muscle or latissimus dorsi provides the tissue bulk to cover the repair or the defect itself, but note that if the latissimus dorsi was transected during the initial operation, this muscle may not be suitable.

Finally, allograft pneumonectomy remains an option of last resort with the possibility of re-transplantation depending upon patient status and organ availability. Colonization with highly resistant bacteria or fungi and unstable clinical status remain relative contraindications to re-transplantation. Individuals requiring re-transplant for airway complication have an overall poorer prognosis.

Conflicts of Interest We declare that we have no conflicts of interest.

References

1. Mughal MM, Gildea TR, Murthy S, Pettersson G, DeCamp M, Mehta AC. Short-term deployment of self-expanding metallic stents facilitates healing of bronchial dehiscence. Am J Respir Crit Care Med. 2005;172(6):768–71.
2. Kshettry VR, Kroshus TJ, Hertz MI, Hunter DW, Shumway SJ, Bolman RM III. Early and late airway complications after lung transplantation: incidence and management. Ann Thorac Surg. 1997;63:1576–83.
3. Kirk AJ, Conacher ID, Corris PA, Ashcroft T, Dark JH. Successful surgical management of bronchial dehiscence after single-lung transplantation. Ann Thorac Surg. 1990;49:147–9.
4. Weder W, Inci I, Korom S, et al. Airway complications after lung transplantation: risk factors, prevention and outcome. Eur J Cardiothorac Surg. 2009;35(2):293–8. discussion 298.
5. Alvarez A, Algar J, Santos F, et al. Airway complications after lung transplantation: a review of 151 anastomoses. Eur J Cardiothorac Surg. 2001;19(4):381–7.
6. Couraud L, Nashef SA, Nicolini P, Jougon J. Classification of airway anastomotic healing. Eur J Cardiothorac Surg. 1992;6(9):496–7. https://doi.org/10.1016/1010-7940(92)90247-u.
7. Santacruz JF, Mehta AC. Airway complications and management after lung transplantation. Proc Am Thorac Soc. 2009;6(1):79–93. https://doi.org/10.1513/pats.200808-094GO. https://www.atsjournals.org/doi/abs/10.1513/pats.200808-094GO.
8. Dutau H, Vandemoortele T, Laroumagne S, et al. A new endoscopic standardized grading system for macroscopic central airway complications following lung transplantation: the MDS classification. Eur J Cardiothorac Surg. 2014;45(2):33. https://doi.org/10.1093/ejcts/ezt499.

9. Crespo MM, McCarthy DP, Hopkins PM, et al. ISHLT consensus statement on adult and pediatric airway complications after lung transplantation: definitions, grading system, and therapeutics. J Heart Lung Transplant. 2018;37(5):548–63. doi: S1053-2498(18)31349-4 [pii].
10. Vigneswaran W, Sakiyalak P, Bhorade S, Bakhos M. Airway complications after isolated lung transplantation. Transplant Rev. 2002;16(2):87–94.
11. Mahajan AK, Folch E, Khandhar SJ, Channick CL, Santacruz JF, Mehta AC, Nathan SD. The diagnosis and Management of Airway Complications Following Lung Transplantation. Chest. 2017;152(3):627–38. https://doi.org/10.1016/j.chest.2017.02.021. Epub 2017 Mar 6.
12. Nathan SD, Shorr AF, Schmidt ME, Burton NA. Aspergillus and endobronchial abnormalities in lung transplant recipients. Chest. 2000;118:403–7.
13. Maloney JD, Weigel TL, Love RB. Endoscopic repair of bronchial dehiscence after lung transplantation. Ann Thorac Surg. 2001;72:2109–11.
14. FitzSullivan E, Gries CJ, Phelan P, et al. Reduction in airway complications after lung transplantation with novel anastomotic technique. Ann Thorac Surg. 2011;92(1):309–15.
15. Shrager JB, Wain JC, Wright CD, Donahue DM, Vlahakes GJ, Moncure AC, Grillo HC, Mathisen DJ. Omentum is highly effective in the management of complex cardiothoracic surgical problems. J Thorac Cardiovasc Surg. 2003;125(3):526–32. https://doi.org/10.1067/mtc.2003.12.
16. Khaghani A, Tadjkarimi S, Al-Kattan K, et al. Wrapping the anastomosis with omentum or an internal mammary artery pedicle does not improve bronchial healing after single lung transplantation: results of a randomized clinical trial. J Heart Lung Transplant. 1994;13(5):767–73.
17. Suh JW, Lee JG, Jeong SJ, Park MS, Kim SY, Paik HC. Risk of bronchial dehiscence in lung transplant recipients with Carbapenemase-producing Klebsiella. Ann Thorac Surg. 2020;110(1):265–71. https://doi.org/10.1016/j.athoracsur.2020.01.076. Epub 2020 Mar 7.
18. Backer E, Dincer EH, Keenan JC, Diaz-Gutierrez I, Cho RJ. Successful treatment of airway dehiscence in a lung transplant patient with radiofrequency ablation. J Bronchology Interv Pulmonol. 2020;27(4):e56–9. https://doi.org/10.1097/LBR.0000000000000668.
19. Ram D. O Carroll M, Sibal AK. Hybrid reconstruction of bronchial dehiscence following lung transplant. J Card Surg. 2020;35(11):3133–5. https://doi.org/10.1111/jocs.15067. Epub 2020 Sep 28.
20. McGiffin D, Wille K, Young K, Leon K. Salvaging the dehisced lung transplant bronchial anastomosis with homograft aorta. Interact Cardiovasc Thorac Surg. 2011;13(6):666–8. https://doi.org/10.1510/icvts.2011.269910. Epub 2011 Sep 13. . PMID: 21920932.
21. Riker A, Vigneswaran W. Management of tracheobronchial strictures and fistulas: a report and review of literature. Int Surg. 2002;87:114–9.
22. Taghavi S, Marta GM, Lang G, Seebacher G, Winkler G, Schmid K, Klepetko W. Bronchial stump coverage with a pedicled pericardial flap: an effective method for prevention of postpneumonectomy bronchopleural fistula. Ann Thorac Surg. 2005;79(1):284–8. https://doi.org/10.1016/j.athoracsur.2004.06.108.
23. Rendina EA, Venuta F, Ricci P, et al. Protection and revascularization of bronchial anastomoses by the intercostal pedicle flap. J Thorac Cardiovasc Surg. 1994;107(5):1251–4. doi: S0022-5223(94)70045-1 [pii].
24. Yserbyt J, Dooms C, Vos R, Dupont LJ, Van Raemdonck DE, Verleden GM. Anastomotic airway complications after lung transplantation: risk factors, treatment modalities and outcome - a single-Centre experience. Eur J Cardiothorac Surg. 2016;49(1):1. https://doi.org/10.1093/ejcts/ezv363.
25. Kumar A, Alraiyes AH, Gildea TR. Amniotic membrane graft for bronchial anastomotic dehiscence in a lung transplant recipient. Ann Am Thorac Soc. 2015;12(10):1583–6. https://doi.org/10.1513/AnnalsATS.201505-265CC. PMID: 26448355.
26. Choong CK, Sweet SC, Zoole JB, et al. Bronchial airway anastomotic complications after pediatric lung transplantation: incidence, cause, management, and outcome. J Thorac Cardiovasc Surg. 2006;131(1):198–203. https://doi.org/10.1016/j.jtcvs.2005.06.053.

27. Varela A, Hoyos L, Romero A, Campo-Cañaveral JL, Crowley S. Management of bronchial complications after lung transplantation and sequelae. Thorac Surg Clin. 2018;28(3):365–75. doi: S1547-4127(18)30047-1 [pii].
28. Krahenbuhl SM, Gonzalez M, Aubert JD, et al. Management of bilateral necrotizing bronchial dehiscence after a double lung transplantation. J Thorac Cardiovasc Surg. 2018;156(1):e29–31. doi: S0022-5223(18)30611-1 [pii].

Chapter 10
Benign Tracheal Stenosis: Medical Versus Surgical Management

Hyun S. Kim, Catherine L. Oberg, Sandeep Khandhar, and Erik E. Folch

Introduction

Tracheal stenosis is a subset of airway diseases that is associated with significant morbidity and mortality. The clinical manifestations include dyspnea, fatigue, chest discomfort, wheezing, and stridor. Tracheal stenosis and to a broader scale central airway obstruction, which includes the stenosis of the trachea, bilateral mainstem bronchi, and the bronchus intermedius, are classically divided into malignant and benign etiologies. Malignant tracheal stenosis is more common than benign etiologies and can be caused by malignancies of the airway or lung parenchyma, as well as metastatic tumors from distant structures or adjacent organs [1, 2]. Benign causes of tracheal stenosis are extremely varied, and include iatrogenic, inflammatory, infiltrative, infectious, and functional causes. The evaluation of tracheal stenosis is comprised of both functional and structural investigative modalities and usually requires a multidisciplinary team that includes chest radiologists, thoracic anesthesiologists, thoracic surgeons, and interventional pulmonologists. With increasingly sophisticated treatment modalities available to the interventional pulmonologists, the outcome of airway procedures is extremely effective in achieving both symptomatic relief and a significant improvement in airway dimension. In this chapter,

H. S. Kim · E. E. Folch (✉)
Massachusetts General Hospital, Harvard Medical School, Boston, MA, USA
e-mail: efolch@mgh.harvard.edu; folch@icloud.edu

C. L. Oberg
David Geffen School of Medicine at the University of California in Los Angeles,
Los Angeles, CA, USA

S. Khandhar
Virginia Cancer Specialists USON, Inova Fairfax, University of Virginia, Fairfax, VA, USA

© The Author(s), under exclusive license to Springer Nature   169
Switzerland AG 2021
J. F. Turner, Jr. et al. (eds.), *From Thoracic Surgery to Interventional
Pulmonology*, Respiratory Medicine,
https://doi.org/10.1007/978-3-030-80298-1_10

the etiology, pathogenesis, diagnostic approaches, available treatment modalities, and future directions of benign tracheal stenosis will be reviewed.

Scope of the Problem

Tracheal Anatomy

The trachea is part of the lower airway and begins at the distal aspect of the cricoid cartilage at the level of the sixth cervical vertebra, ending at the main carina at the level of the intervertebral disc between the T4 and T5 vertebrae. The normal length of the trachea is between 10 and 13 cm in males and is slightly shorter in females [3]. The usual internal diameter ranges between 16 and 20 mm. It is composed of 18–22 C-shaped cartilages that support the anterior and lateral aspect of the trachea, with a posterior membranous wall composed of the trachealis muscle that connects the tracheal cartilages. The upper (cervical) trachea is supplied by the branches of the inferior thyroid artery and thyrocervical trunks that arise from the subclavian arteries, and the lower (thoracic) trachea is supplied by the bronchial arteries directly arising from the aorta. The deoxygenated blood from the trachea is drained by tracheal veins which join the laryngeal vein or drain directly into the left inferior thyroid vein. Stenosis of the trachea can occur anywhere along its longitudinal axis and originate from either the cartilaginous or the membranous walls.

Etiology of Tracheal Stenosis

Benign tracheal stenosis can be categorized into four groups: mechanical, systemic/inflammatory, infectious, and idiopathic. Mechanical causes include post-intubation tracheal stenosis (PITS), post-tracheostomy tracheal stenosis (PTTS), post-surgical tracheal stenosis, stenosis after lung transplantation, airway stent-related stenosis, and compression from an external entity such as mediastinal lymphadenopathy or tumor [4, 5].

PITS and PTTS represent a unique and paradoxical challenge given their iatrogenic nature. The risk factors for tracheal stenosis following intubation and tracheostomy tube placement are prolonged intubation, particularly if exceeding 7 days, and excessive balloon cuff pressure (>20 cm H_2O) [6]. The incidence is estimated to be as high as 21%, though only about 1–2% of these patients develop severe stenosis or symptoms [7, 8]. The stenosis usually takes place at the cuff site for PITS and PTTS and can also occur at the level of the tracheostomy stoma for patients with chronic tracheostomy. The microscopic examination of patients with PITS and PTTS reveals mucosal hemorrhage and ulceration in its early stages and progresses to deeper ulcerations exposing cartilaginous rings, which are then predisposed to dissolution and fragmentation. Further progression of this ischemic injury results in fibrosis and stenosis [9]. High-volume and low-pressure endotracheal and tracheostomy tube cuffs have been developed to more easily adapt to the shape and contour of the trachea without excessive cuff pressures, thereby markedly reducing the incidence of cuff-related ischemic injury [10, 11].

Systemic/inflammatory causes include granulomatous processes such as granulomatosis with polyangiitis (GPA), sarcoidosis, and inflammatory bowel diseases; cartilaginous disorders such as relapsing polychondritis, tracheobronchopathia osteochondroplastica, tracheobronchomalacia (TBM), and excessive dynamic airway collapse (EDAC); and finally, amyloidosis. Infectious etiologies include tuberculosis, fungal infections caused by *Aspergillus* and *Cryptococcus*, recurrent respiratory papillomatosis caused by human papillomavirus (HPV) types 6 and 11, and rhinoscleroma, a rare upper airway disorder caused by *Klebsiella rhinoscleromatis*. Endobronchial tuberculosis is quite common in various parts of the world with the incidence in some studies quoted at over 50% of pulmonary tuberculosis cases [12]. Endobronchial fungal infections are more commonly diagnosed in immunosuppressed patients [13]. The most common causes of benign tracheal stenosis are tumors, PITS, PTTS, and TBM/EDAC [5, 6].

Presentation and Diagnostic Evaluation

Clinical Features

With mild tracheal stenosis, patients may exhibit no signs and symptoms of airway obstruction. The typical symptoms of dyspnea, wheezing, cough, and stridor are dependent on the patient's functional status, cardiopulmonary comorbidities, the degree of the stenosis, the time course over which the stenosis developed, and the sequela of airway obstruction. Although the onset and progression of symptoms depends on multiple factors, one of the key elements contributing to work of breathing stems from turbulent airflow in the trachea [14]. Airway lumen flow is dictated by Poiseuille's law of fluid dynamics; therefore, turbulent flow of air across a stenotic lumen causes an inefficient respiratory cycle, resulting in higher energy expenditure and increased work of breathing. In a study using computational fluid dynamics (CFD), a tracheal obstruction of >75% was associated with a significant pressure drop over the stenosis, which correlated clinically with increased work of breathing [15]. Usually, tracheal narrowing to 8 millimeters (mm) results in dyspnea on exertion, whereas narrowing to 5 mm or less will result in dyspnea at rest. Hypoxemia and/or hypercapnia may be absent in patients with no underlying cardiopulmonary comorbidities.

As the causes of benign tracheal stenosis are very heterogenous, it is crucial to consider the underlying etiology that led to the airway obstruction. Patients with pulmonary sarcoidosis, tuberculosis, and vasculitis may have additional symptoms of excessive cough, wheezing, and hemoptysis unrelated to the tracheal stenosis. Similarly, benign tracheal stenosis from extrinsic compression from mediastinal disease, esophageal disease, or thyroid disease may have signs and symptoms relating to its respective organ dysfunction. Thus, it is imperative to thoroughly assess the patient for comorbidities and approach each case of stenosis with a systematic and logical diagnostic workup while maintaining a high index of suspicion in patients with a history of intubation, tracheostomy, or a known systemic disease that can affect the tracheobronchial tree.

Spirometric Evaluation

There are several diagnostic tools available to assess the severity and location of the tracheal stenosis. The exact sequence and combination of these modalities, however, should be tailored to each individual patient. For example, a patient presenting with acute signs and symptoms of airway obstruction will not be stable enough to undergo a pulmonary function test (PFT) or even a chest computed tomography (CT). Instead, the patient should be managed with airway stabilization first prior to any diagnostic or therapeutic endeavors by the interventional pulmonologist or thoracic surgeon.

   PFTs should be considered in patients with suspected tracheal stenosis who are clinically stable or to follow disease severity clinically once the diagnosis of tracheal stenosis has been made. Spirometric assessment with a flow-volume loop can show defects in the effort-dependent part of the curve in three classic patterns: (1) flattening of both expiratory and inspiratory limbs from fixed airway obstruction (tracheal stenosis, non-dynamic endotracheal tumors, bronchial obstructions), (2) flattening of the expiratory limb from variable intrathoracic obstruction (dynamic tumors of lower trachea, TBM, external compression of lower trachea), and (3) flattening of the inspiratory limb from variable extrathoracic obstruction (vocal cord paralysis, extrathoracic goiter, dynamic tumors of hypopharynx, laryngeal tumors). The advantages of PFTs are objective quantification of the airway disease, assessment of other comorbidities that may be present such as restrictive parenchymal disease, and assessment of pre- and post-procedural spirometric function. However, flow limitation may not be apparent in patients with an airway lumen greater than 8–10 mm [16]; hence, the spirometric diagnosis of tracheal stenosis has poor sensitivity. Moreover, spirometric abnormalities can be confounded by other obstructive lung diseases such as asthma, bronchiolitis, bronchiectasis, or chronic obstructive pulmonary disease (COPD). Thus, isolating the spirometric defect caused by tracheal stenosis can be very difficult. For these reasons, PFTs should not be used exclusively to rule out tracheal stenosis. Also, due to the possibility of inducing respiratory compromise with repeated forced expiratory maneuvers in patients with a tenuous respiratory status, PFTs should not be used in patients with ongoing respiratory distress or severe tracheal stenosis evidenced by imaging studies.

Once the diagnosis of tracheal stenosis has been made via a combination of diagnostic modalities, PFTs can be useful in disease surveillance and as an adjunctive objective diagnostic modality. In a series of 42 patients with idiopathic subglottic stenosis, peak expiratory flow was associated with high sensitivity (84.4%) and specificity (82.0%) for identifying patients who would require surgical intervention within 2 months [17].

Radiographic Evaluation

Chest radiographs are often performed due to convenience, efficiency, portability, and cost-effectiveness. Chest radiographs should be considered in all patients with suspected tracheal stenosis as they may reveal pathology of the airways and the lung parenchyma [18]. The radiographs may show tracheal deviation or mediastinal shift due to mass effect, lung parenchymal consolidation due to complete obstruction of airway or post-obstructive process, or signs of underlying lung disease associated with tracheal stenosis. However, they are rarely diagnostic due to the inherent nature of the study, which does not allow for a full three-dimensional visualization of the tracheal lumen and its nearby structures. In clinical practice, chest radiographs are more readily utilized in assessing complications of airway procedures such as pneumothorax, pneumomediastinum, and atelectasis. They also allow for a quick assessment of metallic stent positioning, change in lung aeration, and as a reference for future assessments.

Computed tomography (CT) imaging of the chest has become an invaluable tool in the diagnostic and pre-procedural phase of any airway disease. It provides a detailed anatomic assessment of the trachea, such as the degree of obstruction, the location of stenosis, anatomic relationship to other key structures, and intraluminal versus extraluminal nature of an obstructing lesion. The information obtained from the CT scan is useful in procedural planning as one can estimate stent sizing, tracheobronchial tree anatomy, and radiographic features that can help determine the chronicity of airway obstruction and distal parenchymal collapse.

CT imaging technology has markedly improved, and imaging protocols allow for (1) an improved resolution, (2) a decrease in motion artifact, and (3) a short breath-hold time required to obtain images. In addition, the cost of CT scans has decreased significantly, allowing patients and physicians to obtain these sophisticated imaging studies more frequently without a prohibitive financial burden to the payer. One of the main advantages of the CT scan as compared to a bronchoscopic evaluation of tracheal stenosis is that CT allows for visualization of the airways, lung parenchyma, and other key structures that are distal to the obstruction, which may not be possible with bronchoscopic evaluation. This distal visualization allows assessment of the feasibility of lung aeration, complexity of the airway lesion, and possible complications that may be encountered during the procedure.

However, there are several limitations of CT scans. In addition to radiation exposure, CT scans cannot differentiate a true airway lesion versus inspissated mucus in the airways. Additionally, with older CT scans that have lower resolutions and thicker slices, thin tracheal webs can often go undetected. Furthermore, a full visualization of complex airway lesions and their relations to nearby key structures is difficult even with multiplanar reconstructed images. Hence, the dynamic airway protocol of the trans-axial CT was developed to counter the "static" nature of the CT evaluation for airway diseases and allows for a luminal assessment of the airway with forced inspiratory and expiratory maneuvers in order to gage dynamic airway collapse. This protocol has shown to have high sensitivity and negative predictive value in pediatric patients with EDAC/TBM [19]. However, CT scans are not sensitive in detecting early or mild airway disease. In order to improve visualization of more complex airway lesions, newer imaging protocols have been developed to allow for a three-dimensional reconstruction of the airways and generate a virtual bronchoscopic view of the trachea, mainstem bronchi, and the bronchial tree down to the fourth order of the airway tree. This virtual bronchoscopy simulates a bronchoscopic evaluation prior to the actual bronchoscopy [20]. Virtual bronchoscopy can further aid the interventional pulmonologist in more comprehensive preoperative planning.

Laboratory Evaluation

Blood work and serologies play a limited, adjunctive role in the workup of tracheal stenosis. In GPA, 80–90% will have a positive antineutrophil cytoplasmic antibody (ANCA) study, with c-ANCA being the most common [21]. Importantly, 10% of patients with GPA are ANCA negative [22]. Patients with relapsing polychondritis may have elevated inflammatory markers, such as erythrocyte sedimentation rate or C-reactive protein; however, these are nonspecific. Serum angiotensin-converting enzyme (ACE) levels are occasionally measured in the evaluation of sarcoidosis; however, they have limited use given poor sensitivity and a nearly 10% rate of false positives [23].

Bronchoscopic Evaluation

Interventional pulmonologists play key roles in diagnostic and therapeutic procedures in patients with suspected tracheal stenosis. Bronchoscopic evaluation should always be considered in patients with tracheal stenosis and central airway obstruction. Direct visualization of the airways allows for characterization of the intraluminal stenosis with respect to the location, degree, extent, and conformation of the stenosis. Additionally, one can evaluate the dynamic nature of the lesion as well as any concerning mucosal abnormalities. Chromoendoscopy using narrow band imaging (NBI) at the time of bronchoscopy may help in assessing malignant features, such as neovascularity and mucosal hyperemia. Compared to traditional white light bronchoscopy, the use of NBI has an increased sensitivity (86% vs. 70%) and specificity (81% vs. 66%) for detecting invasive airway cancer [24].

Bronchoscopic information serves as a crucial step in procedural and operational planning for both interventional pulmonologists and thoracic surgeons. However, flexible bronchoscopy may be difficult and can potentially lead to accelerated respiratory failure in patients with severe tracheal stenosis and airway narrowing. First, the size of the bronchoscope may occlude an already narrowed airway, thus further impeding oxygenation and ventilation. One method to mitigate this risk is by using an ultrathin bronchoscope which has a diameter as small as 3.1 mm. Second, sedation used during bronchoscopy can cause relaxation of the respiratory muscles, which may worsen airway narrowing and lead to respiratory failure.

Performing airway biopsies can help elucidate the histopathologic and microbiologic diagnosis of airway lesions such as hamartomas, endobronchial tuberculosis or aspergillosis, and granulomatous diseases. However, the blood and mucosal edema from the biopsy site can contribute to airway compromise and impaired oxygenation. Thus, it is crucial that the bronchoscopy be performed by an experienced bronchoscopist. Due to the complexity of bronchoscopic evaluation, there is controversy around performing flexible bronchoscopy as a surveillance/planning tool versus deferring the bronchoscopy to the time of definitive treatment [25]. In many clinical practices with a high volume of airway diseases, flexible bronchoscopy is often performed at the time of therapeutic rigid bronchoscopy for the aforementioned reasons.

Classification of Tracheal Stenosis

One of the first classification tools which allowed for a more uniform approach to airway stenosis was developed in 1994 by Myer and Cotton, known as the Myer-Cotton airway grading system. The grading system classifies the degree of subglottic stenosis into four grades: Grade I (<50% luminal obstruction), Grade II (51–70%), Grade III (71–99%), and Grade IV (100%) [26]. Although it was widely adopted in clinical practice, its use was limited as it described only the subglottic region and did not account for the extent, conformation, and dynamic nature of the stenosis.

To augment these limitations, Freitag et al. proposed a classification to standardize (1) the location, (2) degree of stenosis, and (3) type of stenosis which was further subdivided into structural and functional elements to capture dynamic disease [27]. The location of the stenosis is assigned a scoring system of I–V, corresponding to the upper third, middle third, and lower third of the trachea, as well as the right main bronchus and left main bronchus. The degree of the stenosis is given a code ranging from 0 to 5, corresponding to no obstruction, ~25, 50, 75, 90, and 100% obstruction, respectively. Lastly, the type of stenosis is given a 1–4 numerical code in the structural element corresponding to intraluminal, extrinsic, distortion, and scar/stricture type, respectively; a code of 1 or 2 is given in the dynamic evaluation of the stenosis, with 1 describing damaged or malacic cartilage and 2 for a floppy membrane. This classification system was validated in a pilot study that showed a high degree of agreement and strong precision between observers of various training backgrounds. Another classification system was developed by Galluccio et al. in 2009. In their case series studying different morphologies of tracheal stenosis, they categorized the disease into simple versus complex, where a simple tracheal stenosis was defined as (1) <1 cm of endoluminal obstruction, (2) absence of tracheomalacia, and (3) intact cartilaginous support. If the stenosis was >1 cm in length and had either a loss of cartilaginous support or dynamic collapse, the lesion was classified as complex [28]. This classification has been widely accepted due to its simplicity and relative inclusive nature.

Traditional Approach to the Treatment of Tracheal Stenosis

Airway Stabilization

Patients with critical tracheal narrowing can exhibit a very tenuous respiratory status with little to no cardiopulmonary reserve. These patients should be first stabilized by securing an airway via endotracheal tube. Intubation in patients with tracheal stenosis can be challenging, especially if the stenotic area is in the subglottic region or upper third of the trachea, as this will impede the proper passage of the endotracheal tube. Thus, airway management of patients with known or suspected tracheal stenosis should be performed by experienced personnel with readily available backup modalities such as fiber-optic intubation, cricothyroidotomy, and tracheostomy. The latter two modalities can be considered if the known or suspected lesion is at or above the level of the subglottis, with inability to safely endotracheally intubate. A laryngeal mask airway (LMA) may be an acceptable choice to bridge to a definitive airway management if the possibility of traumatic intubation is high due to the proximal location of the stenosis without a critical obstruction. Heliox, a mixture of helium (70–80%) and oxygen (20–30%), can be used to decrease the work of breathing in patients with tracheal stenosis while preparing for definitive airway management and stabilization. Helium is an inert gas with significantly lower density compared to nitrogen and oxygen and allows for lower airflow resistance and increased laminar flow of the inhaled gas through the airway lumen. The efficacy of heliox in tracheal stenosis was studied in a pediatric population where more than 70% of pediatric patients with upper airway obstruction had immediate subjective improvement in work of breathing [29].

Role of Interventional Pulmonology Procedures

Although a significant portion of benign tracheal stenoses are caused by systemic inflammatory disorders with available medical treatments, it is crucial to avoid delays in therapeutic procedures while instituting the most appropriate systemic therapy. Patients who should be evaluated for potential airway procedures by interventional pulmonologists are (1) patients with critical tracheal stenosis who require a prompt stabilization, (2) patients with inoperable or non-severe disease with significant symptoms, and (3) patients with mostly intraluminal lesions rather than extrinsic compression. However, even patients who are good surgical candidates should be evaluated if a "bridge therapy" is needed prior to a definitive surgery or to assess surgical candidacy such as with TBM.

Rigid bronchoscopy is the backbone of many airway procedures for interventional pulmonologists. Rigid bronchoscopy has several key advantages compared to flexible bronchoscopy: (a) it can be used to secure the airway with either a rigid tracheal or bronchial barrel; (b) it allows effective ventilation and oxygenation by both open and closed circuit ventilation; (c) it allows for utilization of different flexible and rigid tools to biopsy, suction, and control bleeding more effectively; and (d) it can be used to provide different therapeutic modalities such as cryodebridement or cryotherapy, thermal ablative techniques such as argon plasma coagulation (APC), laser, radiofrequency ablation (RFA), and electrocautery, mechanical debulking, and stent placement. The choice of flexible versus rigid bronchoscopy should be based on the purpose of the bronchoscopic evaluation (diagnostic vs. therapeutic), the degree of tracheal stenosis, overall clinical stability of the patient, oxygenation/ventilation, and the location of the stenosis. Rigid bronchoscopy is the preferred method if there are any concerns relating to oxygenation, ventilation, and airway bleeding or instability from any cause.

For patients with PITS/PTTS, both simple and complex tracheal stenoses can be treated by interventional pulmonary procedures. Complex tracheal stenoses have significantly higher failure rates compared to simple stenoses and may require a surgical intervention (see Fig. 10.1). Bronchoscopic therapy involves combinations of balloon bronchoplasty, debridement of granulation tissue via thermal energy modes, and cryotherapy [30]. Using the electrocautery knife to make radial cuts in the stenosis followed by balloon bronchoplasty increases the treatment effect compared to balloon bronchoplasty alone [31]. In addition to thermal techniques, endoluminal cryospray therapy with concomitant balloon bronchoplasty has also shown efficacy in improving both symptoms and stenosis severity [32]. Additionally, intraluminal steroid injection has been investigated in proximal tracheal and subglottic stenoses from PITS/PTTS, and increased surgery-free interval by a significant margin (22.6 months vs. 10.1 months) [33]. Mitomycin C, a chemotherapeutic agent with anti-fibroblast properties, has been studied in tracheal stenosis and has also shown to increase interval time between procedures [34]. Stents can be used in

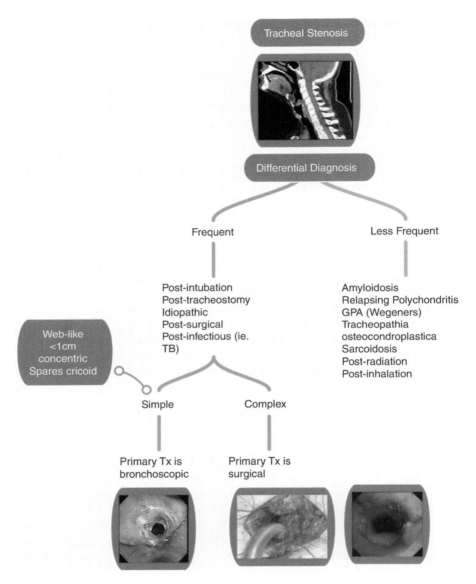

Fig. 10.1 Mind map describing the common and uncommon causes of tracheal stenosis as well as their overall management strategy

certain cases such as patients with recurrent disease despite bronchoscopic interventions who are not surgical candidates and patients who require a "bridge therapy" prior to a definitive surgical resection. Silicone stents are the stents of choice for benign airway conditions and are generally safe and well tolerated [35, 36]. Finally, tracheostomy and/or Montgomery T-tube placement may be helpful in nonsurgical patients who require frequent procedures, have a suboptimal clinical response, and/

or have complicated anatomy. The use of airway prostheses can also be a bridge to definitive surgery or as an adjunct to surgery.

Stent-related tracheal stenosis is another iatrogenic entity that causes significant morbidity. Self-expanding metallic stents (SEMS) in particular have high incidence of granulation tissue and stricture formation [37]. The interventional bronchoscopic management of stent-related stenoses includes balloon bronchoplasty, ablative thermal techniques, cryotherapy, and stent revision if necessary. Stent complications in benign tracheal stenosis can be successfully managed in more than 80% of patients with bronchoscopic techniques [38]. As stents may ignite when using thermal techniques, a high degree of precision must be used when the stent cannot be removed prior to the ablative procedure. High-dose rate brachytherapy also has been used with significant success in patients with stent-related granulation tissue formation that was refractory to multiple bronchoscope interventions [39].

For patients with systemic processes such as GPA, sarcoidosis, and tuberculosis, the first line of therapy should always be systemic treatment targeting the specific disease process. Bronchoscopic interventions serve as a crucial adjunctive therapy for patients with significant symptoms or tracheal narrowing evidenced by imaging studies. The mainstays of bronchoscopic treatment are balloon bronchoplasty with thermal ablative techniques and cryotherapy for webs, focal stenosis, and intraluminal lesions [40, 41]. Endoscopic mitomycin C has been used to complement bronchoscopic therapies with some success in patients with sarcoidosis but with unclear long-term benefits [42]. Other non-granulomatous systemic conditions such as amyloidosis, tracheobronchopathia osteochondroplastica, and relapsing polychondritis are treated similarly with balloon bronchoplasty and thermal techniques for intraluminal lesions. As these conditions are less frequent compared to granulomatous conditions, there are less data for steroids and mitomycin C.

The purposes of interventional pulmonary procedures in the setting of benign tracheal stenosis are severalfold: to stabilize the airway for the procedure, to make the diagnosis of airway obstruction, to find the etiology of the airway disease, and to relieve the airway stenosis if no definitive therapy is available. In addition to providing therapeutic procedures, the interventional pulmonologist plays a central role in delivering multidisciplinary care with general pulmonologists, infectious disease specialists, rheumatologists, radiologists, otolaryngologists, and thoracic surgeons. The information obtained via diagnostic and therapeutic bronchoscopies serves as an important surveillance tool to monitor disease progression and for preoperative optimization.

Outcomes of Interventional Pulmonary Procedures

Most available data from bronchoscopic interventions for tracheal stenosis and central airway obstructions relate to malignant airway obstructions. There is a paucity of high-quality data investigating the outcomes of different benign tracheal stenoses. There are several small case series and retrospective studies across many different entities of benign tracheal disease that show both short-term and long-term improvement in validated quality of life surveys, dyspnea, airway patency, pulmonary function test indices, and exercise capacity as measured by 6-minute walk tests.

Limitations of Interventional Pulmonology Procedures

Although interventional pulmonary procedures are the cornerstones of diagnostic and therapeutic interventions in patients with tracheal stenosis, there are several limitations. The primary limitation is that the procedure is not curative for complex airway stenosis and stenosis related to systemic illnesses. In cases of idiopathic tracheal stenosis and PITS/PTTS, initial success rates as measured by symptomatic improvement and airway patency are as high as 95–100% [43]. Long-term outcomes of these patients are generally quite good with more than 95% of patients maintaining airway patency at 2 years [28]. In contrast, complex stenoses have high failure and recurrence rates of more than 30% and often require multiple bronchoscopic interventions. More than half of patients with complex tracheal stenoses will have recurrence after 2 years, and the majority by 5 years [44]. Finally, bronchoscopic interventions such as stent placement may extend the length of the stenosis, making a curative surgery less feasible.

Role of Thoracic Surgery

Tracheal sleeve resection and reconstruction is the definitive treatment for tracheal stenosis, particularly for complex tracheal stenosis (see Fig. 10.1). The best opportunity for a successful outcome is the initial operation. A detailed plan should be developed, and if there is any doubt, it is better to refer the patient to an institution with experience in the management of airway surgery [45]. Lesions in the upper half of the trachea are frequently approached by cervical collar incision that may be extended to the upper portion of the sternum if access to the mediastinal trachea is needed. The lower third of the trachea and mainstem bronchi are best approached via right posterolateral thoracotomy. It is important to distinguish the exact location of the stenosis and involvement or lack thereof of the cricoid as the choice of tracheal end-to-end anastomosis, cricotracheal anastomosis, and tracheo-cricotracheal anastomosis has increasingly more common complications. The use of release maneuvers to help reduce tension at the tracheal anastomosis is very important and ranges from the simple neck flexion to more complex techniques including proximal and distal mobilization of the pretracheal plane, suprahyoid release, laryngeal release, division of the inferior pulmonary ligament for hilar release, and intrapericardial release including the pericardium around the hilar vessels [46].

Video-assisted thoracoscopic surgery (VATS) tracheal resection/reconstruction has been described as an alternative approach due to its minimally invasive nature as compared to open thoracotomy. Given the limited operating field, some modifications such as employing continuous suturing (versus interrupted) to minimize tangling as well as using high-frequency jet rather than cross-field ventilation are often employed [47].

The overall success rates for tracheal surgery vary with reports between 71% and 95% cited [48]. Large retrospective series of tracheal resection have identified risk factors for anastomotic complications in patients with benign and malignant stenosis [49]. These risk factors include reoperation, diabetes, lengthy resection $> = 4$ cm, laryngotracheal resection, age <17yo, and need for tracheostomy prior to resection. While some of these complications have been attributed to increased anastomotic tension, others remain unclear. Granulation development has been nearly eliminated with the use of absorbable sutures [8]. In a series of 521 tracheal surgeries performed by experienced thoracic surgeons, over 90% of patients had good or satisfactory results. However, there were 20 failures and 12 deaths. Additionally, 49 patients developed granulation tissue, 29 experienced dehiscence or restenosis, 25 had laryngeal dysfunction, and 34 developed infectious complications [8]. Mortality in the surgical literature has been reported as high as 5%, with surgical failure rates between 5% and 15% [50].

It should be noted that these retrospective studies may suffer from selection bias as the patients with the highest risk are frequently excluded. The optimal timing of surgery is unclear, as are the risk factors of bronchoscopic treatment failures for complex tracheal stenoses. Thus, multidisciplinary discussions with the surgical team are imperative after making the diagnosis of complex tracheal stenosis. Other etiologies of tracheal stenosis should be approached in a similar fashion, with local/limited tracheal disease that is refractory to both medical therapy and repeated interventional procedures referred for surgical evaluation.

Recommendations

See Fig. 10.2 for a detailed description of the steps necessary in the evaluation and treatment of benign tracheal stenosis. The implementation of these steps depends on the human and technological capital available at each institution. In many cases, referral to centers with expertise in interventional pulmonology and/or airway surgery may be necessary.

Future Direction

Although the efficacy of balloon bronchoplasty and intraluminal lesion destruction by various thermal techniques has been very positive in majority of the benign tracheal stenoses subtypes, short-term recurrence rate can be significant. Stents provide prolonged artificial structural integrity and can enable remodeling of the

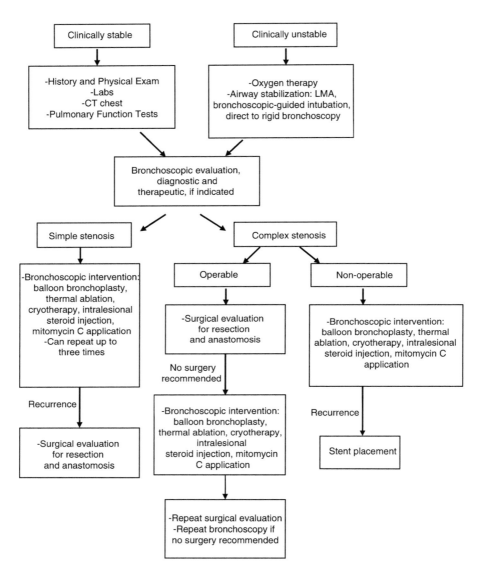

Fig. 10.2 Algorithm for the evaluation and management of benign tracheal stenosis

airways. However, they are also associated with strictures, granulation tissue, migration, fistula formation, and occlusion if left in the long term. Biodegradable stents have been under investigation for several years. These stents are made from polydioxanone, which is a semicrystalline biodegradable polymer with some degree of shape memory. The polymer degrades over time by hydrolysis, making extraction of these stents unnecessary. Biodegradable stents appear to be well tolerated by the tracheal mucosa, retain their mechanical strength for up to 6 weeks, and completely degrade after approximately 15 weeks [51]. Given these properties, these stents can be ideal in patients who require airway procedures while undergoing systemic medical therapy for conditions such as GPA, sarcoidosis, amyloidosis, and relapsing polychondritis. These stents have been used in small number of pediatric and adult patients with improved symptoms [52]. A unique complication of stent fragment expectoration has been described in some patients. However, the remnants of the biodegradable stents are relatively small and are unlikely to cause any significant airway obstruction. As the technology is still in its infancy, there are no robust studies assessing the efficacy and safety in patients with benign tracheal stenoses.

Conclusions

The field of interventional pulmonology is an exciting discipline with a versatile and sophisticated armamentarium of procedures to manage tracheal stenosis and complicated central airways. Rigid bronchoscopy serves as the backbone of therapeutic bronchoscopic procedures, allowing for the application of various procedures ranging from mechanical debulking to thermal ablation. However, there are no clear data assessing the long-term efficacy of bronchoscopic treatment in benign tracheal disease, the efficacy of different bronchoscopic treatment modalities, and most importantly, how bronchoscopic methods compare to surgical resection. Subsequently, consensus on how these inherently complex and morbid conditions are treated continues to evolve. Additionally, the availability and the interplay of interventional pulmonologists, thoracic surgeons, ENT surgeons, and anesthesiologists remain varied. Although there are few studies investigating the efficacy of tracheal resection and reconstruction in benign tracheal stenosis, surgery should remain one of the long-term therapeutic modalities available to all patients with either severe benign tracheal stenosis or recurrent tracheal stenosis despite bronchoscopic interventions. Despite the lack of a standardized approach, interventional pulmonary procedures remain a cornerstone for patients who cannot tolerate surgery due to comorbidities, who have unfavorable anatomy for safe surgical resection, and who have symptomatic non-severe disease.

References

1. Noppen M, Meysman M, D'Haese J, Schlesser M, Vincken W. Interventional bronchoscopy: 5-year experience at the Academic Hospital of the Vrije Universiteit Brussel (AZ-VUB). Acta Clin Belg. 1997;52(6):371–80.
2. Oberg C, Folch E, Santacruz F. Management of malignant airway obstruction. AME Med J. 2018;3:115.
3. Furlow PW, Mathisen DJ. Surgical anatomy of the trachea. Ann Cardiothorac Surg. 2018;7(2):255–60.

4. Oberg CL, Holden VK, Channick CL. Benign central airway obstruction. Semin Respir Crit Care Med. 2018;39(6):731–46.
5. Aravena C, Almeida FA, Mukhopadhyay S, Ghosh S, Lorenz RR, Murthy SC, Mehta AC. Idiopathic subglottic stenosis: a review. J Thorac Dis. 2020;12(3):1100–11.
6. Grenier PA, Beigelman-Aubry C, Brillet P-Y. Nonneoplastic tracheal and bronchial stenoses. Radiol Clin N Am. 2009;47(2):243–60.
7. Sarper A, Ayten A, Eser I, Ozbudak O, Demircan A. Tracheal stenosis after tracheostomy or intubation: review with special regard to cause and management. Tex Heart Inst J. 2005;32(2):154–8.
8. Zias N, Chroneou A, Tabba MK, Gonzalez AV, Gray AW, Lamb CR, et al. Post tracheostomy and post intubation tracheal stenosis: report of 31 cases and review of the literature. BMC Pulm Med. 2008;8:18.
9. Grillo HC, Donahue DM, Mathisen DJ, Wain JC, Wright CD. Postintubation tracheal stenosis. Treatment and results. J Thorac Cardiovasc Surg. 1995;109(3):486–92; discussion 492–493.
10. Cooper JD. Tracheal injuries complicating prolonged intubation and tracheostomy. Thorac Surg Clin. 2018;28(2):139–44.
11. Sue RD, Susanto I. Long-term complications of artificial airways. Clin Chest Med. 2003;24(3):457–71.
12. Jung SS, Park HS, Kim JO, Kim SY. Incidence and clinical predictors of endobronchial tuberculosis in patients with pulmonary tuberculosis. Respirology. 2015;20(03):488–95.
13. Marchioni A, Casalini E, Andreani A, et al. Incidence, etiology, and clinicopathologic features of endobronchial benign lesions: a 10-year consecutive retrospective study. J Bronchology Interv Pulmonol. 2018;25(02):118–24.
14. Barach AL, Eckman M. The effects of inhalation of helium mixed with oxygen on the mechanics of respiration. J Clin Invest. 1936;15(1):47–61.
15. Brouns M, Jayaraju ST, Lacor C, De Mey J, Noppen M, Vincken W, et al. Tracheal stenosis: a flow dynamics study. J Appl Physiol (1985). 2007;102(3):1178–84.
16. Miller RD, Hyatt RE. Evaluation of obstructing lesions of the trachea and larynx by flow-volume loops. Am Rev Respir Dis. 1973;108(3):475–81.
17. Carpenter DJ, Ferrante S, Bakos SR, Clary MS, Gelbard AH, Daniero JJ. Utility of routine sirometry measures for surveillance of idiopathic subglottic stenosis. JAMA Otolaryngol Head Neck Surg. 2019;145(1):21–6.
18. Collins J, Stern EJ. Chest radiology: the essentials [Internet]. Philadelphia: Lippincott Williams & Wilkins; 2008 [cited 2020 Oct 12]. Available from: http://ovidsp.ovid.com/ovidweb.cgi?T=JS&NEWS=n&CSC=Y&PAGE=booktext&D=books&AN=01312096$&XPATH=/PG(0).
19. Ullmann N, Secinaro A, Menchini L, Caggiano S, Verrillo E, Santangelo TP, et al. Dynamic expiratory CT: an effective non-invasive diagnostic exam for fragile children with suspected tracheo-bronchomalacia. Pediatr Pulmonol. 2018;53(1):73–80.
20. De Wever W, Vandecaveye V, Lanciotti S, Verschakelen JA. Multidetector CT-generated virtual bronchoscopy: an illustrated review of the potential clinical indications. Eur Respir J. 2004;23(5):776–82.
21. Guillevin L, Durand-Gasselin B, Cevallos R, et al. Microscopic polyangiitis: clinical and laboratory findings in eighty-five patients. Arthritis Rheum. 1999;42(3):421.
22. Hagen EC, Daha MR, Hermans J. Diagnostic value of standardized assays for anti-neutrophil cytoplasmic antibodies in idiopathic systemic vasculitis. EC/BCR Project for ANCA Assay Standardization. Kidney Int. 1998;53(3):743.
23. Ungprasert P, Carmona EM, Crowson CS, Matteson EL. Diagnostic utility of angiotensin-converting enzyme in sarcoidosis: a population-based study. Lung. 2016;194(1):91–5.
24. Zhu J, Li W, Zhou J, Chen Y, Zhao C, Zhang T, et al. The diagnostic value of narrow-band imaging for early and invasive lung cancer: a meta-analysis. Clinics (Sao Paulo). 2017;72(7):438–48.
25. Ernst A, Feller-Kopman D, Becker HD, Mehta AC. Central airway obstruction. Am J Respir Crit Care Med. 2004;169(12):1278–97.

26. Myer CM, O'Connor DM, Cotton RT. Proposed grading system for subglottic stenosis based on endotracheal tube sizes. Ann Otol Rhinol Laryngol. 1994;103(4 Pt 1):319–23.
27. Freitag L, Ernst A, Unger M, Kovitz K, Marquette CH. A proposed classification system of central airway stenosis. Eur Respir J. 2007;30(1):7–12.
28. Galluccio G, Lucantoni G, Battistoni P, Paone G, Batzella S, Lucifora V, et al. Interventional endoscopy in the management of benign tracheal stenoses: definitive treatment at long-term follow-up. Eur J Cardiothorac Surg. 2009;35(3):429–33; discussion 933–934.
29. Grosz AH, Jacobs IN, Cho C, Schears GJ. Use of helium-oxygen mixtures to relieve upper airway obstruction in a pediatric population. Laryngoscope. 2001;111(9):1512–4.
30. Mehta AC, Lee FY, Cordasco EM, Kirby T, Eliachar I, De Boer G. Concentric tracheal and subglottic stenosis. Management using the Nd-YAG laser for mucosal sparing followed by gentle dilatation. Chest. 1993;104(3):673–7.
31. Bo L, Li C, Chen M, Mu D, Jin F. Application of electrocautery needle knife combined with balloon dilatation versus balloon dilatation in the treatment of tracheal fibrotic scar stenosis. Respiration. 2018;95(3):182–7.
32. Bhora FY, Ayub A, Forleiter CM, Huang C-Y, Alshehri K, Rehmani S, et al. Treatment of benign tracheal stenosis using endoluminal spray cryotherapy. JAMA Otolaryngol Head Neck Surg. 2016;142(11):1082.
33. Bertelsen C, Shoffel-Havakuk H, O'Dell K, Johns MM, Reder LS. Serial in-office intralesional steroid injections in airway stenosis. JAMA Otolaryngol Head Neck Surg. 2018;144(3):203–10.
34. Queiroga TLO, Cataneo DC, Martins RHG, Reis TA, Cataneo AJM. Mitomycin C in the endoscopic treatment of laryngotracheal stenosis: systematic review and proportional meta-analysis. Int Arch Otorhinolaryngol. 2020;24(1):e112–24.
35. Puma F, Ragusa M, Avenia N, Urbani M, Droghetti A, Daddi N, et al. The role of silicone stents in the treatment of cicatricial tracheal stenoses. J Thorac Cardiovasc Surg. 2000;120(6):1064–9.
36. Folch E, Keyes C. Airway stents. Ann Cardiothorac Surg. 2018;7(2):273–83.
37. Gaissert HA, Grillo HC, Wright CD, Donahue DM, Wain JC, Mathisen DJ. Complication of benign tracheobronchial strictures by self-expanding metal stents. J Thorac Cardiovasc Surg. 2003;126(3):744–7.
38. Chung F-T, Chen H-C, Chou C-L, Yu C-T, Kuo C-H, Kuo H-P, et al. An outcome analysis of self-expandable metallic stents in central airway obstruction: a cohort study. J Cardiothorac Surg. 2011;6:46.
39. Rahman NA, Fruchter O, Shitrit D, Fox BD, Kramer MR. Flexible bronchoscopic management of benign tracheal stenosis: long term follow-up of 115 patients. J Cardiothorac Surg. 2010;5:2.
40. Mondoni M, Repossi A, Carlucci P, Centanni S, Sotgiu G. Bronchoscopic techniques in the management of patients with tuberculosis. Int J Infect Dis. 2017;64:27–37.
41. Martinez Del Pero M, Jayne D, Chaudhry A, Sivasothy P, Jani P. Long-term outcome of airway stenosis in granulomatosis with polyangiitis (Wegener granulomatosis): an observational study. JAMA Otolaryngol Head Neck Surg. 2014;140(11):1038.
42. Teo F, Anantham D, Feller-Kopman D, Ernst A. Bronchoscopic management of sarcoidosis related bronchial stenosis with adjunctive topical mitomycin C. Ann Thorac Surg. 2010;89(6):2005–7.
43. Dalar L, Karasulu L, Abul Y, Özdemir C, Sökücü SN, Tarhan M, et al. Bronchoscopic treatment in the management of benign tracheal stenosis: choices for simple and complex tracheal stenosis. Ann Thorac Surg. 2016;101(4):1310–7.
44. Perotin J-M, Jeanfaivre T, Thibout Y, Jouneau S, Lena H, Dutau H, et al. Endoscopic management of idiopathic tracheal stenosis. Ann Thorac Surg. 2011;92(1):297–301.
45. Hammoud ZT, Liptay MJ. Overview of benign disorders of the upper airways, Adult chest surgery. 2nd ed. p. 432–9.
46. Tapias LF. Prevention and management of complications following tracheal resections—lessons learned at the Massachusetts General Hospital. Ann Cardiothorac Surg. 2018;7(2):237–43.

47. Imanishi N, Tanaka F. Thoracoscopic tracheal resection and reconstruction: video-assisted thoracoscopic surgery as a "tool" toward minimally invasive surgery. J Thorac Dis. 2017;9(9):2895–7.
48. Ozemir C, Kocaturk CI, Sokucu SN, et al. Endoscopic and surgical treatment of benign tracheal stenosis: a multidisciplinary team approach. Ann Thorac Cardiovasc Surg. 2018;24(6):288–95.
49. Wright CD. Anastomotic complications after tracheal resection: prognostic factors and management. J Thorac Cardiovasc Surg. 2004;128(5):731–9.
50. Ciccone AM, De Giacomo T, Venuta F, et al. Operative and non-operative treatment of benign subglottic laryngotracheal stenosis. Eur J Cardiothorac Surg. 2004;26:818–22.
51. Novotny L, Crha M, Rauser P, Hep A, Misik J, Necas A, et al. Novel biodegradable polydioxanone stents in a rabbit airway model. J Thorac Cardiovasc Surg. 2012;143(2):437–44.
52. Stehlik L, Hytych V, Letackova J, Kubena P, Vasakova M. Biodegradable polydioxanone stents in the treatment of adult patients with tracheal narrowing. BMC Pulm Med. 2015;15(1):164.

Chapter 11
Hemoptysis

Himanshu Deshwal, Ankur Sinha, Tatiana Weinstein, Amie J. Kent, Jamie L. Bessich, and Samaan Rafeq

Introduction

Hemoptysis is the expectoration of blood from the respiratory tract which can range from clinically insignificant to life-threatening. While hemoptysis is often associated with many serious diseases, it can lead to significant distress to the patient and needs to be evaluated thoroughly. Most cases of hemoptysis are mild and self-limited, but up to 15% of patients can experience a life-threatening bleed [1, 2]. Several definitions have been used to describe massive hemoptysis based on quantity or frequency ranging from 100 cc to 1000 cc over 24 hours [3]. However, hemoptysis of greater than 200 cc/hour in patients with normal lungs or 50 cc/hour in patients with chronic lung disease can be classified as life-threatening hemoptysis [4]. In clinical practice, any amount of hemoptysis that leads to significant respiratory or hemodynamic compromise should be considered life-threatening. Death primarily occurs by asphyxiation rather than exsanguination. Before the advent of

H. Deshwal (✉) · T. Weinstein
Division of Pulmonary, Sleep and Critical Care Medicine, New York University Grossman School of Medicine, New York, NY, USA
e-mail: Himanshu.deshwal@nyulangone.org

A. Sinha
Division of Pulmonary and Critical Care Medicine, Maimonides Medical Center, Brooklyn, NY, USA

A. J. Kent
Department of Cardiothoracic Surgery, New York University Grossman School of Medicine, New York, NY, USA

J. L. Bessich · S. Rafeq
Interventional Pulmonology Program, Division of Pulmonary, Sleep and Critical Care Medicine, New York University Grossman School of Medicine, New York, NY, USA

© The Author(s), under exclusive license to Springer Nature Switzerland AG 2021
J. F. Turner, Jr. et al. (eds.), *From Thoracic Surgery to Interventional Pulmonology*, Respiratory Medicine,
https://doi.org/10.1007/978-3-030-80298-1_11

187

endoscopic interventions, hemoptysis of over 600 cc in 16 hours carried a mortality of 75%; however, the incidence has decreased to 9–38% with the establishment of better protocols, airway protective strategies, and minimally invasive interventional tools such as the bronchoscopy [5–7]. In the pre-bronchoscopic era, surgical interventions were the primary treatment of choice, mortality was as high as 23%, and the patients were primarily treated with surgery [5]. Several factors including acute decompensation leading to emergent surgery as a salvage option may have played a major role in defining such high mortality.

Ever since, several studies have been successful in identifying prognostic and predictive risk factors for recurrence of hemoptysis and in-patient mortality. Chronic alcoholism, lung malignancy, aspergilloma, pulmonary artery bleed, involvement of more than two quadrants on chest radiograph, need for mechanical ventilation, and active bleed or clots seen on bronchoscopy were associated with significantly lower survival [8, 9]. Identifying these factors has helped consolidating decisions on early aggressive intervention to improve survival and outcome in these patients. Over the years, several endoscopic tools have been developed to control active hemoptysis and treat the underlying etiology without further need of surgery and are highlighted in the subsequent sections. Along with interventional pulmonology, surgical techniques have also evolved with minimally invasive, conservative approaches yielding better treatment results, highlighting the importance of a multidisciplinary approach to any case of hemoptysis.

Pulmonary Vascular Anatomy

To identify the etiology of hemoptysis, it is imperative to understand the vascular anatomy of the lungs. The pulmonary vascular anatomy is unique as it comprises a dual blood supply in the form of pulmonary arteries and systemic bronchial arteries. The pulmonary arterial system has high capacitance as it receives 100% of the cardiac output from the right heart with the primary function of oxygenating the blood [10]. The pulmonary arteries follow the bronchial segmental and subsegmental anatomy forming the bronchovascular bundles that divide into a rich capillary bed responsible for lung perfusion and oxygenation [11]. The capillaries drain into pulmonary venules that run along the interlobular septa of the secondary pulmonary lobules [12]. Eventually, the oxygenated blood is carried by the pulmonary veins into the left atrium. The bronchial arteries are a low-capacitance, high-pressure system as they derive oxygenated blood supply from the descending aorta at the level of T5–T6 thoracic vertebrae [13]. The bronchial arteries take up to 1–3% of the total cardiac output and are primarily responsible for providing nourishment, thermoregulation, humidification, and recruitment of inflammatory cells in the lungs [14–16]. The bronchial arteries drain into bronchial veins, majority of which eventually drain into the azygous vein. The bronchial arteries also run alongside the major airways and form perforators to supply the muscular layers of the airways. A part of the bronchial circulation drains into the pulmonary veins due to an extensive anastomosis of pulmonary and bronchial blood supply at capillary level, leading to a physiologic shunt. Despite accounting for 5% of the total pulmonary blood flow, a majority of hemoptysis originates from bronchial artery disruption due to the high-pressure system [17]. In rare occasions such as pulmonary artery aneurysm, large tumor invasion or iatrogenic trauma during right right heart catheterization, pulmonary arteries can be a source of hemoptysis.

Causes of Hemoptysis

The source of hemoptysis depends on the anatomical location of the lesion, namely, the airways, the lung parenchyma, and the adjoining vascular structures. Tracheal tumor, tracheitis, tracheal tear, or tracheoinnominate fistula in a patient with a tracheostomy can be a cause of hemoptysis from the central airways. Bronchial bleed is common in patients with bronchiectasis, bronchopneumonia, chronic bronchitis, endobronchial tumors (particularly neuroendocrine tumors), melanoma, and renal cell carcinoma [3]. Malignant lesions and cavitary lesions are other causes that can lead to significant hemoptysis. Alveolar causes include capillaritis or anticoagulation-induced diffuse alveolar hemorrhage. Other causes include pulmonary venous congestion from causes like mitral stenosis leading to alveolar hemorrhage. In rare instances, especially with a necrotizing infection, a lethal bronchopulmonary artery fistula can lead to significant bleeding. In patients with hereditary hemorrhagic telangiectasia, pulmonary arteriovenous malformations can cause recurrent hemoptysis requiring embolization or surgical resection. Tuberculosis, bronchiectasis, and lung cancer are the leading causes of hemoptysis, accounting for 23–85% of bleeds [1, 18]. Despite a thorough investigation, the etiology of hemoptysis remains unknown in up to 50% of patients [19]. Table 11.1 highlights common causes of hemoptysis.

Diagnosis and Management

Any patient presenting with hemoptysis should be evaluated thoroughly to identify the etiology and risk stratify as the therapeutic approach may change based on risk factors and underlying etiology. A quick history and physical examination with attention to prior episodes of bleeding, underlying malignancy, smoking history, medication history, coagulopathy, and autoimmune disease can narrow the differential diagnosis of hemoptysis. Initial laboratory tests should evaluate for infection, thrombocytopenia, coagulopathy, liver or renal dysfunction, and ongoing vasculitis.

Initial chest radiograph can be performed quickly at bedside and can evaluate common causes such as cavitary lesions, aspergilloma, consolidation, malignancy, and parenchymal disorders such as diffuse alveolar hemorrhage in 35–86% of cases [20, 21]. Despite low sensitivity, initial chest radiograph is essential as it can serve

Table 11.1 Common causes of hemoptysis

Pseudo-hemoptysis	Infectious	Airway	Parenchymal	Vascular
Epistaxis	Tuberculosis	Chronic bronchitis	Adenocarcinoma of the lung	Dieulafoy's lesion
Tonsillitis	Bacterial pneumonia	Bronchiectasis	ANCA vasculitis (granulomatosis with polyangiitis/ eosinophilic granulomatosis with polyangiitis)	Hereditary hemorrhagic telangiectasia/ complex arteriovenous malformations
		Cystic fibrosis		
Tongue malignancy	Necrotizing pneumonia	Endobronchial tumor	Goodpasture syndrome	Rasmussen's aneurysm
Upper gastrointestinal bleed	Fungal pneumonia	Bronchopulmonary artery fistula	IgA vasculitis	Congestive heart failure
Vocal cord lesion	Viral pneumonia	Foreign body	Behcet's disease	Mitral stenosis
Factitious	Lung abscess	Sarcoidosis	Anticoagulation-induced hemorrhage	Pulmonary arterial hypertension
	Aspergilloma	Broncholithiasis		

as a baseline at presentation and a good comparison for further coarse of management (Fig. 11.1). If the patient is hemodynamically stable and able to maintain good oxygenation, a prompt multidetector computed tomography (MDCT) of the chest should be performed, preferably with systemic phase contrast to assess for bronchial artery extravasation. The MDCT carries a high sensitivity of 93% in identifying the source of hemoptysis, which increases to 97% when supplemented by a bronchoscopic airway examination [6]. MDCT can be carried out promptly and is of extreme value in deciding between bronchoscopic intervention, arterial embolization, and surgical intervention. It can also assist in assessing lesions distal to the site of bleed which may otherwise be obscured by active bleeding and poor visualization on bronchoscopy as it can identify both intraluminal and extraluminal etiologies of hemoptysis with good accuracy [19].

Airway compromise is the biggest concern in patients presenting with hemoptysis as the most common cause of death is asphyxiation. Often an episode of mild hemoptysis can be a sentinel episode prior to a life-threatening hemoptysis and should be managed cautiously. A three-tier approach may help stratify treatment plan and activate appropriate pathways to ensure successful resuscitation and therapy.

The first and foremost target is the evaluation and management of a threatened airway. In patients presenting with massive hemoptysis, blood can clot up in the central airways leading to complete obstruction and death. Any sign of respiratory distress, hypoxemia, or large volume hemoptysis should prompt a decision to electively intubate the patient while still hemodynamically stable. Based on initial investigation, if the laterality of hemoptysis is known, the bleeding lung should be placed dependently to prevent aspiration of blood onto the normal side [22]. It is imperative to protect yourself with a gown, a face mask, and a face shield to prevent exposure to the patient's blood during intubation. Fiber-optic bronchoscopy can

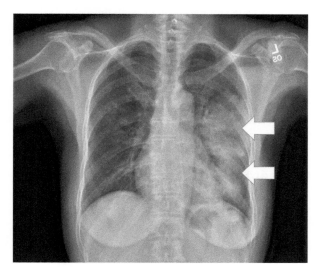

Fig. 11.1 A posterior-anterior view of the chest radiograph demonstrating dense infiltrates in the left lung in a patient with massive hemoptysis (arrows)

help visualize any source of posterior pharyngeal or upper airway bleed and can assist in successful intubation [23]. A size 8.0- or 8.5-mm endotracheal tube (ETT) should be utilized for intubation as it allows for bronchoscopic management of hemoptysis. The bed of the head can be kept elevated (up to 20 degrees) to prevent aspiration of blood and aid visualization of vocal cords as the blood moves down with gravity [24, 25]. The most experienced provider should pursue intubation to minimize duration and any complications related to intubation. If on initial assessment, the location of the source of hemoptysis is identified, a selective bronchial intubation can be attempted. In an emergent situation, once the ETT has passed beyond the vocal cords, the tube can be rotated by 90 degrees in the direction of the unaffected lung and advanced further to achieve selective bronchial intubation [26]. Alternatively, for a more definitive approach, isolation and intubation of unaffected lung can be achieved using a portable bronchoscope. This technique also provides the opportunity to have a first look to identify or confirm the location of the bleed. A double-lumen intubation has been described but can be technically challenging given need for advanced expertise and a lengthier process of placement [27].

Alongside, airway protection, assessment, and prompt treatment of any hemodynamic decompensation are important during a life-threatening bleeding. If there is any concern for hypovolemic shock or end-organ hypoperfusion, prompt resuscitation with intravenous fluid, vasopressors, and O negative packed red blood cell transfusion should be given to stabilize the patient.

The final approach to the treatment of hemoptysis includes identifying the etiology and controlling the source of bleeding. In emergent situations, several initial therapies can be utilized to temporize the bleeding before considering a more definitive treatment. Initial noninvasive measures include reversal of coagulopathy using fresh frozen plasma, vitamin K, or specific antidote to an offending anticoagulant the patient may be taking. In cases of severe thrombocytopenia, prompt transfusion of platelets can be lifesaving. Patients with liver and renal failure may have dysfunctional platelets and may benefit from intravenous desmopressin [28].

Once temporizing measures have been performed, a multidisciplinary discussion should be held with the intensivists, interventional pulmonologists, interventional radiologists, and cardiothoracic surgeons regarding the best approach for more definitive management of hemoptysis.

An early flexible bronchoscopy for airway examination can still be valuable to identify the source of bleed and provides opportunity to perform therapeutic procedures or decide on surgical versus arterial embolization methods.

Current Role of Interventional Pulmonology

Interventional pulmonology (IP) has evolved as an exciting field in thoracic medicine and revolutionized the management of hemoptysis, offering several less invasive techniques and procedures with good accuracy and outcome. To highlight the importance of various avenues offered by IP, it is helpful to classify bronchoscopic approach for hemoptysis into diagnostic and therapeutic roles.

Diagnostic Utility of Bronchoscopy

Bronchoscopy can be a pivotal tool in the management of hemoptysis. The timing and utility of the procedure remains a matter of debate. The amount of bleeding and the hemodynamic status of the patient should be considered prior to making a decision. While a CT is comparable to bronchoscopy in identifying the site of the bleeding, it is far superior to bronchoscopy in diagnosing the cause of the bleeding [29]. Millar et al. demonstrated, while studying 40 cases of hemoptysis with a negative bronchoscopy, that a CT scan was able to visualize an abnormality in 50% of cases [30]. However, in cases of large volume hemoptysis, the sensitivity of radiological modalities suffers due to spillover of blood to non-bleeding segments of the lung as well as the contralateral lung. A visual examination by bronchoscopy can play a key role in localizing the site of the bleed as well as provide therapeutic interventions (Fig. 11.2).

Modini et al. performed a multicenter study involving 486 patient with hemoptysis requiring bronchoscopy, and concluded that early bronchoscopy performed within 48 hours of presentation had a higher chance of localizing a bleeding site [31]. Under the care of an experienced team performing the bronchoscopy, the rate of complications arising from the bronchoscopy itself was fairly low (<4%), as demonstrated by Ost et al. in their study of over 1100 encounters of bronchoscopy

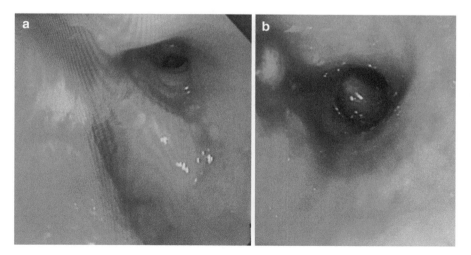

Fig. 11.2 Bronchoscopic images of a patient presenting with hemoptysis. (**a**) Trail of bleeding visualized on inspection of the airway leading to site of bleeding. (**b**) Bleeding endobronchial lesion visualized on direct inspection in the right lower lobe

in patients with complex central airway obstruction [32]. In cases of ongoing bleed which qualifies as life-threatening hemoptysis, an early initial examination of the airway can help institute lifesaving measures with the use of lung isolation techniques. It can also help clear the airway and improve oxygenation in addition to locating the source of the bleeding. Bronchoscopy plays a key role in patients with hemoptysis without a discernible causative source identified on CT [33]. Sources of bleeding that are poorly differentiated on a CT include mucosal lesions, small endobronchial lesions, and immunologic/vasculopathic causes of bleeding [34].

Diffuse alveolar hemorrhage (DAH) is a life-threatening emergency that can be caused by a multitude of disorders, and presents with hemoptysis with diffuse pulmonary infiltrates on chest radiology (Fig. 11.3). Early bronchoscopy plays a key role in the diagnosis of diffuse alveolar hemorrhage. Sequential aliquots of bronchoalveolar lavage (BAL) are obtained from the same subsegment of the lung, and a rising red blood cell (RBC) count is diagnostic of DAH. Microscopic evaluation can reveal hemosiderin-laden macrophages. Bronchoscopy also provides specimens for excluding infectious causes, and can help provide tissue diagnosis if a biopsy is performed. However, performing a transbronchial biopsy in a patient with DAH remains controversial, and is rarely performed because of the risks involved with disruption of the mechanical architecture of the lung with ongoing bleeding [35].

Bronchoscopy can help visualize vascular abnormalities like Dieulafoy's lesions, which are dilated tortuous arteries that project into the mucosa, and can cause significant hemoptysis. Similar dilated and tortuous vessels in the bronchial mucosa from underlying pathology like vasculitis, or tumors, can be visualized on bronchoscopic evaluation. The advent of advanced high-definition (HD) bronchoscopy equipment with narrow band imaging (NBI) in addition to the standard white light

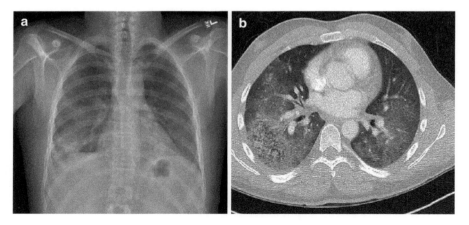

Fig. 11.3 (a) Chest radiograph (posterior-anterior view) demonstrating bilateral basal infiltrates in a patient with persistent hemoptysis. (b) Computed tomography of the chest (axial cuts) depicting areas of diffuse ground glass opacities in bilateral lower lobes suggestive of diffuse alveolar hemorrhage in a patient with systemic vasculitis

imaging can help differentiate between inflammation and vascularization by optimizing light wavelengths at 415 nm and 540 nm [36].

Therapeutic Bronchoscopy

In addition to the diagnostic bronchoscopy, the major role of interventional pulmonology is in the bronchoscopic management of hemoptysis. With the advent of newer tools and technologies, a majority of cases with hemoptysis can be treated using a flexible or rigid bronchoscope, bypassing the need for an invasive surgical intervention. Several temporizing and definitive treatments can be applied endoscopically. Rigid bronchoscopy also plays a significant role in managing central airway bleeding and massive hemoptysis and needs an interventional pulmonologist or thoracic surgeon expertise to perform the procedure (Fig. 11.4). The rigid bronchoscope provides several advantages compared to flexible bronchoscopy and can be considered as a first-choice tool if expertise is available for management of hemoptysis [3]. It provides a secure airway and route for effective ventilation, thus preventing asphyxiation. The larger port allows for effective large volume suctioning of blood and application for various endobronchial tools to control the bleeding [37]. A flexible bronchoscope can be introduced through it to examine a distal bleeding site and allows for bronchial blocker to be placed. In addition, it has the advantage of isolating the unaffected lung while hemostasis in the affected lung is achieved. A cryoprobe or argon plasma photocoagulation probe can be introduced through the rigid bronchoscope to treat tumoral obstruction and achieve prompt hemostasis and removal of blood clot. In cases of recurrent hemoptysis where alternate methods fail to control the bleeding from central airway, modified Y-shaped silicone stents can be

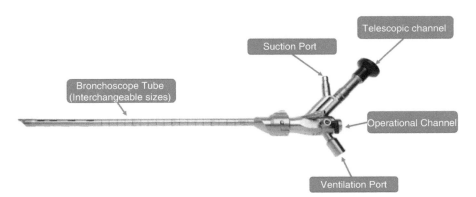

Fig. 11.4 A rigid bronchoscope depicting the suction port, the telescopic channel, the ventilation port, and the operational channel. The operational channel can be used to insert a variety of instruments including a flexible bronchoscope for distal airway visualization

placed via rigid bronchoscope to achieve successful hemostasis with a technical success rate of almost 100% and a clinical success rate of 85.7% [38].

While a rigid bronchoscope is an excellent tool, it has its limitations. It cannot be used to inspect segments with an abrupt upward takeoff like the right upper lobe. Its functionality is improved when used with a fiber-optic bronchoscope inserter through its operational channel. It requires skill and training in the field of interventional pulmonology. Many centers may not have experienced providers to utilize this tool. There is also a significant variation in training and competency in using rigid bronchoscopy in interventional pulmonology training programs [39].

Vasoconstrictors

Direct bronchoscopic vasoconstrictor therapy is a common modality for hemoptysis or procedure-related bleeding. One liter of iced saline cooled at 4 degrees Celsius is often a part of the preparation for any bronchoscopic procedure. Instillation of iced saline in aliquots of 5 cc to 50 cc can achieve hemostasis by inducing vasoconstriction and is often the first-line modality for minor bleeding [40]. Occasionally, instillation of iced saline can cause bradycardia or transient heart block due to vagal stimulation, but this is usually transient and self-limited. Such patients need closer monitoring post bronchoscopy [41]. In addition to iced saline, diluted epinephrine (1:10,000 to 20,000) in 2 cc aliquots is often used to achieve hemostasis in persistent oozing [42]. Ideally, a dose over 0.6 mg should be avoided due to risk of arrhythmias, and often alternate methods of hemostasis are warranted in persistent bleeding. In certain high-risk patients such as lung transplant recipients undergoing surveillance transbronchial biopsies, prophylactic epinephrine is often instilled at the biopsy site to minimize the risk of bleeding and trials are underway to assess its efficacy [43]. Vasopressin analogues such as ornipressin and terlipressin can also be used for topical instillation for biopsy-associated bleeding. While both are equally efficacious, terlipressin tends to have more systemic effect on hemodynamics compared to ornipressin and closer monitoring is required [44].

Bronchial Blocker

Bronchial blockers have been approved for lung isolation in thoracic surgeries but have been frequently used as a temporizing method in case of massive hemoptysis. A bronchial blocker is an easily available tool that can be used with flexible bronchoscopy to isolate the bleeding segment and allow for hemostasis to occur. A Fogarty® balloon catheter has a nylon loop at its tip that latches onto the bronchoscope and can be easily directed to the site of bleed. Once the catheter is successfully placed in the bleeding segment, using normal saline, the balloon is inflated till complete cessation of blood spillage is noted (Fig. 11.5). The advantage of

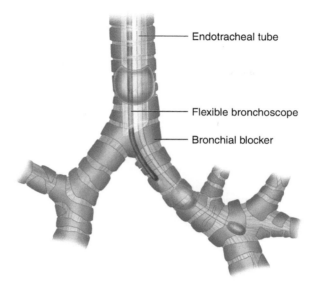

Endotracheal tube

Flexible bronchoscope

Bronchial blocker

Fig. 11.5 Schematic diagram of a bronchial blocker in place to isolate the bleeding segment of the lung

bronchial blockers is that multiple blockers can be placed simultaneously while a more definitive treatment is sought. In most cases, the bronchial blocker is left in situ for 24–48 hours before consideration of removal if hemostasis is achieved [45]. In addition, continued ventilation of aerated segments can be continued, thus preventing hypoxemia. Overinflation of the balloon should be avoided to prevent pressure injury. In certain instances, migration of the balloon can lead to central obstruction and should be considered if acute hypoxemia, decreased tidal volume, or elevated airway pressures is observed on mechanical ventilation. Alternatively, endobronchial embolization with a silicone spigot has been described as a successful method for hemostasis [46]. In rare instances, if a Fogarty® balloon is not instantly available, one can improvise and use a pulmonary artery catheter to occlude the bleeding segment endobronchially [47].

Procoagulants

Several procoagulants can be used to achieve temporary hemostasis. After initial cold saline and epinephrine instillation, fibrinogen-thrombin combination can be instilled into the bleeding segment to augment clotting. To further stabilize, the clot factor XIII has also been used in addition to the fibrinogen-thrombin complex [48]. This method can be used for hemostasis in patients who have a contraindication to bronchial artery embolization. The studies on the endobronchial use of fibrinogen-thrombin are limited to case series, and there is a risk of early recurrence. Therefore, this method should be considered only as a temporizing technique while a more definitive plan is being contemplated. Alternatively, oxidized regenerated cellulose fabric mesh can be used with direct tamponade for immediate cessation of bleeding [49]. Using a biopsy forceps, the mesh can be advanced into any bleeding segment or subsegment to achieve hemostasis. The advantage of this technique is that a peripheral bleeding subsegment can be reached with flexible bronchoscope and hemostasis can be achieved. However, similar to fibrinogen-thrombin complex, oxidized regenerating cellulose is also a temporizing method to prevent further bleeding and better prepare the patient for definitive treatment.

Intravenous tranexamic acid (TXA) has been used for hemostasis in cases of massive hemoptysis. Pooled systematic meta-analysis demonstrated no significant differences in bleeding duration with TXA compared to control groups. However, there was a significant reduction in hemoptysis volume [50]. Intravenous TXA can be utilized in patients with massive hemoptysis from a cavitary lesion such as an aspergilloma, while the patient is being prepared for a bronchial artery embolization [51]. Being a procoagulant, the risk of venothromboembolism has to be considered with intravenous TXA; therefore, some authors suggest nebulized TXA as a safer alternative [52].

Laser Photocoagulation

Bronchoscopic laser therapy using neodymium-doped yttrium aluminum garnet (Nd:YAG) laser therapy is a safe and effective treatment modality for malignant obstruction of larger airways. Laser therapy is frequently utilized for treatment of hemoptysis related to tumoral obstruction [53]. The neodymium crystal produces a light with 1064 nm continuous wavelength that is not completely absorbed by water and tissue, allowing to penetrate deeper (up to 5–10 mm) into the bronchial tissue. Since the Nd:YAG laser light wave is not visible to the human eye, therefore an additional wavelength of visible light is added to assist the operator to target the lesion [54]. The laser works on the principle of molecular agitation leading to the generation of thermal energy and coagulation. It leads to immediate coagulation necrosis of the tumor known as photoresection, thus helping improve airway patency and treating the source of bleeding definitively [55, 56]. In the next 6–8 weeks, healing occurs with deposition of granulation and fibrosis of the surrounding structures, thus reducing the risk of recurrence. Improvement in hemoptysis can occur in up to 94% of patients, while complete cessation of bleeding can occur in 60–74% patients treated with Nd:YAG laser photocoagulation [57]. Several factors play into the success or failure of Nd:YAG laser therapy. Laser therapy can be used with curative intent in certain tumors such as the endobronchial carcinoid tumors [58].

The risk of bleeding recurrence or incomplete therapy is higher in cases of extrinsic tracheobronchial obstruction, primarily submucosal lesions, lesions greater than 4 cm, abnormal coagulation profile, and bleeding not directly visible bronchoscopically [58]. Further, laser therapy is best avoided in complete or near-complete airway obstruction as failure to visualize distal lumen can increase the risk of perforation.

Argon Plasma Coagulation

Argon plasma coagulation (APC) is a method of noncontact transfer of electrical energy leading to tissue desiccation and coagulation. The argon gas is insufflated into the airway in pulses, and the electricity is conducted in the form of monopolar current via the ionized gas plasma [59] (Fig. 11.6). Blood and tissue are good conductors of electricity, making APC a good choice for superficial and endobronchial bleeds. As the tissue desiccation and coagulation occurs, the conductance of electricity reduces, preventing deeper penetration and perforation. It also leads to a more uniform tissue desiccation compared to laser and is superior in controlling bleeds located in anatomic corners, not in direct line of vision. Malignant airway obstruction, endobronchial hemangiomas, or Dieulafoy's lesions tend to bleed profusely and can be treated promptly with APC [60]. Immediate cessation of bleeding occurs and has a long-lasting effect with decreased incidence of recurrence of up to a mean follow-up of 97 days. Any malignant airway obstruction can be simultaneously treated with immediate and sustained symptomatic improvement [61]. Robust functioning suction and route for gas to escape is a necessity as fatal complications such as gas embolization can occur in rare cases [62]. APC is preferred in central and larger airways as it is essential to avoid touching the airway surface, as tissue coagulation can occur via direct contact rather than ionized plasma leading to deeper penetration and potential perforation.

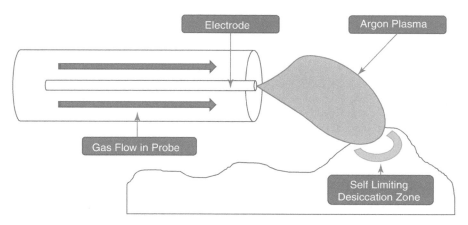

Fig. 11.6 Schematic diagram demonstrating mechanism of action of an argon plasma coagulation probe depicting the formation of plasma, leading to a self-limited zone of desiccation in the diseased mucosa

Cryotherapy

Bronchoscopic cryotherapy has been utilized to manage central airway obstruction from malignant tumors and hemoptysis. Cryotherapy utilizes Joule-Thomson principle of thermodynamics where a pressurized liquified gas undergoes rapid expansion to gaseous form that leads to a rapid drop in temperature [63]. A rapid freeze-thaw cycle at the cryoprobe tip leads to rapid coagulation of blood and formation of a thrombus that sticks to the probe and is easily retrievable [64]. The cryoprobe (generally 1.9-mm outer diameter) is introduced through the working channel of the bronchoscope and adhered to the blood clot in the central airway. The probe tip is then rapidly cooled for 15–30 seconds and passively thawed. This leads to tight adherence of the clot to the cryoprobe which can then be retrieved along with the clot in its entirety.

The temperature change also leads to strong vasoconstriction and minimizes further bleeding. In cases of malignant tumors, rapid decline in temperature leads to intracellular and extracellular crystallization leading to cell death and tissue necrosis [65]. Therefore, in addition to prompt bleeding control, it serves as a definitive treatment of the source of hemoptysis. Since the cryotherapy depends on the intracellular water content of the tissue, fat, nerve sheaths, fibrosis, and cartilaginous tissues are relatively cryoresistant in contrast to nerves, granulation tissue, endothelium, and mucus membranes which are cryosensitive [65]. Cryoprobes are available for both rigid and flexible bronchoscopy and are an economic option for emergent use in life-threatening hemoptysis where central airway obstruction is a concern. The medical intensive care team and bronchoscopy suite should have a cryoprobe in their armamentarium for prompt use in emergent situations.

Procedure-Related Bleeding

Bleeding is a common complication during a bronchoscopic procedure but rarely life-threatening. In general, the risk has been reported between 0.26% and 5% [66]. There are, however, certain patient and procedural risk factors that can change individual bleeding risk.

Underlying coagulopathy, renal dysfunction, liver dysfunction, heart failure, mitral stenosis, and pulmonary hypertension are independent risk factors for bronchoscopy-related bleeding [66]. Immunocompromised patients and lung transplant recipients are also at increased risk of procedure-related bleeding and have a higher likelihood of early termination of a procedure due to bleeding [67]. Inflamed and hypervascular tissues such as carcinoid tumors, renal cell carcinoma, thyroid cancer, and metastatic melanoma tend to bleed more during bronchoscopic biopsies, and preventive measures should be anticipated before any intervention on such tissue [68] (Fig. 11.7).

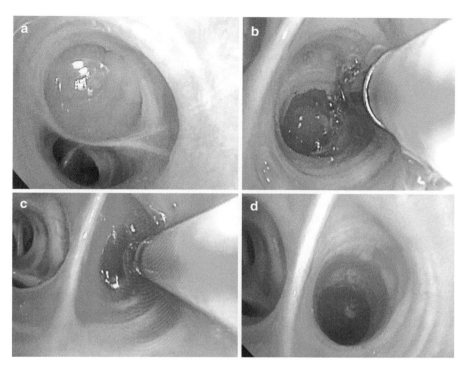

Fig. 11.7 (**a**) Bronchoscopic images of a highly vascular metastatic thyroid nodule visualized on diagnostic bronchoscopy. (**b**) Bleeding observed in the tumor on gentle probing. (**c**) Brisk bleeding was noted during the endobronchial biopsy. (**d**) Successful control of bleeding after instillation of 50 cc of cold saline solution

Certain procedures carry higher risk of bleeding compared to others. Transbronchial lung cryobiopsies and regular transbronchial biopsy of a peripheral lesion are at the highest risk of bleeding-related complications [69, 70]. The risk of clinically significant bleeding with cryobiopsy is 16% compared to 4% with a forceps biopsy [70]. Occasionally, a tamponade balloon/bronchial blocker is prophylactically inflated at the time of biopsy to achieve hemostasis.

To mitigate intrinsic bleeding risk, the British Thoracic Society recommends assessment of coagulation studies, platelet count, and hemoglobin pre-procedurally when clinical risk factors are present [71]. It is suggested that platelet counts should be >75,000 and INR <1.4 to reduce the possibility of significant bleeding. In addition, patients should hold their antiplatelet agents (aside from acetylsalicylic acid) and anticoagulation, although this recommendation is largely based on a discussion of individualized risk benefit ratio. For example, if a patient is at a high or very high risk for thrombotic complications from holding anticoagulation, procedures should be postponed until thromboembolic risk is low to moderate. If pursued, this should be done with bridging therapy using short-acting reversible anticoagulation.

Table 11.2 Grades of procedure-related bleeding [72]

Grade I	Suctioning of bleed required for less than 1 minute
Grade II	Suctioning of more than 1 minute required or repeat wedging of the bronchoscope for persistent bleeding or instillation of cold saline, diluted vasoactive substances, or thrombin
Grade III	Selective intubation with ETT or balloon/bronchial blocker for less than 20 minutes or premature interruption of the procedure
Grade IV	Persistent selective intubation >20 minutes or new admission to the ICU or PRBC transfusion or need for bronchial artery embolization or resuscitation

ETT endotracheal tube, *ICU* intensive care unit, *PRBC* packed red blood cells

When bleeding is encountered, application of a bleeding scale developed by Delphi consensus can assist in quantifying the severity of the bleeding, and it facilitates communication among team members and helps anticipate the next course of action [72]. The scale grades bleeding from 1 to 4 and is based on procedural findings and interventions as well as specific clinical outcome measures (i.e., need for PRBC transfusion or higher level of care) (Table 11.2) [72].

Most procedure-related bleeding events are self-limited, and hemostasis can be achieved by simply wedging the bronchoscope into the bleeding segment and allowing for clot formation. Similar bronchoscopic approach can be followed for control of endobronchial bleeding using cold saline, vasoconstrictor, or a cryoprobe.

Bronchial Artery Embolization

As the bronchial arteries run in the bronchovascular bundle and comprise a high-pressure circulation, majority of hemoptysis originates from the bronchial arteries. In most situations with brisk bleeding, bronchial artery embolization (BAE) by an experienced interventional radiologist is paramount to the treatment of hemoptysis [73]. While most literature on BAE arises from cystic fibrosis (CF) and bronchiectasis literature, BAE is commonly used for multiple other etiologies such as bleeding cavitary lesions, malignancy, and arteriovenous malformations [74]. BAE is generally not used in neoplasm-related bleeding as the failure rates are higher due to the progressive nature of the disease [75].

This modality highlights the importance of a multidisciplinary treatment approach to hemoptysis as an early consultation with interventional radiologist and cardiothoracic surgeons becomes imperative to make a graded approach to patient care. Once the patient's hemodynamics and airway are stabilized, the patient can be brought to an interventional radiology suite that is equipped with digital subtraction radiography and other necessary equipment. A thoracic aortogram is performed to identify the site of bronchial artery extravasation and any aberrant vascular anatomy [76]. In most instances, the microcatheter is inserted below the spinal artery to prevent neurologic complications. In rare cases, the artery of Adamkiewicz supplying the anterior spinal region may originate from the intercostal branches and may lead to paraplegia if not identified before embolization [77].

Once the site of extravasation is identified, the bleeding vessel can be embolized using gel foams, cyanoacrylate, polyvinyl alcohol, and several other available sealants [78] (Fig. 11.8). In cases of large cavitary lesions, multiple branches may need to be embolized to control the bleeding. In most cases, BAE can lead to long-term cessation of bleeding, allowing for a definitive surgical planning to treat the etiology of the bleed; however, recurrence can occur in up to 46% patients in 12-month time needing repeat BAE, especially in CF patients [79]. The success rate of BAE is

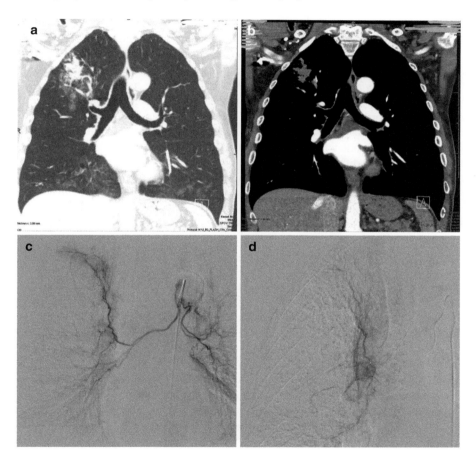

Fig. 11.8 (**a**, **b**) Coronal reformatted CT scan of the chest demonstrating a nodular consolidative opacity with surrounding ground glass opacities in a patient with known aspergilloma who presented with massive hemoptysis. (**c**) Fluoroscopic thoracic aortogram demonstrating a blush in the right upper bronchial artery branch suggestive of active extravasation of blood in the known aspergilloma cavity. (**d**) Post-embolization fluoroscopic thoracic aortogram demonstrating complete cessation of extravasation suggesting successful bronchial artery embolization

75%, 89%, and 93% in the first, second, and third BAE, respectively [79]. In most instances, BAE is a safe procedure; however, catheter insertion site bleeding or thrombosis, transverse myelitis or paraplegia, bronchial infarction, ischemic colitis, and rarely strokes have been described in the literature [80]. The most common complication is transient chest pain which usually resolves in few hours post procedure [81].

Current Role of Thoracic Surgery

In life-threatening hemoptysis, surgical management is an essential facet of therapy. An early consultation with thoracic surgeon becomes imperative to design a plan of action in the treatment of massive hemoptysis. Prior to the 1980s, a devastating 78–86% mortality was reported for patients with massive hemoptysis who were eligible for surgery and surgery was not pursued [5]. However, with advancements in critical supportive care, bronchoscopic interventions, and interventional radiology over the past 40+ years, the scope of surgical involvement has shifted from an emergent need to a fine balance between stabilization and definitive management of the underlying condition. It has become clear that the most appropriate surgical approach and timing is essential in determining outcomes.

In fact, most cases of life-threatening hemoptysis should be managed first with supportive measures and simultaneous bronchoscopic intervention or interventional radiology bronchial artery embolization [3, 73]. Outcomes can change dramatically when surgical lung resection is pursued in the stabilized patient. One series looking at surgical intervention in severe hemoptysis reported a 35% mortality in patients operated during active bleeding versus 4% in those operated on after control of bleeding [82]. Emergent surgery, pneumonectomy, and surgical resection of mycetoma are independent predictors of postoperative complications, while chronic alcoholism, need for mechanical ventilation or vasopressors, and blood transfusion are independent predictors of mortality in surgical patients [82]. Though bronchial artery embolization can aid in immediate control of bleeding, recurrence occurs in 10–57% of cases [83]. Thus, the indications for emergent surgical interventions are reserved for those who cannot undergo BAE, those with uncontrolled bleeding after embolization, and specific clinical situations and life-threatening conditions where surgery is the only option, for example, an aortobronchial fistula [84]. Even in these necessary circumstances, the mortality remains high. More recently, an endovascular approach in combination with surgery has been successful in treatment of aortobronchofistula [85]. Other major indications for surgical treatment (Table 11.3) include vascular anomalies (tracheoinnominate fistula, pulmonary artery rupture, and complex arteriovenous malformations), cavitary lesions with recurrent hemoptysis, chest trauma, and catamenial hemoptysis (Figs. 11.9 and 11.10). In many cases, surgery is the only curative option to manage the underlying condition and prevent recurrence. While hormonal therapy is the first-line treatment for

Table 11.3 Indications for surgical management of hemoptysis

Indications for surgical management of hemoptysis
Failed embolization or bronchoscopic therapies
Stage I–IIIA lung malignancy without metastasis

Cavitary lesion greater than 6 cm with recurrent bleeding
  Mycobacterium tuberculosis
  Atypical mycobacteria
  Aspergilloma
  Lung abscess
  Sarcoidosis

Catamenial hemoptysis
Aortobronchofistula
Arteriovenous malformation (AVMs) with failed embolization
Tracheoinnominate fistula
Pulmonary artery rupture
Traumatic lung injury
Severe focal bronchiectasis

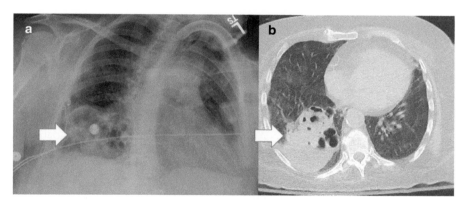

Fig. 11.9 (a) Radiograph anterior-posterior view of a patient with a dense right lower lobe cavitary lesion leading to hemoptysis (arrow). (b) CT scan, axial cuts of the chest depicting dense cavitary lesion leading to hemoptysis (arrow)

catamenial hemoptysis, surgical resection may become imperative in patients not responding to conservative management [86, 87]. Though there are nuanced avenues that exist, the general surgical approach remains lung resection, and as noted previously, optimizing surgical conditions is critical for patient outcomes. Therefore, every effort should be made to stabilize the patient prior to surgery, emergent or not. An airway should be secured, oxygenation and hemodynamic support provided. The patient should be transfused as appropriate and prompt reversal of any coagulopathy should be completed. Management of hemoptysis continues to be multidisciplinary, and the key to successful treatment lies in early involvement of surgical and interventional specialists.

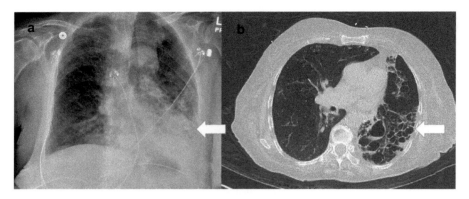

Fig. 11.10 (**a**) Chest radiograph (anterior-posterior view) of a patient with left lower lobe severe bronchiectasis presenting with hemoptysis (arrow). (**b**) CT scan of the chest (axial cuts) depicting left lower lobe severe bronchiectasis (arrow)

Permissions All appropriate literature used to develop this manuscript has been appropriately cited. No images were requested from pre-existing literature, and hence permission was not required. Tables based on guidelines have been cited appropriately in the manuscript.

References

1. Knott-Craig CJ, Oostuizen JG, Rossouw G, Joubert JR, Barnard PM. Management and prognosis of massive hemoptysis. Recent experience with 120 patients. J Thorac Cardiovasc Surg. 1993;105:394–7.
2. Ong TH, Eng P. Massive hemoptysis requiring intensive care. Intensive Care Med. 2003;29:317–20.
3. Sakr L, Dutau H. Massive hemoptysis: an update on the role of bronchoscopy in diagnosis and management. Respiration. 2010;80:38–58.
4. Mal H, Rullon I, Mellot F, et al. Immediate and long-term results of bronchial artery embolization for life-threatening hemoptysis. Chest. 1999;115:996–1001.
5. Crocco JA, Rooney JJ, Fankushen DS, DiBenedetto RJ, Lyons HA. Massive hemoptysis. Arch Intern Med. 1968;121:495–8.
6. Hirshberg B, Biran I, Glazer M, Kramer MR. Hemoptysis: etiology, evaluation, and outcome in a tertiary referral hospital. Chest. 1997;112:440–4.
7. Abdulmalak C, Cottenet J, Beltramo G, et al. Haemoptysis in adults: a 5-year study using the French nationwide hospital administrative database. Eur Respir J. 2015;46:503.
8. Choi J, Baik JH, Kim CH, et al. Long-term outcomes and prognostic factors in patients with mild hemoptysis. Am J Emerg Med. 2018;36:1160–5.
9. Fartoukh M, Khoshnood B, Parrot A, et al. Early prediction of in-hospital mortality of patients with hemoptysis: an approach to defining severe hemoptysis. Respiration. 2012;83:106–14.
10. Rizzo AN, Fraidenburg DR, Yuan JXJ. Pulmonary Vascular Anatomy. In: Lanzer P, editor. PanVascular Medicine. Berlin, Heidelberg: Springer Berlin Heidelberg; 2015. p. 4041–56.
11. Sealy WC, Connally SR, Dalton ML. Naming the bronchopulmonary segments and the development of pulmonary surgery. Ann Thorac Surg. 1993;55:184–8.
12. Gil J. The normal lung circulation. State of the art. Chest. 1988;93:80s–2s.

13. Kandathil A, Chamarthy M. Pulmonary vascular anatomy & anatomical variants. Cardiovasc Diagn Ther. 2018;8:201–7.
14. Wagner E. Bronchial vasculature: the other pulmonary circulation. In: Rounds NFVaS, editor. The pulmonary endothelium; 2009. p. 217–27.
15. Deffebach ME, Charan NB, Lakshminarayan S, Butler J. The bronchial circulation. Small, but a vital attribute of the lung. Am Rev Respir Dis. 1987;135:463–81.
16. Serikov VB, Fleming NW. Pulmonary and bronchial circulations: contributions to heat and water exchange in isolated lungs. J Appl Physiol (Bethesda, MD: 1985). 2001;91:1977–85.
17. Khalil A, Parrot A, Nedelcu C, Fartoukh M, Marsault C, Carette MF. Severe hemoptysis of pulmonary arterial origin: signs and role of multidetector row CT angiography. Chest. 2008;133:212–9.
18. Reisz G, Stevens D, Boutwell C, Nair V. The causes of hemoptysis revisited. A review of the etiologies of hemoptysis between 1986 and 1995. Mo Med. 1997;94:633–5.
19. McGuinness G, Beacher JR, Harkin TJ, Garay SM, Rom WN, Naidich DP. Hemoptysis: prospective high-resolution CT/bronchoscopic correlation. Chest. 1994;105:1155–62.
20. Lee S, Chan JW, Chan SC, et al. Bronchial artery embolisation can be equally safe and effective in the management of chronic recurrent haemoptysis. Hong Kong Med J = Xianggang yi xue za zhi. 2008;14:14–20.
21. Serasli E, Kalpakidis V, Iatrou K, Tsara V, Siopi D, Christaki P. Percutaneous bronchial artery embolization in the management of massive hemoptysis in chronic lung diseases. Immediate and long-term outcomes. Int Angiol. 2008;27:319–28.
22. Jean-Baptiste E. Clinical assessment and management of massive hemoptysis. Crit Care Med. 2000;28:1642–7.
23. Dellinger RP. Fiberoptic bronchoscopy in adult airway management. Eur Clin Respir J. 1990;18:882–7.
24. Turner JS, Ellender TJ, Okonkwo ER, et al. Feasibility of upright patient positioning and intubation success rates at two academic EDs. Am J Emerg Med. 2017;35:986–92.
25. Lane S, Saunders D, Schofield A, Padmanabhan R, Hildreth A, Laws D. A prospective, randomised controlled trial comparing the efficacy of pre-oxygenation in the 20 degrees head-up vs supine position. Anaesthesia. 2005;60:1064–7.
26. Bair AE, Doherty MJ, Harper R, Albertson TE. An evaluation of a blind rotational technique for selective mainstem intubation. Acad Emerg Med. 2004;11:1105–7.
27. Campos JH. Which device should be considered the best for lung isolation: double-lumen endotracheal tube versus bronchial blockers. Curr Opin Anaesthesiol. 2007;20:27–31.
28. Pea L, Roda L, Boussaud V, Lonjon B. Desmopressin therapy for massive hemoptysis associated with severe leptospirosis. Am J Respir Crit Care Med. 2003;167:726–8.
29. Radchenko C, Alraiyes AH, Shojaee S. A systematic approach to the management of massive hemoptysis. J Thorac Dis. 2017;9:S1069–s86.
30. Millar AB, Boothroyd AE, Edwards D, Hetzel MR. The role of computed tomography (CT) in the investigation of unexplained haemoptysis. Respir Med. 1992;86:39–44.
31. Mondoni M, Carlucci P, Cipolla G, et al. Bronchoscopy to assess patients with hemoptysis: which is the optimal timing? BMC Pulm Med. 2019;19:36.
32. Ost DE, Ernst A, Grosu HB, et al. Complications following therapeutic bronchoscopy for malignant central airway obstruction: results of the AQuIRE registry. Chest. 2015;148:450–71.
33. Lee YJ, Lee SM, Park JS, et al. The clinical implications of bronchoscopy in hemoptysis patients with no explainable lesions in computed tomography. Respir Med. 2012;106:413–9.
34. Larici AR, Franchi P, Occhipinti M, et al. Diagnosis and management of hemoptysis. Diagn Interv Radiol (Ankara, Turkey). 2014;20:299–309.
35. Schnabel A, Holl-Ulrich K, Dalhoff K, Reuter M, Gross WL. Efficacy of transbronchial biopsy in pulmonary vaculitides. Eur Respir J. 1997;10:2738–43.
36. Muthreja D, Swarnakar R, Sontakke A. Narrow band imaging: advantages over white light bronchoscopy; single center experience of 500 patients. Eur Respir J. 2018;52:PA4179.

37. Diaz-Mendoza J, Peralta AR, Debiane L, Simoff MJ. Rigid bronchoscopy. Semin Respir Crit Care Med. 2018;39:674–84.
38. Zeng J, Wu X, Zhang M, Lin L, Ke M. Modified silicone stent for difficult-to-treat massive hemoptysis: a pilot study of 14 cases. J Thorac Dis. 2020;12:956–65.
39. Pastis NJ, Nietert PJ, Silvestri GA. Variation in training for interventional pulmonary procedures among US pulmonary/critical care fellowships: a survey of fellowship directors. Chest. 2005;127:1614–21.
40. Conlan AA, Hurwitz SS. Management of massive haemoptysis with the rigid bronchoscope and cold saline lavage. Thorax. 1980;35:901–4.
41. Sagar A-ES, Cherian SV, Estrada-Y-Martin RM. Complete heart block following cold saline lavage during bronchoscopy. J Bronchol Interv Pulmonol. 2017;24:41–2.
42. Lee P, Mehta AC, Mathur PN. Management of complications from diagnostic and interventional bronchoscopy. Respirology (Carlton, VIC). 2009;14:940–53.
43. Kalchiem-Dekel O, Iacono A, Pickering EM, et al. Prophylactic epinephrine for the prevention of transbronchial lung biopsy-related bleeding in lung transplant recipients (PROPHET) study: a protocol for a multicentre randomised, double-blind, placebo-controlled trial. BMJ Open. 2019;9:e024521.
44. Tuller C, Tuller D, Tamm M, Brutsche MH. Hemodynamic effects of endobronchial application of ornipressin versus terlipressin. Respiration. 2004;71:397–401.
45. Freitag L, Tekolf E, Stamatis G, Montag M, Greschuchna D. Three years experience with a new balloon catheter for the management of haemoptysis. Eur Respir J. 1994;7:2033–7.
46. Dutau H, Palot A, Haas A, Decamps I, Durieux O. Endobronchial embolization with a silicone spigot as a temporary treatment for massive hemoptysis: a new bronchoscopic approach of the disease. Respiration. 2006;73:830–2.
47. Jolliet P, Soccal P, Chevrolet J-C. Control of massive hemoptysis by endobronchial tamponade with a pulmonary artery balloon catheter. Crit Care Med. 1992;20
48. de Gracia J, de la Rosa D, Catalán E, Alvarez A, Bravo C, Morell F. Use of endoscopic fibrinogen-thrombin in the treatment of severe hemoptysis. Respir Med. 2003;97:790–5.
49. Valipour A, Kreuzer A, Koller H, Koessler W, Burghuber OC. Bronchoscopy-guided topical hemostatic tamponade therapy for the management of life-threatening hemoptysis. Chest. 2005;127:2113–8.
50. Tsai YS, Hsu LW, Wu MS, Chen KH, Kang YN. Effects of tranexamic acid on hemoptysis: a systematic review and meta-analysis of randomized controlled trials. Clin Drug Investig. 2020;40:789–97.
51. Alastruey-Izquierdo A, Cadranel J, Flick H, et al. Treatment of chronic pulmonary aspergillosis: current standards and future perspectives. Respiration. 2018;96:159–70.
52. Wand O, Guber E, Guber A, Epstein Shochet G, Israeli-Shani L, Shitrit D. Inhaled tranexamic acid for hemoptysis treatment: a randomized controlled trial. Chest. 2018;154:1379–84.
53. Hermes A, Heigener D, Gatzemeier U, Schatz J, Reck M. Efficacy and safety of bronchoscopic laser therapy in patients with tracheal and bronchial obstruction: a retrospective single institution report. Clin Respir J. 2012;6:67–71.
54. Unger M. Bronchoscopic utilization of the Nd:YAG laser for obstructing lesions of the trachea and bronchi. Surg Clin North Am. 1984;64:931–8.
55. Patel A. Chapter 40 – Anesthesia for laser airway surgery. In: Hagberg CA, editor. Benumof and Hagberg's airway management. 3rd ed. Philadelphia: W.B. Saunders; 2013. p. 824–58.e4.
56. Bolliger CT, Sutedja TG, Strausz J, Freitag L. Therapeutic bronchoscopy with immediate effect: laser, electrocautery, argon plasma coagulation and stents. Eur Respir J. 2006;27:1258.
57. Han CC, Prasetyo D, Wright GM. Endobronchial palliation using Nd:YAG laser is associated with improved survival when combined with multimodal adjuvant treatments. J Thorac Oncol. 2007;2:59–64.
58. Khemasuwan D, Mehta AC, Wang K-P. Past, present, and future of endobronchial laser photoresection. J Thorac Dis. 2015;7:S380–S8.
59. Zenker M. Argon plasma coagulation. GMS Krankenhhyg Interdiszip. 2008;3:Doc15-Doc.

60. Dalar L, Sökücü SN, Özdemir C, Büyükkale S, Altın S. Endobronchial argon plasma coagulation for treatment of Dieulafoy disease. Respir Care. 2015;60:e11.
61. Morice RC, Ece T, Ece F, Keus L. Endobronchial argon plasma coagulation for treatment of hemoptysis and neoplastic airway obstruction. Chest. 2001;119:781–7.
62. Reddy C, Majid A, Michaud G, et al. Gas embolism following bronchoscopic argon plasma coagulation: a case series. Chest. 2008;134:1066–9.
63. Amoils SP. The Joule Thomson Cryoprobe. Arch Ophthalmol. 1967;78:201–7.
64. Sehgal IS, Dhooria S, Agarwal R, Behera D. Use of a flexible cryoprobe for removal of tracheobronchial blood clots. Respir Care. 2015;60:e128.
65. DiBardino DM, Lanfranco AR, Haas AR. Bronchoscopic cryotherapy. Clinical applications of the cryoprobe, cryospray, and cryoadhesion. Ann Am Thorac Soc. 2016;13:1405–15.
66. Bernasconi M, Koegelenberg CFN, Koutsokera A, et al. Iatrogenic bleeding during flexible bronchoscopy: risk factors, prophylactic measures and management. ERJ Open Res. 2017;3
67. Diette GB, Wiener CM, White P Jr. The higher risk of bleeding in lung transplant recipients from bronchoscopy is independent of traditional bleeding risks: results of a prospective Cohort Study. Chest. 1999;115:397–402.
68. Dixon RK, Britt EJ, Netzer GA, et al. Ten-year single center experience of pulmonary carcinoid tumors and diagnostic yield of bronchoscopic biopsy. Lung. 2016;194:905–10.
69. Cordasco EM Jr, Mehta AC, Ahmad M. Bronchoscopically induced bleeding. A summary of nine years' Cleveland clinic experience and review of the literature. Chest. 1991;100:1141–7.
70. Hetzel J, Eberhardt R, Petermann C, et al. Bleeding risk of transbronchial cryobiopsy compared to transbronchial forceps biopsy in interstitial lung disease – a prospective, randomized, multicentre cross-over trial. Respir Res. 2019;20:140.
71. Du Rand IA, Barber PV, Goldring J, et al. British Thoracic Society guideline for advanced diagnostic and therapeutic flexible bronchoscopy in adults. Thorax. 2011;66 Suppl 3:iii1–21.
72. Folch EE, Mahajan AK, Oberg CL, et al. Standardized definitions of bleeding after transbronchial lung biopsy: a Delphi consensus statement from the Nashville Working Group. Chest. 2020;158:393–400.
73. Marshall TJ, Jackson JE. Vascular intervention in the thorax: bronchial artery embolization for haemoptysis. Eur Radiol. 1997;7:1221–7.
74. Martin LN, Higgins L, Mohabir P, Sze DY, Hofmann LV. Bronchial artery embolization for hemoptysis in cystic fibrosis patients: a 17-year review. J Vasc Interv Radiol. 2020;31(2):331–5.
75. Hayakawa K, Tanaka F, Torizuka T, et al. Bronchial artery embolization for hemoptysis: immediate and long-term results. Cardiovasc Intervent Radiol. 1992;15:154–8; discussion 8–9.
76. Piola FPF, Nogueira-Barbosa MH, Maranho DAC, Martins AA, Barbosa MF, Herrero C. Identification of the Artery of Adamkiewicz using multidetector computed tomography angiography (MCTA). Rev Bras Ortop. 2020;55:70–4.
77. Taterra D, Skinningsrud B, Pękala PA, et al. Artery of Adamkiewicz: a meta-analysis of anatomical characteristics. Neuroradiology. 2019;61:869–80.
78. Hahn S, Kim YJ, Kwon W, Cha S-W, Lee W-Y. Comparison of the effectiveness of embolic agents for bronchial artery embolization: gelfoam versus polyvinyl alcohol. Korean J Radiol. 2010;11:542–6.
79. Brinson GM, Noone PG, Mauro MA, et al. Bronchial artery embolization for the treatment of hemoptysis in patients with cystic fibrosis. Am J Respir Crit Care Med. 1998;157:1951–8.
80. Lorenz J, Sheth D, Patel J. Bronchial artery embolization. Semin Intervent Radiol. 2012;29:155–60.
81. Cohen AM, Doershuk CF, Stern RC. Bronchial artery embolization to control hemoptysis in cystic fibrosis. Radiology. 1990;175:401–5.
82. Andréjak C, Parrot A, Bazelly B, et al. Surgical lung resection for severe hemoptysis. Ann Thorac Surg. 2009;88:1556–65.
83. Panda A, Bhalla AS, Goyal A. Bronchial artery embolization in hemoptysis: a systematic review. Diagn Interv Radiol (Ankara, Turkey). 2017;23:307–17.

84. Sakai M, Ozawa Y, Nakajima T, Ikeda A, Konishi T, Matsuzaki K. Thick lung wedge resection for acute life-threatening massive hemoptysis due to aortobronchial fistula. J Thorac Dis. 2016;8:E957–e60.
85. Canaud L, D'Annoville T, Ozdemir BA, Marty-Ané C, Alric P. Combined endovascular and surgical approach for aortobronchial fistula. J Thorac Cardiovasc Surg. 2014;148:2108–11.
86. Kim CJ, Nam HS, Lee CY, et al. Catamenial hemoptysis: a nationwide analysis in Korea. Respiration. 2010;79:296–301.
87. Channabasavaiah AD, Joseph JV. Thoracic endometriosis: revisiting the association between clinical presentation and thoracic pathology based on thoracoscopic findings in 110 patients. Medicine. 2010;89

Chapter 12
Role of Interventional Pulmonology in Miscellaneous Conditions

Prasoon Jain, Sarah Hadique, Rajeev Dhupar, and Atul C. Mehta

In this chapter, we discuss the emerging role and current status of interventional pulmonology techniques in management of several conditions that have traditionally required more invasive interventions. We first discuss the current role of bronchoscopy in diagnosis and management of broncholithiasis, bronchogenic cysts, and lung abscess. Finally, we discuss current role of bronchoscopy in diagnosis and management of central carcinoid tumors.

At the outset, it is important to point out that bronchoscopic procedures have not replaced thoracic surgery in majority of the entities covered herein. However, these techniques are providing a less invasive adjunct or alternative to more invasive procedures in a carefully selected group of patients with results that are nearly equivalent to the traditional treatments. It is important is to make sure that long-term outcome is not compromised in any way when bronchoscopic treatment modality is

P. Jain (✉)
Pulmonary and Critical Care, Louis A Johnson VA Medical Center, Clarksburg, WV, USA

S. Hadique
Department of Pulmonary and Critical Care, West Virginia University, Morgantown, WV, USA
e-mail: shadique@hsc.wvu.edu

R. Dhupar
University of Pittsburgh School of Medicine, Pittsburgh, PA, USA

VAPHS, Pittsburgh, PA, USA
e-mail: dhuparr2@upmc.edu

A. C. Mehta
Buoncore Family Endowed Chair in Lung Transplantation, Respiratory Institute, Cleveland Clinic, Cleveland, OH, USA

© The Author(s), under exclusive license to Springer Nature Switzerland AG 2021
J. F. Turner, Jr. et al. (eds.), *From Thoracic Surgery to Interventional Pulmonology*, Respiratory Medicine,
https://doi.org/10.1007/978-3-030-80298-1_12

chosen over surgery. In fact, due to emergence of bronchoscopic treatments, a close collaboration between the bronchoscopist and the thoracic surgeon has become more critical than ever before.

Broncholithiasis

Broncholithiasis is an uncommon condition in which calcified peribronchial lymph nodes erode into the airway lumen [1]. The calcified material within the airways is called a broncholith. Intraluminal broncholiths and associated granulation tissue cause endobronchial obstruction and a variety of clinical symptoms. Calcified perihilar or mediastinal lymph nodes are nearly always found in patients diagnosed to have broncholithiasis. Some authors have included bronchial compression or distortion within the working definition of broncholithiasis [2]. However, an overwhelming majority of such calcified lymph nodes never cause any symptoms. Our discussion is limited to the cases in which a free or partially eroded broncholith is visible to the operator during bronchoscopy.

The majority of calcified mediastinal lymph nodes that cause broncholithiasis result from healed granulomatous infections. Histoplasmosis is the most common cause in the United States [3].

In the rest of the world including Europe, tuberculosis is the leading cause of broncholithiasis [4, 5].

Silicosis is the most common noninfectious cause of broncholithiasis [6]. Intraluminal calcified foreign body and endobronchial actinomycosis infection are also identified as causes of broncholiths in rare instances [7, 8].

Calcified lymph nodes compress and gradually erode adjacent bronchi due to their movement with respiratory activity and cardiac pulsations. Invariably, the presence of calcified material in endobronchial tree causes irritation and evokes chronic inflammatory changes. Granulation tissue is a universal finding on airway inspection. In some instances, granulomatous reaction is so pronounced that it becomes difficult to differentiate it from endobronchial malignancy. Bronchoscopic biopsies are needed to exclude malignancy in these cases. In some cases, broncholiths are entirely intrabronchial, loosely attached to the airway wall. In other cases, only a small part of calcified lymph node is present within the airway lumen. In these cases, the endobronchial component only represents the tip of the iceberg with the majority of calcified mass outside the airways. In many instances, broncholiths are firmly embedded or even entirely covered with the granulation tissue. Such broncholiths are easily missed on airway examination.

Many broncholiths are asymptomatic and are discovered as an incidental finding on chest computed tomography (CT) or bronchoscopy [9]. In symptomatic patients, chronic cough and hemoptysis are the most common symptoms. Hemoptysis is usually mild and intermittent, but broncholithiasis is known to cause massive and life-threatening airway bleeding in some patients. Endobronchial obstruction due to broncholith and granulation tissue causes atelectasis and recurrent pneumonia in some patients. Focal bronchiectasis may also develop due to obstruction and repeated bronchial infections. Spontaneous expectoration of broncholiths, called lithoptysis, is an uncommon symptom, reported in 3 (16%) patients in a series of 19 cases [10]. Lithoptysis is often ignored and is rarely self-reported by patients unless directly inquired by physician [11].

Broncholithiasis is an important cause of right middle lobe syndrome (Fig. 12.1). Therefore, chest CT and bronchoscopy must be performed to exclude broncholithiasis in any patient with recurrent right middle lobe atelectasis. Other symptoms include dyspnea, chest pain, and wheezing. Since clinical presentation is rather nonspecific, the majority of patients remain undiagnosed for an extended period of time. It is not unusual for some patients to be treated for a mistaken diagnosis of difficult asthma for years before the correct underlying pathology is identified.

Chest radiographs may disclose calcified hilar or mediastinal lymph nodes in close proximity to the major airways. Chest CT is more sensitive than plain radiography for this purpose. A high-resolution chest CT is advised in every patient suspected to have broncholithiasis (Fig. 12.2). Administration of intravenous contrast is not needed. In one study, CT showed calcified lymph node in all 15 cases of broncholithiasis [12]. In ten patients proven to have intraluminal broncholiths on bronchoscopy in this study, the lymph nodes on CT appeared to erode the airways in six patients and appeared peribronchial in four patients. Atelectasis was detected in six patients, focal bronchiectasis in four patients, post-obstructive pneumonia in four patients, and air trapping in one patient. Broncholiths are more often seen on the right side.

Chest CT provides additional information that is helpful in treatment planning. Important findings in this context are presence of fistulous connections with surrounding mediastinal structures such as the esophagus and proximity of calcified lymph node to the pulmonary artery. It is important to determine whether the eroding lymph node is attached to the surrounding vessels or other mediastinal

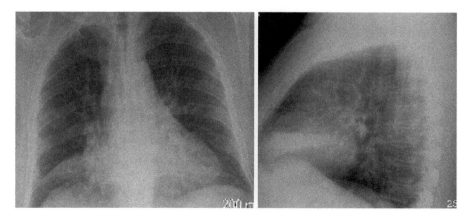

Fig. 12.1 PA and lateral chest radiographs showing right middle lobe atelectasis in a patient with recurrent episodes of cough, purulent sputum, and minor hemoptysis

Fig. 12.2 Chest computed
tomography in the same
patient showed right
middle lobe atelectasis and
calcified material in right
middle lobe bronchus

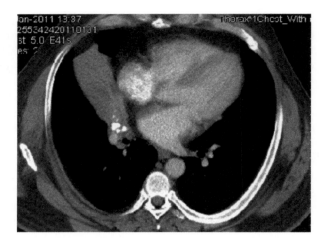

structures. Any attempts at bronchoscopic extraction of such broncholiths may lead
to catastrophic airway bleeding or injury to the mediastinal structures. Worsening of
broncho-esophageal fistula has been observed after extraction of broncholiths in
one report [13].

Management

Broncholithiasis is rare and there are no clinical guidelines for management. The
majority of practicing physicians have no firsthand experience in managing these
cases. It may be worthwhile to consider an early referral to a tertiary care center.
Bronchoscopy is the usual next step in patients suspected to have broncholithiasis
on the basis of clinical and radiological findings in order to confirm the diagnosis.
Early consultation with a thoracic surgeon is strongly recommended to determine
the best long-term management strategy, which may involve extraction by rigid
bronchoscopy or surgery.

Role of Bronchoscopy

Bronchoscopy has a key diagnostic role in patients with broncholithiasis.
Bronchoscopy is more sensitive than CT in these patients. An important goal of bronchoscopy is to determine whether the entire broncholith is freely located within the
airway lumen or whether only a part of calcified lymph node is eroding through the
bronchial wall. Airways must be carefully examined for any suggestions of fistulous
connection with the esophagus or other mediastinal structures.

Bronchoscopy in broncholithiasis is a difficult procedure. First, excessive cough-ing during the procedure is very common. Second, the correct diagnosis may not be possible because some broncholiths are fully covered with granulation tissue and surrounding inflammation (Fig. 12.3). The bronchoscopic findings closely mimic endobronchial tumor in many instances. Third, some patients with broncholithiasis have tendency to bleed excessively after endobronchial biopsies, which can be mas-sive and life-threatening in some instances. A prior history of hemoptysis is thought to be associated with a greater risk of bleeding during bronchoscopy in these patients. Caution is warranted when excessive bleeding is observed with initial biopsies or minimal manipulation of the broncholith. It should alert the operator to a possibility of large volume airway bleeding with further attempts at broncho-scopic extraction of the broncholith.

Bronchoscopy has important therapeutic role in selected patients with broncho-lithiasis. In a retrospective review from Mayo Clinic, bronchoscopic extraction was attempted in 71 of 127 (56%) broncholiths [14]. Bronchoscopic removal was attempted in 46% (48 of 104) of partially eroding broncholiths and 100% (23 of 23) of loose broncholiths. Successful extraction was feasible in 48% (23 of 48) of par-tially eroding broncholiths and 100% (23 of 23) of loose broncholiths. Significant complications included severe dyspnea in one patient due to obstruction of the tra-chea with a large broncholith and massive airway bleeding in another patient requir-ing urgent surgical intervention.

Fig. 12.3 Bronchoscopy in patient with broncholithiasis showing marked inflammation and swelling of opening of middle lobe bronchus. Broncholith was not visible but grating was felt when probed with biopsy forceps. Patient underwent right middle lobectomy with complete resolution of symptoms

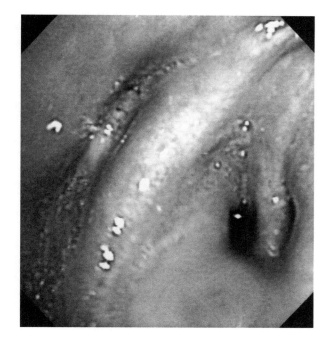

In a more recent series, Cerfolio and associates performed rigid bronchoscopy in 34 patients with broncholiths [15]. All 29 mobile broncholiths were successfully retrieved via bronchoscopic route. Surgery was needed in three patients with fixed broncholiths and two patients with broncho-esophageal fistula. No procedure-related complications were encountered. Only three patients required additional bronchoscopic extraction over a median follow-up period of 4.2 years. A similar experience was reported in a Korean study in which flexible ($n = 2$) or rigid ($n = 13$) bronchoscopy was successful in removing all 15 intraluminal broncholiths. However, bronchoscopic removal failed in every case of mixed broncholith where the calcified lymph node was partly located within and partly outside the airway lumen [16]. These and several other short reports establish the feasibility and safety of removing mobile broncholiths with bronchoscopy [17, 18]. The main danger with bronchoscopic removal of broncholiths is major bleeding, but this is fortunately a rare occurrence. [19]

An important question when contemplating removal of broncholiths is whether to use a flexible or rigid bronchoscope. Several studies have established feasibility using a flexible bronchoscope for this purpose. A flexible bronchoscope is also used to retrieve distal broncholiths that are beyond the reach of a rigid bronchoscope. However, there can be little doubt about superior ability of a rigid bronchoscope in removing broncholiths compared to the flexible bronchoscopes. As expected, Olson and associates reported a 67% success with rigid scope compared to 30% success with flexible bronchoscope for complete extraction of broncholiths [14]. The same can be said about the usefulness of a rigid bronchoscope to control brisk airway bleeding that is sometimes encountered during bronchoscopic extraction of broncholiths. A rigid bronchoscope is also more effective than a flexible scope in extracting a large broncholith that is acutely obstructing the central airways. Due to these reasons, having rigid bronchoscopy readily available is a necessity rather than an option in this situation.

Some broncholiths are too large to be removed via bronchoscopic route. A majority of these patients require surgical treatment. In highly selected cases, Nd:YAG laser can be used to dislodge or break the broncholith into smaller fragments to facilitate bronchoscopic extraction. [20, 21]

Laser treatment has also been used to remove obstructing granulation tissue surrounding the broncholiths [22]. Restoration of the airway lumen with this approach is helpful in controlling post-obstructive pneumonia and distal atelectasis. A further application of Nd:YAG laser in these patients is in control of spontaneous or post-biopsy airway bleeding.

There are isolated reports of using cryotherapy for management of broncholithiasis [23, 24]. Granulation tissue is particularly suitable for removal using a cryorecanalization technique. Large broncholiths firmly attached to airways cannot be removed using this technique.

Surgery for Broncholithiasis

Surgery is needed in many patients with symptomatic broncholiths who are not suitable for bronchoscopic therapies. Indications for surgery are large broncholiths that cannot be removed via bronchoscope, suspected adhesions with the mediastinal structures, esophageal fistula, recurrent pneumonia and atelectasis, symptomatic focal bronchiectasis, and massive hemoptysis [18]. Surgery is also needed in some patients to exclude an underlying malignancy. Surgery can be technically challenging due to extensive mediastinal adhesions, but a successful operation provides lasting relief from symptoms [25].

Surgical options for broncholithiasis include bronchotomy and broncholithectomy with removal of calcified lymph nodes. Lung-sparing surgery, such as a segmentectomy, is recommended when feasible [26]. Lobectomy and rarely, pneumonectomy are needed in some cases [14, 27]. Incision and curettage without removing the outer shell may be the most suitable intervention if lymph nodes are firmly adhered to the mediastinal structures. Clearly, surgery is more invasive than bronchoscopic interventions, but sometimes it is the best option. Postoperative complications can include pneumonia, prolonged air leak, and bronchopleural fistula. Thus, the decision for the best approach should be made after a detailed multi-specialty evaluation.

Conclusions

Appropriate management of broncholithiasis is not easy. Asymptomatic broncholiths may be followed with interval symptom assessment and radiography. While bronchoscopy is successful in many carefully selected patients, an ill-advised attempt to remove broncholiths during bronchoscopy can lead to serious hemorrhage and poor patient outcome. Surgical treatment can also have challenges due to adhesions, fibrosis, and fistulae. Optimal results require a close collaboration between an interventional pulmonologist and thoracic surgeon from the outset.

Bronchogenic Cysts

Bronchogenic cysts are rare congenital disorders of the tracheobronchial tree. Cystic lesions constitute around 15–20% of all mediastinal disorders. Bronchogenic cysts account for 40–50% of all mediastinal cysts [28]. Overall, bronchogenic cysts account for about 5–10% of all mediastinal pathologies [29]. Appropriate diagnosis and treatment of this disorder requires experience and expertise of a multidisciplinary team consisting of a thoracic surgeon, pulmonologist, and thoracic radiologist.

Bronchogenic cysts arise from abnormal budding of primitive foregut [30]. Development of human lungs starts around the fourth week of gestation with formation of a diverticulum from the ventral wall of primitive foregut. The distal end of lung bud divides into two parts forming right and left mainstem bronchi for each lung. Abnormal separation of a part of lung bud during this process leads to formation of bronchogenic cysts [31].

The cysts are located along tracheobronchial tree when the separation of bud occurs in early gestation. Nearly 75% of bronchogenic cysts are found in the mediastinum, most commonly in subcarinal and paratracheal locations [32]. Delayed separation of the lung bud is associated with the remaining 25% of bronchogenic cysts that develop within the lung parenchyma. Indeed, bronchogenic cysts are known to develop anywhere along the developmental route of the primitive foregut. Unusual locations for bronchogenic cysts include the pericardium, diaphragm, abdomen, stomach, pancreas, and skin. Bronchogenic cysts in the lung parenchyma need to be differentiated from lung abscess, hydatid cyst, infected emphysematous bulla, traumatic cyst, and tuberculosis. The treatment of parenchymal bronchogenic cysts is surgical resection. There is no role of interventional bronchoscopy procedures in these patients. Such is not the case with bronchogenic cysts located in the mediastinum. Our subsequent discussion will mainly focus on patients with mediastinal bronchogenic cysts.

While a majority is unilocular, some bronchogenic cysts are multi-loculated. Histological examination reveals ciliated pseudostratified columnar epithelial lining, similar to normal human airways. The cyst wall contains variable amounts of hyaline cartilage, smooth muscles, elastic fibers, fibrous connective tissue, nerve trunks, and bronchial glands [33]. It is not unusual for the cyst wall to have fibrous attachments with surrounding structures such as the esophagus, trachea, pleura, and pericardium. The majority of mediastinal cysts have no direct connection with an airway lumen. Infection and attempts at needle aspiration may lead to development of communication between the bronchogenic cyst and the tracheobronchial tree. The gross appearance of fluid in bronchogenic cysts is highly variable. It may appear milky and gelatinous; green and mucoid; brown, white, and translucent; and yellow and pus-like and serous [34]. In some instances, the cyst fluid is described as milk of calcium. Cytology reveals nonhemorrhagic fluid with bronchial epithelial cells and mucus. There are no neutrophils, lymphocytes, acid-fast bacilli, or malignant cells in uncomplicated cysts.

The clinical presentation of bronchogenic cysts is highly variable. The majority of pediatric patients experience symptoms of cough, stridor, acute respiratory distress, and respiratory infection [35, 36]. Compression of mediastinal structures such as central airways, pulmonary arteries, and cardiac chambers is a major concern in these patients. In adults, 30–70% of bronchogenic cysts are asymptomatic, discovered as an incidental radiological finding in the second to fourth decade of life [37].

Nevertheless, a majority of asymptomatic patients managed conservatively can be expected to develop symptoms at a future date. For instance, in one series, 24 of 37 (65%) of adults with a bronchogenic cyst developed new symptoms while being watched without any specific intervention [38]. Symptoms of bronchogenic cysts in adults are nonspecific and include chest pain, cough, dyspnea, dysphagia, and recurrent lung infections.

Complications of bronchogenic cysts among adult patients are reported in up to 25% of patients. These include central airway compression, superior vena cava syndrome, superimposed infection, airway fistula formation, and hemorrhage. Compression of mediastinal structures is more often seen in pediatric patients than in adults with bronchogenic cysts. The potential for future complications is the main argument for early surgical intervention in bronchogenic cysts in asymptomatic patients. An additional concern is malignant transformation of bronchogenic cysts [39, 40]. In an extensive review of literature, 5 of 683 (0.7%) of bronchogenic cysts were found to have malignant cells [41]. Though opinions may vary, such low risk of malignant transformation of bronchogenic cysts may not be clinically as important as previously thought [42].

Bronchogenic cysts are often detected as an incidental radiological finding [43, 44]. Chest radiographs may show round or oval densities in right paratracheal or subcarinal areas. However, plain radiographs have a low sensitivity and computed tomography is often needed for further evaluation. On CT, bronchogenic cysts are seen as circumscribed homogeneous masses with thin and smooth walls (Fig. 12.4a). The majority of mediastinal cysts are located in the middle mediastinum. Nearly one-half of these have a water density with CT attenuation values of 0–20 Hounsfield units [34]. Remaining cysts have a higher soft tissue attenuation values due to presence of mucus, protein, and calcium oxalate [45]. Superimposed infection and hemorrhage may also cause attenuation values as high as 120 Hounsfield units on CT in bronchogenic cysts. [46, 47]

Soft tissue density raises a concern for malignancy at the first sight. A contrast-enhanced chest CT is helpful in these patients. Soft tissue masses show inhomogeneous enhancement, whereas the uncomplicated bronchogenic cysts remain unchanged after administration of contrast agent. This is different for infected bronchogenic cysts that may demonstrate peripheral and sometimes inhomogeneous enhancement on post-contrast CT images. An air-fluid level in bronchogenic cysts indicates presence of infection or fistulous connection with the airway. Overall, a confident diagnosis of uncomplicated mediastinal cysts can be made with chest CT in up to two-thirds of all cases.

Magnetic resonance imaging (MRI) is also useful in patients suspected to have bronchogenic cysts. A marked increase in signal density similar to cerebrospinal fluid on T2-weighted images establishes the cystic nature of the lesion. Cysts containing serous fluid have a low density, and those with high protein fluid have a high signal density on T1-weighted images [48]. Gadolinium administration is not required. In one study, MRI correctly identified bronchogenic cysts in all nine patients previously thought of having solid or indeterminate lesions on CT imaging. This suggests that MRI may be superior to CT in assessment of bronchogenic cysts. However, for all practical purposes, CT remains the most widely used initial imaging modality in these patients.

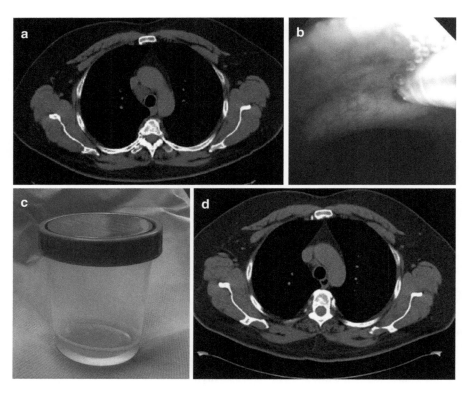

Fig. 12.4 (**a–d**): Chest CT (**a**) showing bronchogenic cyst in an asymptomatic patient. Patient initially declined surgery. He underwent a transbronchial needle aspiration (**b**) that yielded about 20 ml of straw-colored fluid (**c**). A repeat CT after the procedure showed a significant decrease in size of the cyst. After a few months, patient underwent successful surgery due to re-accumulation of fluid

A confident diagnosis on the basis of radiological findings cannot be made in every patient. In fact, in some series, a correct diagnosis on preoperative imaging was suspected in less than one-half of patients confirmed to have bronchogenic cysts after the surgery.

Management

Complete surgical removal is the most definitive therapy. There is limited role of bronchoscopic treatment in highly selected situations. Early consultation with a thoracic surgeon is strongly recommended.

Surgery for Bronchogenic Cysts

Complete surgical excision is recommended for all symptomatic bronchogenic cysts. Although there is some debate, most experts would also recommend surgical resection for asymptomatic bronchogenic cysts discovered incidentally. There are several arguments for recommending surgery in every case of bronchogenic cyst. These are (1) surgical exploration and excision of a cyst removes any doubts regarding accuracy of the underlying diagnosis; (2) most asymptomatic patients would develop symptoms and surgery would eliminate the future development of symptoms; (3) surgery is curative and eliminates any future risk of complications such as enlargement of the cyst, compression of mediastinal structures, infection, hemorrhage, and malignant transformation; and (4) surgery is easier and less complicated in asymptomatic patients than in symptomatic patients who have already developed a cyst-related complication such as infection, adhesions, and airway fistula [37, 38, 44, 49].

Thoracic surgeons approach mediastinal bronchogenic cysts located in paratracheal and subcarinal locations through either posterolateral thoracotomy or minimally invasively. Alternative approaches may be required for cysts located elsewhere in the mediastinum. The goal is to perform total enucleation of the cyst because delayed recurrence has been reported after incomplete excision. Stripping and removal of epithelial lining is an acceptable alternative when adhesions with the surrounding structures preclude total enucleation of the cyst.

Video-assisted thoracoscopic surgery (VATS) or robotic-assisted thoracic surgery (RATS) provides a less invasive approach to surgical removal of bronchogenic cysts and has become the preferred approach in many advanced medical centers [50, 51]. Complete excision was feasible in up to 95% of patients in some series. Conversion to formal thoracotomy is reported in a small proportion of patients [52]. The advantages of VATS or RATS approach are less postoperative pain, shorter hospital stay, lower complication rate, and better cosmetic results.

Role of Bronchoscopy

Bronchoscopic transbronchial aspiration is feasible for many mediastinal bronchogenic cysts [53, 54] (Fig. 12.4b–d). Successful aspiration can be achieved both with standard "blind" transbronchial needle aspiration (TBNA) and endobronchial ultrasound-guided transbronchial needle aspiration (EBUS-TBNA). One review on this subject identified 32 patients from 26 different studies who underwent TBNA procedure for bronchogenic cysts [55]. Nineteen of 32 patients were symptomatic at presentation. Cyst was located in paratracheal location in 14 patients. Aspiration was performed with therapeutic intent in 19 patients and diagnostic or palliative purpose in the remaining patients. Thirty-one cysts were drained using either conventional TBNA ($n = 16$) or EBUS-TBNA ($n = 15$). Complications were reported in five (16.1%) patients. Infection of mediastinal cysts was encountered in two patients. No recurrence was reported during a median follow-up period of 14 months.

On its face value, transbronchial needle aspiration may look like an attractive treatment option for mediastinal bronchogenic cysts. The procedure is technically straightforward and can be accomplished without much difficulty under conscious sedation. However, it would be a grave mistake to consider bronchoscopic aspiration as an alternative to surgery for definitive management other than in cases in which there is a contraindication to surgery. Transbronchial aspiration is not curative. Re-accumulation of fluid has been reported in prior reports. There is no information on incidence of future recurrence after bronchoscopic aspiration because long-term follow-up studies are not available. Most importantly, there is potential for introduction of infection in the cyst and mediastinitis that can be life-threatening. [56–58] Some investigators recommend routine administration of antibiotics prior to aspiration of mediastinal cysts to prevent this complication [59]. However, the efficacy of prophylactic antibiotics for aspiration of bronchogenic cyst has not been studied. In this regard, it is also important to stress that a routine practice of aspirating a bronchogenic cyst prior to surgical intervention to "confirm diagnosis" is ill-advised, and there is nothing to be gained with this practice.

So, what could be the role of bronchoscopic TBNA in bronchogenic cysts? We can think of three situations in which bronchoscopic TBNA could be offered to these patients. First, a rapid decompression of cyst with TBNA may provide immediate relief in distressing symptoms due to airway or cardiac compression by a large or enlarging bronchogenic cyst [60–62]. Acting as a bridge, bronchoscopic TBNA may allow definitive surgery in a more controlled setting in these patients. Second, bronchoscopic TBNA can be used for draining an infected mediastinal bronchogenic cyst [63, 64]. Effective drainage and antimicrobial therapy may control sepsis and pave the way for future resection of the cyst. Finally, bronchoscopic TBNA can also be offered to symptomatic patients who decline or are medically unfit to undergo surgery. A case can also be made for management of recurrent bronchogenic cyst with bronchoscopic aspiration after an incomplete prior surgical excision [65]. At least, a short-term relief from symptoms can be expected with bronchoscopic aspiration in a majority of these patients.

We cannot emphasize enough that extreme caution is needed before choosing bronchoscopic treatment over surgery. A particularly difficult situation arises when an asymptomatic cyst is detected in a patient who declines surgery or cannot undergo surgery for medical reasons. Bronchoscopic drainage can be offered to these patients. However, our recommendation is to watch these patients with serial imaging for a few months and perform bronchoscopic drainage only if the cyst increases in size or the patient develops symptoms.

Conclusion

Surgical removal is recommended for the majority of patients with mediastinal bronchogenic cysts. Surgery is diagnostic and curative in these patients. In highly selected situations, a temporary relief in symptoms can be accomplished with bronchoscopic aspiration of the cyst. Although the bronchoscopic approach is technically simple, it cannot be considered a viable alternative to surgery due to the potential for introducing infection and lack of information on long-term outcome with this therapy.

Lung Abscess

Lung abscess is a result of destruction of the lung parenchyma that leads to development of cavities filled with pus or necrotic material [66]. Patients with lung abscess present with cough, fever, and purulent sputum. Radiological imaging reveals air-fluid level in a cavity surrounded by variable degree of consolidation (Fig. 12.5). The majority of lung abscesses are due to aspiration of oropharyngeal secretions into the lung. Important predisposing causes are altered mental status, chronic alcoholism, poor dental hygiene, uncontrolled diabetes, malnutrition, swallowing disorders, and immunocompromised state. Airway obstruction due to lung cancer is also an important cause of lung abscess. An inhaled foreign body may also cause endobronchial obstruction and lung abscess in certain situations. The majority of primary lung abscesses due to aspiration of oropharyngeal contents are polymicrobial in nature. Oral anaerobic organisms are most often implicated [67]. Other important

Fig. 12.5 Chest radiograph showing a lung abscess in a patient presenting with cough, fever, and purulent sputum. All abnormalities resolved with a 4-week treatment with amoxicillin-clavulanic acid

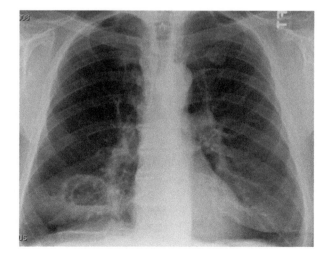

etiological agents include *Klebsiella pneumoniae*, *Staphylococcus aureus*, *Pseudomonas aeruginosa*, group A streptococcus, enteric gram-negative rods, and *Streptococcus pneumoniae*. Mycobacterium tuberculosis, endemic fungal infections, and parasitic infections should also be considered in certain epidemiological settings.

Lung abscess is a serious infection [68]. A review of 184 lung abscess cases in 1983 showed an overall mortality of 25% [69]. More recent experience suggests an improvement in survival, but a mortality of 5–10% can be expected in patients with lung abscess [70].

Antimicrobial therapy, postural drainage, and nutritional support are the mainstays of lung abscess treatment. The majority of lung abscess patients show clinical and radiological improvement with appropriate antimicrobial agents and supportive care [65]. Subjective improvement and resolution of fever can be expected in 7–10 days. However, 10–20% of patients fail to show clinical response. Suboptimal clinical and radiological response with 2 weeks of appropriate medical therapy should prompt a review of management strategy. Resistant or unusual organism, ineffective cough reflex, immunocompromised state, and endobronchial obstruction are the leading causes of treatment failure and poor outcomes in such patients [71].

Antimicrobial therapy must be reviewed and altered if resistant organisms are suspected or isolated. Drainage of lung abscess and surgical resection are important considerations in patients who are not responding to the therapy [72–74]. Drainage of lung abscess can be accomplished via percutaneous or bronchoscopic routes. Failure of drainage procedure is an indication for surgical treatment. Choosing the most appropriate intervention is a complex clinical decision. A multidisciplinary discussion is very helpful in selecting the most effective therapeutic approach.

CT-Guided Drainage in Lung Abscess

An important reason of treatment failure is inability to expectorate purulent contents of abscess cavity due to endobronchial obstruction secondary to inflammatory edema. CT-guided percutaneous drainage can be useful in such patients.

Several case series have reported usefulness of CT-guided drainage of abscess cavity in patients with poor response to antibiotics. In one study, CT-guided catheters were placed in 19 lung abscess patients who had persistent sepsis despite appropriate antimicrobial therapy. Clinical and radiological response was observed in all patients. However, three patients still required surgery. The procedure was complicated by hemothorax in one patient [75]. In another study, 40 patients with failed response to antibiotics underwent a CT-guided drainage [76]. Lung abscess resolved completely in 33 (83%) patients. Remaining seven patients required surgical intervention. The procedure was complicated by pneumothorax in five (12.5%) patients.

In a literature review that included 21 studies, data from 124 lung abscess patients undergoing percutaneous drainage were examined [77]. Treatment success was defined by control of sepsis, avoidance of surgical therapy, and improvement in radiological findings. Overall, 104/124 (83.9%) of study subjects has a successful treatment outcome with percutaneous drainage. Complication rate was 16.1%. Pneumothorax was the most common complication. Other complications included bleeding, hemothorax, and empyema. The overall mortality in this series was 4%. This is lower than 14–18% mortality reported after surgical therapy [78]. However, the mortality comparison between percutaneous drainage and surgical treatment is not valid because surgery is performed in more complicated and sicker patients, often after percutaneous drainage has already failed to achieve the desired clinical outcome.

Percutaneous drainage also provides specimens for microbiological studies which are helpful in choosing appropriate antimicrobial therapy. Antimicrobial therapy was modified in 43% and 56% of patients who underwent a percutaneous drainage of lung abscess in two separate studies [79, 80].

Unfortunately, in the absence of any controlled trials, the indications and timing of percutaneous drainage of lung abscess remain poorly defined. Failure of clinical response with 2 weeks of antimicrobial therapy, persistence of worsening of sepsis, and size of abscess >4–8 cm are accepted indications for consideration of CT-guided drainage. Similarly, how long to continue percutaneous drainage is uncertain and needs to be determined on case-by-case basis. Percutaneous drainage can be accompanied by persistent broncho-cutaneous fistula, which can result in the need for a prolonged drainage tube or the need for surgical procedures such as a Clagett window. Therefore, consultation with a thoracic surgeon prior to percutaneous drainage may facilitate long-term success and potentially avoid complications. Successful outcome in multi-loculated and thick-walled cavities is less likely, and in the absence of prompt clinical response, a surgical referral is indicated in these patients.

Bronchoscopy in Lung Abscess

Bronchoscopy was frequently performed for drainage of lung abscess in pre-antibiotic era [81, 82]. However, with availability of effective antimicrobial agents, a routine bronchoscopy is no longer indicated in all cases of lung abscess. In fact, extreme caution is warranted during bronchoscopy due to risk of sudden flooding of airways with purulent material in patients with lung abscess [83]. Nonetheless, in carefully selected patients, bronchoscopy has important diagnostic role in management of lung abscess. Less often bronchoscopy may also be used for drainage of lung abscess, especially in cases where an obstruction is present.

Diagnostic Role of Bronchoscopy

Bronchoscopy is indicated in patients with lung abscess when endobronchial obstruction due to tumor or airway foreign body is suspected. In a series of 184 patients with lung abscess, 7.6% of patients had proximal obstructing tumor [69]. In some instances, bronchoscopy is needed for collecting specimens for microbiological studies. Mostly, this is needed when patients are not responding to antimicrobial therapy and there is suspicion for tuberculosis and fungal or parasitic infections. Bronchoscopy is also indicated in lung abscess patients with significant hemoptysis. We also advise bronchoscopy in any patient who is being considered for percutaneous drainage or surgical therapy for lung abscess.

The most common findings on bronchoscopy in lung abscess are inflammation, swelling, and edema of the segmental bronchus leading to the abscess cavity. Purulent material may be seen in endobronchial tree. Mucosal friability and some granulomatous changes may be observed. In some patients, differentiating these changes from submucosal and endobronchial spread of tumor may not be possible without biopsies and careful follow-up.

Therapeutic Role of Bronchoscopy

There are limited data on the role of bronchoscopic drainage of lung abscess. As such, the concept of bronchoscopic drainage of lung abscess is not new. Several short series and case reports in the 1970s established feasibility of bronchoscopic drainage of lung abscess [84, 85]. However, in the absence of controlled studies, the indication and timing of such intervention remains poorly defined. Still, in carefully selected patients, bronchoscopic drainage of lung abscess provides an effective and minimally invasive approach to drainage of lung abscess not responding to antibiotic therapy (Fig. 12.6a–f).

Several studies have established technical feasibility of bronchoscopic drainage of lung abscess. For example, Rowe and associates used brush forceps and angiographic catheters to drain ten patients with lung abscesses [86]. Rapid clinical response was observed in all patients. Multiple microbial agents were cultured from the pus drained from abscess cavity. The complete resolution of abscess was observed in seven patients on radiological imaging 3 months after the procedure. No procedure-related complications were encountered. Similarly, Jeong and associates performed bronchoscopic drainage of lung abscess in 11 patients who did not show expected clinical and radiological improvement with antimicrobial therapy [87]. The cavity sizes ranged from 4 to 15 cm. The investigators introduced a flexible polyethylene catheter into the abscess cavity and aspirated pus with a 30-cc syringe. Six patients had significant clinical and radiological improvement. In those who

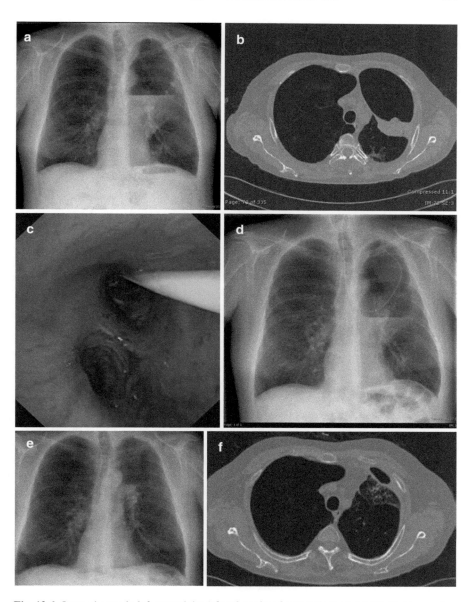

Fig. 12.6 Lung abscess in left upper lobe (after 6 weeks of antibiotic therapy) (**a**). Corresponding CT from the same patient (**b**). Bronchoscopic image of the pigtail catheter entering the left upper lobe (**c**). Chest radiograph showing the pigtail catheter within the abscess cavity (**d**). Chest radiograph (**e**) and CT (**f**) 6 weeks after bronchoscopic drainage. (Reprinted with permission from Herth [147])

responded, the abscess was larger than 8 cm, and air-fluid level was higher than 2/3 of abscess cavity. The amount of aspirate in these patients ranged from 20 to 110 ml. Useful diagnostic information was obtained in two additional patients. No complications were noted. In another report, Schmitt and associates described bronchoscopic placement of an intracavitary indwelling catheter prolonged irrigation and drainage of lung abscess in three patients [88]. The procedure was performed under fluoroscopic guidance. Resolution of infection was achieved in all three cases.

In the largest study on this subject, Herth and associates performed transbronchial drainage in 42 patients who were failing medical therapy for lung abscess [89]. The investigators placed pigtail catheters over guide wire into the cavity during bronchoscopy. The procedure was successful in 38 patients. The abscess cavity was flushed with gentamicin twice a day. All patients responded to therapy after a mean of 6.2 days. Two patients required transient mechanical ventilation. There were no other complications.

In a recent case series from Israel, 15 patients underwent 16 bronchoscopy procedures during which pigtail catheters were placed under fluoroscopy guidance [90]. An adequate drainage could be accomplished in 13 cases. The catheter was kept in the abscess cavity for a median of 4 days. Most patients responded clinically. One patient developed pneumothorax and empyema requiring chest tube drainage. Emergent surgery was needed in another patient who developed significant bleeding after the procedure.

There are isolated reports of using Nd:YAG laser to facilitate placement of catheter into abscess cavity. The experience is very limited and at present, this approach cannot be recommended due to potential risk of bleeding complications [91]. In one case report, argon plasma coagulation was applied to restore patency of airway that facilitated the bronchoscopic drainage of lung abscess [92]. Of great interest are recent reports of aspirating lung abscess using radial probe endobronchial ultrasound (R-EBUS) technology during bronchoscopy [93–96]. The technique is rather simple. After lung abscess is located with R-EBUS, the ultrasound probe is removed and the guide sheath is used to drain the pus from the abscess cavity. Microbiological analysis of drained material in these studies was found to be helpful in identification of causative organisms and choice of appropriate antimicrobial agents. All patients treated using this approach made full recovery without any procedure-related complications. In addition, the recent introduction of robotic bronchoscopy has facilitated the ability to place a scope into very distal airways under visualization, which has potential to allow for easier drainage and sampling. It remains to be seen if this is a practical application of the technology.

Based on review of current literature, it can be concluded that bronchoscopic drainage of lung abscess is technically feasible and clinically useful in many patients. The bronchoscopic approach is most suitable for patients who have a centrally located abscess with a bronchus leading to the abscess cavity. A decision to proceed with bronchoscopic drainage can be made after a multidisciplinary discussion in patients who are failing medical therapy.

Surgical Treatment of Lung Abscess

Surgery was the mainstay of lung abscess treatment before availability of antimicrobial agents [97]. In post-antibiotic era, surgery is needed in less than 10% of patients with lung abscess [69]. Surgery is most often performed when there is failure of both medical therapy and nonsurgical drainage procedures. Immediate surgery may be needed for patients with persistent bronchial obstruction due to lung cancer or embedded foreign body, major hemoptysis, and extension of infection to the pleural space [74]. Lobectomy is the most common surgery for lung abscess [98]. Some patients can be treated with segmentectomy. However, general medical condition, pulmonary reserves, and the very inflamed state of the thoracic cavity may not allow any form of resection in some patients. Cavernostomy can be considered in these patients. In this operation, the abscess cavity is opened and all purulent and infected material is removed. This is followed by immediate closures or marsupialization of cavity. In a cohort of lung abscess patients who required surgical intervention, 28 patients underwent surgical resection and 32 underwent surgical drainage (cavernostomy) [78]. The drainage procedure was performed in sicker patients who could not tolerate resection due to general medical condition. Drainage was also chosen over surgical resection due to technical reasons such as severe adhesions. The complication rate and mortality were 36.3% and 18.2%, respectively, in drainage group compared to 32.1% and 14.3%, respectively, in resection group.

When surgery is a consideration for suppurative lung disease, it is important to differentiate a lung abscess with a single large cavity filled with pus from necrotizing pneumonia and pulmonary gangrene. Lung abscess patients should have a trial of nonsurgical drainage if initial antibiotic therapy is not effective, as discussed above. A clinical and radiological response with this approach would obviate the need for surgery and over the next few weeks. Surgery should be considered when there is failure of clinical response to percutaneous or bronchoscopic drainage. Gangrene of the lung should be approached differently [99]. Radiological imaging in necrotizing pneumonia and pulmonary gangrene shows multiple abscesses within necrotic sloughing of the lung parenchyma [100, 101]. Clinical deterioration despite adequate antimicrobial therapy is a strong indication for surgical consultation in these patients [100]. CT-guided or bronchoscopic drainage has no role in such cases. Appropriate timing of surgery in these cases is a matter of clinical judgment, but it should be performed before development of septic shock or pleural extension of infection as much as possible [102, 103]. Emergent surgery including pneumonectomy has a lifesaving value in these patients [104].

Conclusions

Antimicrobial therapy remains the mainstay of treatment. However, 10–20% of patients who do not respond to the initial therapy require a drainage procedure. Percutaneous drainage is most often used initially, but recent experience has shown bronchoscopic approach to be as effective but safer in properly selected patients. There is an emerging role of R-EBUS in this regard. Nonsurgical drainage of lung abscess using these techniques has potential to reduce the need for surgical interventions and to improve patient outcomes.

Bronchial Carcinoid

Carcinoid tumors are a low-grade malignancy of neuroendocrine origin [105]. Overall, carcinoid tumors account for 2–3% of all malignant tumors of the lung [106]. The majority of carcinoid tumors arise from large central airways. About 10–15% of carcinoid tumors are peripheral in location [107].

Small localized peripheral carcinoids are most often discovered as an incidental finding on radiological imaging in asymptomatic patients. On chest CT, these are seen as smooth or lobulated solitary nodules in the lung parenchyma with a significant enhancement after administration of intravenous contrast. Central carcinoid tumors account for the remaining 85–90% of cases. As opposed to peripheral carcinoids, the majority of patients with central carcinoid tumors are symptomatic with recurrent post-obstructive pneumonia, cough, hemoptysis, wheezing, or atelectasis [108, 109]. Symptoms of carcinoid syndrome such as flushing, diarrhea, sweating, palpitations, and dizziness are very uncommon, seen in <2–5% of patients [110]. CT imaging in central carcinoids shows endobronchial tumor with or without additional findings such as distal atelectasis, or localized hyperinflation. In many instances, the tumor has a dumbbell shape with the main part of the tumor in the lung parenchyma and a smaller component within the airway lumen.

Histologically, carcinoid tumors are classified into typical carcinoid and atypical carcinoid [111]. Typical carcinoid tumors have 0–1 mitosis/mm^2 without necrosis. Atypical carcinoids are pathologically defined by ≥ 2 mitosis/mm^2 with associated focal necrosis. Atypical carcinoid tumors demonstrate a more aggressive biological behavior with greater tendency of metastasis to regional lymph nodes and other distal locations. Typical carcinoids are more indolent and have lower incidence of distal metastatic disease. At the time of diagnosis, up to 20% of patients with atypical carcinoid tumors have evidence of distant metastasis as opposed to less than 5% of patients with typical bronchial carcinoids.

In a recent review of data on 4111 patients with biopsy-proven lymph node-negative typical carcinoid tumor of the lung, 5-year overall survival after lobectomy, sub-lobar resection, and no surgery was 93%, 94%, and 69% respectively. Corresponding disease-specific survival was 97%, 98%, and 88%, respectively [112]. It is important to note that the distinction between typical and atypical carcinoid is possible only in surgically removed tumors. A confident distinction may not be possible on small biopsy obtained with bronchoscopy, as discussed below.

Role of Bronchoscopy in Diagnosis

Peripheral carcinoid tumors are most often diagnosed on histological examination of surgical specimen. A CT-guided biopsy has provided diagnosis in a handful of cases. Bronchoscopy is not helpful in diagnosis of peripheral carcinoids.

In contrast, bronchoscopy is most often used for diagnosis of central carcinoid tumors (Fig. 12.7). Airway inspection reveals a pink to red smooth and glistening endobronchial tumor partially or totally occluding the airway lumen. Some tumors are only loosely attached to the airway wall. Tumors are typically located in main-stem, lobar, or segmental bronchi. Carcinoid tumors are highly vascular. There are reports of excessive bleeding spontaneously or after endobronchial biopsies from carcinoid tumors [113]. The risk of bleeding with bronchoscopic biopsies has varied widely in different studies. For instance, in a series of 23 patients, moderate to severe hemorrhage was observed in 6 (26%) of patients after bronchoscopic biop-sies [114]. In another report, excessive bleeding was observed in 12 of 25 (48%) of patients with bronchial carcinoid after endobronchial biopsies. One patient required blood transfusion [115]. Due to this reason, there is some reluctance to perform endobronchial biopsies in suspected carcinoid tumors [116]. However, recent expe-rience indicates that the bleeding risk may not be as great as previously thought. For example, in a recent study, moderate to severe bleeding was encountered in 2 of 35 (5.6%) of patients undergoing bronchoscopic biopsies for central carcinoid tumors [117]. No patient required blood transfusion or emergency thoracotomy for uncon-trolled bleeding. The incidence of bleeding after biopsy in this study was very simi-lar to 5.9% bleeding risk in 454 similar patients reported in medical literature [117]. Most experts now agree that bleeding risk should not preclude attempts to obtain tissue diagnosis from suspected carcinoid tumors during bronchoscopy [110]. Nevertheless, it is prudent to have equipment and expertise readily available to man-age a large post-biopsy airway bleeding in these patients.

Diagnosis cannot be confirmed with bronchoscopy in every patient with bron-chial carcinoid. Diagnostic yield of bronchoscopy has varied from 50 to 70% in different studies [118]. In one series, incorrect diagnosis was given on initial bron-choscopic biopsies in 50% of patients later proven to have carcinoid tumors on surgical specimens [119]. In some instances, carcinoid tumor is mistaken for a small cell lung cancer due to presence of crush artifacts. Ki-67 cell proliferation labeling index is helpful in differentiating small cell lung cancers from carcinoid tumors [120]. In small cell lung cancer, the Ki-67 index is >50%, whereas it is $\leq$20% in carcinoid tumors. Small size of biopsy specimens also precludes a pathological dis-tinction between atypical and typical carcinoid tumors. Staining for Ki-67 is not helpful in this situation [121, 122]. It is particularly difficult to interpret biopsies from atypical carcinoid tumors. In one study, the majority of tumors identified to be atypical carcinoids after surgery were initially thought to be some other tumor on

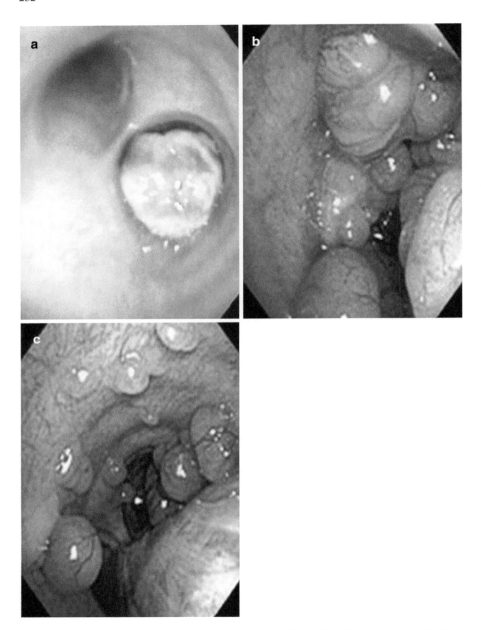

Fig. 12.7 Endobronchial carcinoid tumor completely blocking right main bronchus (**a**). Multiple atypical carcinoid tumorlets involving the trachea in another patient (**b, c**)

preoperative bronchoscopic biopsies [123]. There is interest in improving diagnostic yield of bronchoscopy using cryobiopsies in which the tissue specimen is larger than that obtained with usual forceps biopsies. In a small series, cryobiopsies provided diagnostic tissue in all five patients with bronchial carcinoids [124]. Excessive bleeding was not observed in any patient. The results from this study suggest a future role of cryobiopsies in bronchial carcinoids but more work is needed in this area. Clinical presentation in conjunction with a multidisciplinary discussion with a pulmonologist, thoracic surgeon, radiologist, and pathologist can facilitate treatment planning in cases where the diagnosis is unclear.

Treatment of Bronchial Carcinoid Tumors

Surgical resection is the current standard of treatment for localized bronchial carcinoid tumors. An important goal of surgery is to preserve as much lung parenchyma as feasible [119]. Systematic lymph node dissection or sampling is indicated to ensure appropriate staging and complete anatomic resection. Lymph node involvement is reported in up to 25% of patients with typical and 50% of patients with atypical bronchial carcinoids. Lobectomy and bi-lobectomy are the most common surgical procedures in many large case series [123, 125]. Pneumonectomy is performed in 3–10% of patients. Bronchial sleeve resection or a sleeve lobectomy to preserve the lung parenchyma is strongly preferred over pneumonectomy. A 5-year survival of >90% and a 10-year survival of >80–85% can be expected after surgery in patients with typical carcinoid tumors [116, 123, 126, 127]. Corresponding survival rates are 70% and 50%, respectively, for patient with atypical carcinoids. A multidisciplinary decision-making in diagnostic and therapeutic choices from the outset is associated with better patient outcomes.

Role of Therapeutic Bronchoscopy

There is interest in exploring interventional bronchoscopy procedures for definitive treatment of bronchial carcinoids strictly limited to endoluminal location without evidence of extra-luminal tumor, or mediastinal lymph node involvement. Several studies published over a span of more than two decades have explored this treatment option. Generally speaking, despite considerable progress in this area, bronchoscopic therapies have not replaced surgery for definitive therapy of bronchial carcinoids. There is little doubt that bronchoscopy has much to offer in symptom palliation in these patients. However, the idea of choosing interventional bronchoscopy over surgery as a stand-alone therapy in these patients has not gained widespread acceptance. In the following section, we examine the current literature on this subject.

In 1995, Sutedja and associates from the Netherlands used bronchoscopic therapies in 11 patients with intraluminal typical bronchial carcinoid tumors [128]. Six patients received Nd:YAG laser, one patient received Nd:YAG and photodynamic therapy, and four patients had mechanical debulking using rigid bronchoscope. Six patients who underwent surgical therapy after initial bronchoscopic therapies showed no residual tumor. Remaining five patients remained free of carcinoid over a median follow-up period of 47 months (range 27–246 months). Treatment-related bronchostenosis developed in one patient.

In a subsequent report, the same group highlighted the importance of high-resolution chest CT (HRCT) in selection of patients suitable for bronchoscopic therapies [129]. In this study, 18 patients underwent HRCT prior to bronchoscopic therapy. Nine of ten patients without evidence of peribronchial disease on CT remained free of tumor after bronchoscopic therapy. In five patients, HRCT showed peribronchial disease. Salvage surgery was needed in three of these patients after initial bronchoscopic therapy. HRCT findings were inconclusive in three patients. Absence of peribronchial invasion on HRCT was felt to be useful in selecting patients suitable for bronchoscopic therapy.

Cavaliere and associates reported treating 38 intraluminal carcinoid tumors without mediastinal lymph node enlargement with laser therapy [130]. Selection criteria in this study required tumor to be small (<4–5 cm^2), pedunculated or with implantation base <1.5 cm, and minimum or no infiltration of bronchial wall. Treatment was highly successful in 92% of patients over a median follow-up of 24 months.

In a study from the UK, 28 patients had mechanical removal of endobronchial carcinoid using a rigid bronchoscope [131]. An average of five treatment sessions was needed for complete eradication of the tumor. Patients were followed for a median of 8.8 years. One and 10-year disease-free survival was 100% and 94%, respectively. One patient had a recurrence 80 months after initial treatment and underwent a successful surgical resection. Significant hemorrhage was encountered in one patient but it could be controlled with local measures.

Bertoletti and associates used bronchoscopic cryotherapy to treat 11 patients with isolated endobronchial carcinoid tumors [132]. Both rigid and flexible bronchoscopes were used. Median follow-up period was 55 months. Only one patient had recurrence 7 years after initial therapy. No treatment-related complications such as bronchial stenosis were encountered. Several additional case series have reported similar experience with bronchoscopic therapy of bronchial carcinoids [133–136]. It is important to point out that initial bronchoscopic therapy does not seem to interfere with success of future resectional surgery in these patients.

Brokx and associates have recently reported an update on 112 patients with central carcinoids treated with bronchoscopic treatments [137]. Twenty nine (26%) of subjects had atypical carcinoid tumor. The minimal follow-up period was 5 years. Bronchoscopic treatment was curative in 42% of patients. Emergency pneumonectomy for uncontrolled bleeding was needed in one case. Five-year survival was 97%. Disease-specific 5-year survival was 100%. Overall and disease-specific 10-year survival was 80% and 97%, respectively. Recurrence on long-term follow-up was encountered in 7.8% of patients initially treated with bronchoscopic treatment. Salvage surgery was not adversely affected by prior bronchoscopic treatment in these patients. In a related report, a tumor diameter of <1.5 cm and the tumor strictly located within the bronchial lumen on computed tomography predicted treatment success on multivariate analysis [138].

Advocates of bronchoscopic therapy have made many pleas to consider it as an initial treatment in selected patients with central bronchial carcinoids [139, 140]. However, many experts and practice guidelines in this area do not agree with their view and continue to recommend surgical treatment for every patient with bronchial carcinoid [108, 109]. Whether bronchoscopic therapy is non-inferior to surgery in at least some of these patients can only be settled with a prospective randomized trial with a long-term follow-up [141]. Such a trial is not a realistic possibility anytime soon. It is worthwhile to recall that a majority of data on surgical therapy for this disease also comes from retrospective case series.

The experience with bronchoscopic treatments accumulated for over more than two decades is difficult to ignore. At a minimum, these data provide enough justification to pursue bronchoscopic therapies in patients who have localized endobronchial carcinoid but cannot tolerate lung surgery due to limited pulmonary reserves or associated comorbidities. Patient preference must also be taken into account with shared decision-making. One might add the caveat that bronchoscopic therapy must only be offered by experienced interventional pulmonologists after a thorough planning, multidisciplinary discussions, thoracic surgery backup, and detailed informed consent. Serious complications are uncommon but an occasional patient has needed emergency thoracotomy to manage severe bleeding. We have reported a case of cardiac arrest due to carcinoid crisis and coronary spasm in one such patient undergoing laser bronchoscopy [142].

The role of bronchoscopic treatment as an adjunct to definitive surgery has also been explored. For example, in one study, nine patients underwent bronchoscopic resection followed by surgical therapy [143]. Removal of endobronchial obstruction led to clearing of distal pneumonia in five study patients. Bronchoscopic treatment was also felt to improve pre-surgical status and allowed a less extensive lung resection in these patients. Similar experience was recently reported in 25 patients with endobronchial carcinoids [144]. Initial endobronchial resection of tumor allowed successful bronchoplasty in all study patients without needing any lung resection. High success with two-stage surgery in this report suggests an interesting future role of bronchoscopy alongside surgical treatment for central carcinoid tumors.

There cannot be much disagreement that bronchoscopy has a role in palliative therapy of central airway obstruction due to inoperable central carcinoid. Many inoperable patients have undergone bronchoscopic treatment with good control of symptoms. Bronchoscopic therapies can also be useful for disease recurrence in patients who had prior surgical therapy [145, 146].

In our view, bronchoscopic therapy for bronchial carcinoids is an important component of overall treatment paradigm, and it should be considered an adjunct or alternative rather than a replacement for surgical resection.

Conclusions

Bronchial carcinoids are low-grade malignant tumors of neuroendocrine origin. At presentation, the majority of bronchial carcinoids are localized to central airways. Surgery is the current standard of care for eligible patients. Bronchoscopic treatments may be considered in carefully selected patients after appropriate multidisciplinary discussion and detailed planning. A careful long-term follow-up including serial bronchoscopies and chest CT must also be established if bronchoscopic therapy with curative intent is chosen. Bronchoscopy also has an important role in palliation of symptoms in advanced and inoperable disease.

References

1. Seo JB, Song KS, Lee JS, et al. Broncholithiasis: review of the causes with radiologic-pathologic correlation. Radiographics. 2002;22:S199–213.
2. Arrigoni MG, Bernatz PE, Donoghue FE. Broncholithiasis. J Thorac Cardiovasc Surg. 1971;62:231–7.
3. Baum GL, Bernstein IL, Schwarz J. Broncholithiasis produced by histoplasmosis. Am Rev Tuberc. 1958;7:162–7.
4. Weeds LA, Andersen HA. Etiology of broncholithiasis. Dis Chest. 1960;37:270–7.
5. Galdermans D, Verhaert J, Van Meerbeeck J, et al. Broncholithiasis: present clinical spectrum. Respir Med. 1990;84:155–6.
6. Antao VC, Pinheiro GA, Jansen JM. Broncholithiasis and lithoptysis associated with silicosis. Eur Respir J. 2002;20:1057–9.
7. Kim TS, Han J, Koh WJ, et al. Endobronchial actinomycosis associated with broncholithiasis: CT findings in nine patients. AJR. 2005;185:347–53.
8. Henry NR, Hinze JD. Broncholithiasis secondary to pulmonary actinomycosis. Respir Care. 2014;59:e27–30.
9. Anwer M, Venkatram S. Broncholithiasis: incidental finding during bronchoscopy- case report and review of the literature. J Bronchol Intervent Pulmonol. 2011;18:181–3.
10. Dixon GF, Donnerberg RL, Schonfeld SA, Whitcomb ME. Advances in the diagnosis and treatment of broncholithiasis. Am Rev Respir Dis. 1984;129:1028–30.
11. Samson IM, Rossoff LJ. Chronic lithoptysis with multiple bilateral broncholiths. Chest. 1997;112:563–5.
12. Conces DJ, Traver RD, Vix VA. Broncholithiasis: CT features in 15 patients. AJR Am J Roentgenol. 1991;157:249–53.
13. Shaaban AM, Mann H, Morell G, et al. A case of broncholithiasis and esophagobronchial fistula. J Thorac Imaging. 2007;22:259–62.
14. Olson EJ, Utz JP, Prakash UBS. Therapeutic bronchoscopy in broncholithiasis. Am J Respir Crit Care Med. 1999;160:766–70.
15. Cerfolio RJ, Bryant AS, Maniscalco L. Rigid bronchoscopy and surgical resection for broncholithiasis and calcified mediastinal lymph nodes. J Thorac Cardiovasc Surg. 2008;136:186–90.
16. Lim SY, Lee KJ, Jeon K, et al. Classification of broncholiths and clinical outcomes. Respirology. 2013;18:637–42.
17. Noleff AS, Vansteenkiste JF, Demedts MG. Broncholithiasis: rare but still present. Respir Med. 1998;92:963–5.
18. Menivale F, Deslee G, Vallerand H, et al. Therapeutic management of broncholithiasis. Ann Thorac Surg. 2005;79:1774–6.

19. Brantigan CO. Endoscopy for broncholithiasis. JAMA. 1978;240:1483.
20. Ferguson JS, Rippentrop JM, Fallon B, et al. Management of obstructing pulmonary broncholithiasis with three dimensional imaging and Holmium laser lithotripsy. Chest. 2006;130:909–12.
21. Morris MJ, Anders GT, Cohen DJ. Management of recurrent broncholithiasis using the Nd:YAG laser. J Bronchol. 1999;6:25–8.
22. Snyder RW, Unger M, Sawicki RW. Bilateral partial bronchial obstruction due to broncholithiasis treated with laser therapy. Chest. 1998;113:240–2.
23. Reddy AJ, Govert JA, Sporn TA, Wahidi MM. Broncholith removal using cryotherapy during flexible bronchoscopy. A case report. Chest. 2007;132:1661–3.
24. Lee JH, Ahn JH, Shin AY, et al. A promising treatment for broncholith removal using cryotherapy during flexible bronchoscopy: two case reports. Tuberc Respir Dis. 2012;73:282–7.
25. Cole FH, Cole FH Jr, Khandekar A, Watson DC. Management of broncholithiasis: is thoracotomy necessary? Ann Thorac Surg. 1986;42:255–7.
26. Faber LP, Jensik RJ, Chawla SK, Kittle CF. The surgical implication of broncholithiasis. J Thorac Cardiovasc Surg. 1975;70:779–89.
27. Trastek VF, Pairolero PC, Ceithaml EL, et al. Surgical management of broncholithiasis. J Thorac Cardiovasc Surg. 1985;90:842–8.
28. Takeda S, Miyoshi S, Minami M, et al. Clinical spectrum of mediastinal cysts. Chest. 2003;124:125–32.
29. Bower RJ, Kiesewetter WB. Mediastinal masses in infants and children. Arch Surg. 1977;112:1003–9.
30. O'Rahilly R, Muller F. Chevalier Jackson Lecture. Respiratory and alimentary relations in staged human embros: new embryological data and congenital anomalies. Ann Otol Rhinol Laryngol. 1984;93:421–9.
31. Zylak CJ, Eyler WR, Spizarny DL, Stone CH. Developmental lung anomalies in the adult: radiologic-pathologic correlation. Radiographics. 2002;22:S25–43.
32. Patel SR, Meeker DP, Biscotti CV, et al. Presentation and management of bronchogenic cysts in the adults. Chest. 1994;106:79–85.
33. Limaiem F, Ayadi-Kaddour A, Djilani H, et al. Pulmonary and mediastinal bronchogenic cysts: a clinicopathologic study of 33 cases. Lung. 2008;186:55–61.
34. McAdams HP, Kirejczyk WM, Rosedo-de-Christensen ML, Matsumoto S. Bronchogenic cysts: imaging features with clinical and histolopathologic correlations. Radiology. 2000;217:441–6.
35. Ribet ME, Copin MC, Gosselin BH. Bronchogenic cysts of the lung. Ann Thorac Surg. 1996;61:1636–40.
36. Eraklis AJ, Griscom MT, McGovern JB. Bronchogenic cysts of the mediastinum in infancy. N Engl J Med. 1969;281:1150–5.
37. Cuypers P, Leyn PD, Cappelle L, et al. Bronchogenic cysts: a review of 20 cases. Eur J Cardiothorac Surg. 1996;10:393–6.
38. St. George R, Deslauriers J, Duranceau A, et al. Clinical spectrum of bronchogenic cysts of mediastinum and lung in the adults. Ann Thorac Surg. 1991;52:6–13.
39. Okada Y, Mori H, Maeda T, Obashi A, Itoh Y, Doi K. Congenital mediastinal bronchogenic cyst with malignant transformation: an autopsy report. Pathol Int. 1996;46:594–600.
40. Miralles Lozano F, Gonzalez Martínez B, Luna More S, Valencia RA. Carcinoma arising in a calcified bronchogenic cyst. Respiration. 1981;42:135–7.
41. Kirmani B, Kirmani B, Sogliani F. Should asymptomatic bronchogenic cysts in adults be treated conservatively or with surgery. Interact Cardiovasc Thorac Surg. 2010;11:649–59.
42. Ponn RB. Simple mediastinal cysts: resect them all? Chest. 2003;124:4–6.
43. Maier HC. Bronchogenic cysts of mediastinum. Ann Surg. 1948;127:476–502.
44. Aktogu A, Yuncu G, Halilcolar H, et al. Bronchogenic cysts: clinicopathological presentation and treatment. Eur Respir J. 1996;9:2017–21.

45. Nakata H, Nakayama C, Kimoto T, et al. Computed tomography of mediastinal bronchogenic cysts. J Comput Assist Tomogr. 1982;6:733–8.
46. Kuhlman JE, Fishman EK, Wang KP, et al. Mediastinal cysts: diagnosis by CT and needle aspiration. AJR. 1988;150:75–8.
47. Mendelson DS, Rose JS, Efremidis SC, et al. Bronchogenic cysts with high CT numbers. AJR. 1983;140:463–5.
48. Suen HC, Mathisen DJ, Grillo HC, et al. Surgical management and radiological characteristics of bronchogenic cysts. Ann Thorac Surg. 1993;55:476–81.
49. Sirivella S, Ford WB, Zikria EA, et al. Foregut cysts of the mediastinum: result in 20 consecutive surgically treated cases. J Thorac Cardiovasc Surg. 1985;90:776–82.
50. De Giacomo T, Diso D, Anile M, et al. Thoracoscopic resection of mediastinal bronchogenic cysts in adults. Eur J Cardiothorac Surg. 2009;36:357–9.
51. Guo C, Mei J, Liu C, et al. Video-assisted thoracoscopic surgery compared with posterolateral thoracotomy for mediastinal bronchogenic cysts in adult patients. J Thorac Dis. 2016;8:2504–11.
52. Jung HS, Kim DK, Lee GD, et al. Video-assisted thoracoscopic surgery for bronchogenic cysts: is this the surgical approach of choice? Interact Cardiovasc Thorac Surg. 2014;19:824–9.
53. Schwartz DB, Beals TF, Wimbish KJ, Hammersley JR. Transbronchial fine needle aspiration of bronchogenic cysts. Chest. 1985;88:573–5.
54. Schwartz AR, Fishman EK, Wang KP. Diagnosis and treatment of bronchogenic cysts using transbronchial needle aspiration. Thorax. 1986;41:326–7.
55. Maturu VN, Dhooria S, Agarwal R. Efficacy and safety of transbronchial needle aspiration in diagnosis and treatment of mediastinal bronchogenic cysts. Systematic review of case reports. J Bronchol Intervent Pulmonol. 2015;22:195–203.
56. Wildi SM, Hoda RS, Fickling W, et al. Diagnosis of benign cysts of the mediastinum: the role and risks of EUS and FNA. Gatroinest Endosc. 2003;58:362–8.
57. Gamrekeli A, Kalweit G, Schafer H, et al. Infection of a bronchogenic cyst after ultrasonography guided fine needle aspiration. Ann Thorac Surg. 2013;95:2154–5.
58. Onuki T, Kuramochi M, Inagaki M. Mediastinitis of bronchogenic cyst caused by endobronchial ultrasound. Respirol Case Rep. 2014;2:73–5.
59. Annema JT, Veselic M, Versteegh MI, et al. Mediastinitis caused by EUS-FNA of a bronchogenic cyst. Endoscopy. 2003;35:791–3.
60. McDougall JC, Fromme GA. Transcarinal aspiration of a mediastinal cyst to facilitate anesthetic management. Chest. 1990;97:1490–7.
61. Aragaki-Nakahodo AA, Guitron-Roig J, Eshenbacher W, et al. Endobronchial ultrasound guided needle aspiration of a bronchogenic cyst to liberate from mechanical ventilation. Case report and literature review. J Bronchol Intervent Pulmonol. 2013;20:152–4.
62. Nakajima T, Yasufuku K, Shibuya K, Fugisawa T. Endobronchial ultrasound guided transbronchial needle aspiration for treatment of central airway stenosis caused by mediastinal cyst. Eur J Cardiothorac Surg. 2007;32:538–40.
63. Casal RF, Jimenez CA, Mehran RJ, et al. Infected mediastinal bronchogenic cyst successfully treated by endobronchial ultrasound guided fine needle aspiration. Ann Thorac Surg. 2010;90:e52–3.
64. Bukamur HS, Alkhankan E, Mezughi HM, et al. The role and safety of endobronchial ultrasound guided transbronchial needle aspiration in the diagnosis and management of infected bronchogenic mediastinal cysts in adults. Respir Med Case Rep. 2018;24:46–9.
65. Gulluccio G, Lucantoni G. Mediastinal bronchogenic cyst's recurrence treated with EBUS-FNA with a long term follow up. Eur J Cardiothorac Surg. 2006;29:627–9.
66. Kuhajda I, Zarogoulidis Z, Tsirgogianni K, et al. Lung abscess-etiology, diagnostic and treatment options. Ann Transl Med. 2015;3:183.
67. Bartlett JG, Gorbach SL, Finegold SM. The bacteriology of aspiration pneumonia. Am J Med. 1974;56:202–7.

68. Harber P, Terry PB. Fatal lung abscesses: review of 11 years' experience. South Med J. 1981;74:281–3.
69. Hagan JL, Hardy JD. Lung abscess revisited. A survey of 184 cases. Ann Surg. 1983;197:755–62.
70. Moreira JS, Camargo JP, Felicetti JC, et al. Lung abscess: an analysis of 252 consecutive cases diagnosed between 1968 and 2004. J Bras Pneumol. 2006;32:136–43.
71. Hirshberg B, Sklair-Levi M, Nir-Paz R, et al. Factors predicting mortality of patients with lung abscess. Chest. 1999;115:746–50.
72. Wali SO, Shugaeri A, Samman YS, et al. Percutaneous drainage of pyogenic lung abscess. Scand J Infect Dis. 2002;34:673–9.
73. Raymond D. Surgical intervention for thoracic infections. Surg Clin N Am. 2014;94:1283–303.
74. Merritt RE, Shrager JB. Indications for surgery in patients with localized pulmonary infection. Thorac Surg Clin. 2012;22:325–32.
75. vanSonnenberg E, D'agostino HB, Casola G, et al. Lung abscess: CT-guided drainage. Radiology. 1991;178:347–51.
76. Kelogrigoris M, Tsagouli P, Stathopoulos K, et al. CT-guided percutaneous drainage of lung abscesses: review of 40 cases. JBR-BTR. 2011;94:191–5.
77. Wali SO. An update on the drainage of pyogenic lung abscesses. Ann Thorac Med. 2012;7:3–7.
78. Lee CH, Liu YH, Lu MS, et al. Pneumonotomy: an alternative way for managing lung abscess. ANZ J Surg. 2007;77:852–4.
79. Yang PC, Luh KT, Lee YC, Chang DB, et al. Lung abscesses: US examination and US-guided transthoracic aspiration. Radiology. 1991;180:171–5.
80. Duncan C, Nadolski GJ, Gade T, Hunt S. Understanding the Lung Abscess Microbiome: outcomes of percutaneous lung parenchymal abscess drainage with microbiologic correlation. Cardiovasc Intervent Radiol. 2017;40:902–6.
81. Clerf LH. Bronchoscopy in the treatment of pulmonary abscess and bronchiectasis. N Engl J Med. 1934;210:1319–21.
82. Pinchin AJ, Morlock HV. The Bronchoscope in the diagnosis and treatment of pulmonary diseases. Postgrad Med J. 1932;8:337–41.
83. Hammer DL, Aranda CP, Galati V, Adams FV. Massive intrabronchial aspiration of contents of pulmonary abscess after fiberoptic bronchoscopy. Chest. 1978;74:306–7.
84. Connors JP, Roper CL, Ferguson TB. Transbronchial catheterization of pulmonary abscess. Ann Thorac Surg. 1975;19:254–60.
85. Groff DB, Marquis J. Treatment of lung abscess by transbronchial catheter drainage. Radiology. 1973;107:61–2.
86. Rowe LD, Keane WM, Jafek BW, Atkins JP. Transbronchial drainage of pulmonary abscess with the flexible fiberoptic bronchoscopy. Laryngoscope. 1979;89:122–8.
87. Jeong MP, Kin WS, Han SK, Shim YS, Kim KY, Han YC. Transbronchial catheter drainage via fiberoptic bronchoscope in intractable lung abscess. Korean J Intern Med. 1989;4:54–8.
88. Schmitt GS, Ohar JM, Kanter KR, Naunheim KS. Indwelling transbronchial catheter drainage of pulmonary abscess. Ann Thorac Surg. 1988;45:43–7.
89. Herth F, Ernst A, Becker HD. Endoscopic drainage of lung abscesses: technique and outcome. Chest. 2005;127:1378–81.
90. Unterman A, Fruchter O, Rosengarten D, et al. Bronchoscopic drainage of lung abscesses using a pigtail catheter. Respiration. 2017;93:99–105.
91. Shlomi D, Kramer MR, Fuks L, Peled N, Shitrit D. Endobronchial drainage of lung abscess: the use of laser. Scand J Infect Dis. 2010;42:65–8.
92. Goudie E, Kazakov J, Poirier C, Liberman M. Endoscopic lung abscess drainage with argon plasma coagulation. J Thorac Cardiovasc Surg. 2013;146:e35–7.
93. Yaguchi D, Ichikawa M, Inoue N, et al. Transbronchial drainage using endobronchial ultrasonography with guide sheath for lung abscess: a case report. Medicine (Baltimore). 2018;97(20):e10812.

94. Izumi H, Kodani M, Matsumoto, et al. A case of lung abscess successfully treated by trans-bronchial drainage using a guide sheath. Respirol Case Rep. 2017;5:e00228.
95. Takaki M, Tsuyama N, Ikeda E, et al. The transbronchial drainage of a lung abscess using endobronchial ultrasonography with a modified guide sheath. Intern Med. 2019;58:97–100.
96. Miki M. Standard and novel additional (optional) therapy for lung abscess by drainage using bronchoscopic endobronchial ultrasonography with a guide sheath (EBUS-GS). Intern Med. 2019;58:1–2.
97. Schweigert M, Dubecz A, Stadlhuber RJ, Stein HJ. Modern history of surgical management of lung abscess: from Harold Neuhof to current concepts. Ann Thorac Surg. 2011;92:2293–7.
98. Hagan R, Delarue NC, Pearson FG, Nelems JM, et al. Lung abscess: surgical implications. Can J Surg. 1980;23:297–302.
99. Penner C, Maycher B, Long R. Pulmonary gangrene. A complication of bacterial pneumonia. Chest. 1994;105:567–73.
100. Catha N, Fortin D, Bosma KJ. Management of necrotizing pneumonia and pulmonary gangrene: a case series and review of literature. Can Respir J. 2014;21:239–45.
101. Curry CA, Fishman EK, Buckley JA. Pulmonary gangrene: radiologic and pathologic correlations. South Med J. 1998;91:957–60.
102. Reimel BA, Krishnadasen B, Cuschieri J, et al. Surgical management of acute necrotizing lung infection. Can Respir J. 2006;13:369–73.
103. Schweigert M, Dubecz A, Beron M, et al. Surgical therapy for necrotizing pneumonia and lung gangrene. Thorac Cardiovasc Surg. 2013;61:636–41.
104. Schweigert M, Giraldo Ospina CF, Solymosi N, et al. Emergent pneumonectomy for lung gangrene: does the outcome warrant the procedure. Ann Thorac Surg. 2014;98:265–70.
105. Wolin EM. Advances in the diagnosis and management of well-differentiated and intermediated differentiated neuroendocrine tumors of the lung. Chest. 2017;151:1141–6.
106. Rekhtman N. Neuroendocrine tumors of lung: an update. Arch Pathol Lab Med. 2010;134:1628–38.
107. Gustafsson BI, Kidd M, Chan A, et al. Bronchopulmonary neuroendocrine tumors. Cancer. 2008;113:5–21.
108. Caplin ME, Baudin E, Ferolla P, et al. Pulmonary neuroendocrine (carcinoid) tumors: European neuroendocrine society expert consensus and recommendations for best practice for typical and atypical carcinoids. Ann Oncol. 2015;26:1604–20.
109. Hendifar AE, Marchevsky AM, Tuli R. Neuroendocrine tumors of the lung: current challenges and advances in the diagnosis and management of well-differentiated disease. J Thorac Oncol. 2016;12:425–36.
110. Detterbeck FC. Management of carcinoid tumors. Ann Thorac Surg. 2010;89:998–1005.
111. Travis WD. Pathology and diagnosis of neuroendocrine tumors: lung endocrine. Thorac Surg Clin. 2014;24:257–66.
112. Raz DJ, Nelson RA, Grannis FW, Kim JY. Natural history of typical pulmonary carcinoid tumors. A comparison of non-surgical and surgical treatment. Chest. 2015;147:1111–7.
113. Ayache M, Donatelli C, Roncin K, et al. Massive hemorrhage after inspection bronchoscopy for carcinoid tumor. Respir Med Case Rep. 2018;24:125–8.
114. Todd TR, Cooper JD, Weissberg D, et al. Bronchial carcinoid tumors: twenty years experience. J Thorac Cardiovasc Surg. 1980;79:532–6.
115. Thomas R, Christopher DJ, Balamugesh T, Shah A. Clinico-pathologic study of pulmonary carcinoid tumors- a retrospective analysis and review of literature. Respir Med. 2008;102:1611–4.
116. Marty-Ane CH, Costes V, Pujol JL, et al. Carcinoid tumors of the lung: do atypical features require aggressive management. Ann Thorac Surg. 1995;59:78–83.
117. Dixon RK, Britt EJ, Netzer GA, et al. Ten-year single center experience of pulmonary carcinoid tumors and diagnostic yield of bronchoscopic biopsy. Lung. 2016;194:905–10.
118. Fink G, Krelbaum T, Yellin A, et al. Pulmonary carcinoid. Presentation, diagnosis, and outcome in 142 cases in Israel and review of 640 cases from the literature. Chest. 2001;119:1647–51.

119. El Jamal ME, Nicholson AG, Goldstraw P. The feasibility of conservative resection for carcinoid tumors: is pneumonectomy ever necessary for uncomplicated cases? Eur J Cardiothorac Surg. 2000;18:301–6.
120. Pelosi G, Rodriguez J, Viale G, Rosai J. Typical and atypical pulmonary carcinoid tumor overdiagnosed as small cell carcinoma on biopsy specimens: a major pitfall in the management of lung cancer patients. Am J Surg Pathol. 2005;29:179–87.
121. Pelosi G, Papotti M, Rindi G, Scrapa A. Unraveling tumor grading and genomic landscape in lung neuroendocrine tumors. Endcr Pathol. 2014;25:151–64.
122. Travis WD, Brambilla E, Nicholson AG, et al. The 2015 World Health Organization classification of lung tumors: impact of genetic, clinical and radiologic advances since 2004 classification. J Thorac Oncol. 2015;10:1243–60.
123. Schrevens L, vansteenkiste J, Deneffe G, et al. Clinical-radiological presentation and outcome of surgically treated pulmonary carcinoid tumors: a long term single institution experience. Lung Cancer. 2004;43:39–45.
124. Boyd M, Sahebazamani M, Ie S, Rubio E. The safety of cryobiopsy in diagnosing carcinoid tumors. J Bronchol Interv Pulmonol. 2014;21:234–6.
125. Bagheri R, Mashhadi MTR, Haghi SZ, et al. Tracheobronchopulmonary carcinoid tumors: analysis of 40 patients. Ann Thorac Cardiovasc Surg. 2011;17:7–12.
126. Filosso PL, Guerrera F, Evangelista A, et al. Prognostic model of survival for typical bronchial carcinoid tumors: analysis of 1109 patients on behalf of the European Association of thoracic surgeons (ESTS) neuroendocrine tumors working group. Eur J Cardiothorac Surg. 2015;48:441–7.
127. Machuca TN, Cordoso PFG, Camargo SM, et al. Surgical treatment of bronchial carcinoid tumors: a single center experience. Lung Cancer. 2010;70:158–62.
128. Sutedja TG, Schreurs AJ, Vanderschueren RG, et al. Bronchoscopic therapy in patients with intraluminal typical bronchial carcinoid. Chest. 1995;107:556–8.
129. Van Boxem TJ, Golding RP, Venmans BJ, et al. High-resolution CT in patients with intraluminal typical bronchial carcinoid tumors treated with bronchoscopic therapy. Chest. 2000;117:125–8.
130. Cavaliere S, Foccoli P, Toninelli C. Curative bronchoscopic laser therapy for surgically resectable tracheobronchial tumors: personal experience. J Bronchol. 2002;9:90–5.
131. Luckraz H, Amer K, Thomas L, et al. Long-term outcome of bronchoscopically resected endobronchial typical carcinoid tumors. J Thorac Cardiovasc Surg. 2006;132:113–5.
132. Bertoletti L, Elleuch R, Kaczmarek D, et al. Bronchoscopic cryotherapy treatment of isolated endoluminal typical carcinoid tumor. Chest. 2006;130:1405–11.
133. Brokx HAP, Risse EK, Paul MA, et al. Initial bronchoscopic treatment for patients with intraluminal bronchial carcinoids. J Thorac Cardiovasc Surg. 2007;133:973–8.
134. Fuks L, Fruchter O, Amital A, et al. Long term follow up of flexible bronchoscopic treatment for bronchial carcinoids with curative intent. Diagn Ther Endosc. 2009;2009:782961.
135. Neyman K, Sundest A, Naalsund A, et al. Endoscopic treatment of bronchial carcinoids in comparison to surgical resection: a retrospective study. J Bronchol Interv Pulmonol. 2012;19:29–34.
136. Dalar L, Ozdemir C, Abul Y, et al. Endobronchial treatment of carcinoid tumors of the lung. Thorac Cardiovasc Surg. 2016;64:166–71.
137. Brokx HAP, Paul MA, Postmus PE, Sutedja TG. Long-term follow up after first line bronchoscopic therapy in patients with bronchial carcinoids. Thorax. 2015;70:468–72.
138. Reuling EMBP, Dickhoff C, Plaisier PW, et al. Endobronchial treatment for bronchial carcinoid: patient selection and predictors of outcome. Respiration. 2018;95:220–7.
139. Reuling EMBP, Dickhoff C, Daniels JMA. Treatment of bronchial carcinoid tumors: is surgery really necessary? J Thorac Oncol. 2017;12:e57–8.
140. Van der Heijden EHFM. Bronchial carcinoid? Interventional pulmonologist first! Respiration. 2018;95:217–9.

141. Machuzak M. Can bronchial carcinoid be managed primarily with a bronchoscope? J Bronchol Interv Pulmonol. 2012;19:88–90.

142. Mehta AC, Rafanan AL, Bulkley R, et al. Coronary spasm and cardiac arrest from carcinoid crisis during laser bronchoscopy. Chest. 1999;115:598–600.

143. Guarino C, Mazzarella G, De Rosa N, et al. Pre-surgical bronchoscopic treatment for typical endobronchial carcinoids. Int J Surg. 2016;33:S30–5.

144. Pikin O, Ryabov A, Sokolov V, et al. Two-stage surgery without parenchyma resection for endobronchial carcinoid tumor. Ann Thorac Surg. 2017;104:1846–51.

145. Orino K, Kawai H, Ogawa J. Bronchoscopic treatment with argon plasma coagulation for recurrent typical carcinoids: report of a case. Anticancer Res. 2004;24:4073–8.

146. Katsenos S, Rojas-Solano J, Schuhmann M, Becker HD. Bronchoscopic long term palliation of a recurrent atypical carcinoid tumor. Respiration. 2011;81:345–50.

147. Herth FJF. Endoscopic lung abscess drainage. In: Ernst A, Herth FJF, editors. Principles and practice of Interventional Pulmonology. New York: Springer Science; 2012. p. 449–54.

Chapter 13
Undiagnosed Exudative Effusion: Thoracoscopy Vs. Pleuroscopy

Pyng Lee

Abbreviations

CXR   Chest radiograph
CT   Computed tomography
PET   Positron emission tomography
MRI   Magnetic resonance imaging
PF   Pleural fluid
CEA   Carcinoembryonic antigen
Cyfra Cytokeratin fragment
CNB   Closed pleural biopsy

Introduction

Medical thoracoscopy (MT), pleuroscopy, and video-assisted thoracic surgery (VATS) are terms used interchangeably to describe a minimally invasive procedure that provides the physician a window into the pleural space. They differ only in the approach to anesthesia. Stapled lung biopsy, resection of pulmonary nodules, lobectomy, pneumonectomy, esophagectomy, and pericardial windows are performed in the operating room with single-lung ventilation and rigid instruments, while others

P. Lee (✉)
Division of Respiratory and Critical Care Medicine, Department of Medicine, National University Hospital, Singapore

Yong Loo Lin Medical School, National University of Singapore, Singapore
e-mail: mdclp@nus.edu.sg

© The Author(s), under exclusive license to Springer Nature   243
Switzerland AG 2021
J. F. Turner, Jr. et al. (eds.), *From Thoracic Surgery to Interventional Pulmonology*, Respiratory Medicine,
https://doi.org/10.1007/978-3-030-80298-1_13

Table 13.1 VATS versus pleuroscopy

Procedure	VATS	Pleuroscopy
Where	Operating room (OR)	Endoscopy suite or OR
Who	Surgeons	Trained non-surgeons
Anesthesia	General anesthesia Double-lumen intubation Single-lung ventilation	Local anesthesia Conscious sedation Spontaneous respiration
Indications	Parietal pleural biopsy, pleurodesis, decortication, stapled lung biopsy, lung nodule resection, lobectomy, pneumonectomy, pericardial window, esophagectomy lung	Parietal pleural biopsy, pleurodesis, chest tube placement under direct visualization

have performed VATS wedge resection under regional anesthesia [1, 2]. Pleuroscopy is conducted by non-surgeon pulmonologist in an endoscopy suite under local anesthesia and conscious sedation (Table 13.1) [3, 4].

In 1910, Hans Christian Jacobaeus, a Swedish internist, described examination of the thoracic cavity using a rigid cystoscope attached to an electric lamp. His first two patients had exudative pleuritis and the procedure was referred to as "thorakoskopie." Jacobaeus later detailed lysis of pleural adhesions by galvanocautery that collapsed the underlying tuberculous lung also known as Jacobaeus operation for the lack of effective antituberculous drugs [5–7].

Pleural Effusion of Unknown Etiology

The first step toward investigating pleural effusion is thoracentesis. More than half of exudative effusions are due to malignancy [8], and although pleural fluid cytology is the simplest definitive method, its diagnostic yield depends on the extent of disease and nature of the primary malignancy [9]. Cytologic examination of the pleural fluid may be positive in 62% of patients with metastatic disease and less than 20% for mesothelioma [8, 9]. Repeated large volume thoracentesis increases the yield by 27% with a second aspiration, and a further 5% with a third [10]. The addition of closed pleural biopsy merely improves the yield by 10%, and is of little value for tumors confined to the diaphragmatic, visceral, or mediastinal pleura [11].

Contrast-enhanced CT is better than standard CT for the evaluation of the pleura, and features such as nodularity, irregularity, and pleural thickness greater than 1 cm are highly suggestive of malignancy [12, 13]. Higher diffusion coefficient values are also observed in epithelioid mesothelioma compared with sarcomatoid or biphasic types when dynamic contrast-enhanced MR imaging is performed [14]. Positron emission tomography (PET) with 18-fluorodeoxyglucose (18-FDG) is helpful for the detection of malignancy in patients with preexisting benign pleural pathologies so long as there is no infection, inflammation, or prior talc pleurodesis [15, 16]. Imaging of the pleura can be performed at the patient's bedside using US, and US is increasingly utilized to guide pleural procedures, particularly in the selection of appropriate sites for thoracentesis, tube thoracostomy, and thoracoscopy [17].

Ultrasonography (US) features of pleural thickening >10 mm, pleural nodularity, and diaphragmatic thickening >7 mm are diagnostic of malignancy with 73% sensitivity and 100% specificity [18]. "Echogenic swirling pattern" during respiratory or cardiac movements may be another US sign of malignant pleural effusion [19].

Pleural fluid (PF) biomarker carcinoembryonic antigen (CEA) conferred 94% specificity but poor sensitivity (54%) for malignancy [20]. Cytokeratin fragment (Cyfra) 21–1 combined with CEA increased sensitivity and specificity >90% [21], while Cyfra 21–1 and telomerase demonstrated 86.9% accuracy for malignancy [22]. BIRC5 mRNA and CEA appeared promising but would require clinical validation [23]. PF cytology has a poor diagnostic yield (32%) if mesothelioma is suspected [9]. PF and serum osteopontin levels showed low sensitivity and specificity for mesothelioma [24–26]. Serum-soluble mesothelin-related protein was also not useful in differentiating malignant mesothelioma from lung cancer and asbestosis [27]. In tuberculosis-prevalent areas, routine pleural fluid analysis might not reveal the underlying etiology of a lymphocyte-rich pleural effusion. VEGF and endostatin at cutoff values of 1.60 ng/ml and 4.00 ng/ml, respectively, might discriminate malignancy from tuberculous pleurisy with good sensitivity and specificity [28].

"Blind" or closed pleural biopsy (CNB) is the next step in investigating a cytology-negative exudate. CNB is cheap and still used in many institutions, but it is less sensitive than image-guided (CT or US) pleural biopsy or pleuroscopy due to patchy pleural involvement observed in malignancy, which also tends to affect inaccessible sites for biopsy (costophrenic recess and diaphragm). CNB increases the yield by 7–27% when combined with PF cytology. PF cytology and CNB increase the diagnostic yield for mesothelioma from 32% to 50% [29, 30].

In a randomized trial, CT-guided biopsy of pleural thickening >5 mm (Fig. 13.1) achieved 87% yield for malignancy versus 47% with Abrams needle [31]. US-guided biopsy of pleural lesions >20 mm with 14-gauge cutting needle gave 85.5% yield for malignancy, 100% for malignant mesothelioma, and 4% pneumothorax rate [32]. The type of needle appeared important: for malignancy, Tru-cut needle was superior over modified Menghini needle (95.4% vs. 85.8%) [33], and for tuberculous effusions, the Abrams needle was better than Tru-cut [34].

Fig. 13.1 Pleural nodularity due to metastases

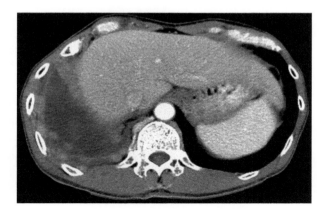

In cytology-negative pleural effusion, contrast-enhanced thoracic CT is recommended [29], but abnormal pleural appearances are not always seen on CT and biopsies can be negative. In a study where histological results obtained via medical thoracoscopy were compared against CT reported diagnoses, sensitivity for CT report of malignancy was 68% suggesting that a significant number of patients had malignancy despite negative CT report. Using CT alone to determine who should undergo invasive pleural biopsies must be re-evaluated, and studies defining the diagnostic pathway are now required [35].

Despite repeated thoracentesis, CNB, or image-guided needle biopsy, 20% of pleural effusions remain undiagnosed [36]. The primary advantage of thoracoscopy is to enhance our diagnostic capabilities when other minimally invasive tests fail [37]. If a neoplasm is strongly suspected, the diagnostic sensitivity of thoracoscopic exploration and biopsy approaches 90–100% [3, 4, 37–40]. Certain endoscopic characteristics, such as nodules, polypoid masses, and "candle wax drops," are highly suggestive of malignancy (Fig. 13.2); however, early stage mesothelioma can resemble pleural inflammation (Fig. 13.3) [3, 4, 36–38]. Additional image modalities may supplement pleuroscopic evaluation. Janssen and coworkers added autofluorescence to white light thoracoscopy for the evaluation of 24 patients with exudative pleural effusions [41]. The aims were to determine if the autofluorescence mode could differentiate early malignant lesions from nonspecific inflammation, aid in selecting appropriate sites for biopsy, and better delineate tumor margins for more precise staging. A color change from white/pink to red was demonstrated in all cases of malignant pleuritis (sensitivity: 100%). These lesions were more easily located and their margins more precisely delineated with autofluorescence thoracoscopy. In two cases of chronic pleuritis, a color change from white/pink to orange/red was also observed, giving a specificity of 75%. Although the authors concluded that there was little value of autofluorescence thoracoscopy in clinical practice, since most patients with malignant pleural effusions had extensive pleural involvement which was easy to diagnose with white light thoracoscopy, the autofluorescence

Fig. 13.2 Talc poudrage

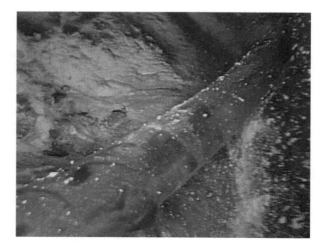

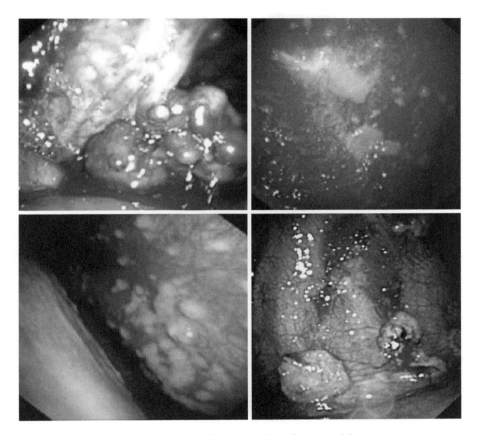

Fig. 13.3 Endoscopic findings of polypoid masses and candle wax nodules

mode might be useful when early pleural malignancies are studied. Similar conclusions were derived from a recent study that evaluated narrow band imaging (NBI) incorporated into the flex-rigid videopleuroscope (prototype Olympus XLTF 160). NBI technology uses unfiltered narrow bands in the blue (415 nm) and green (540 nm) light wavelengths that coincide with the peak absorption of oxyhemoglobin. By applying these wavelengths, NBI enhances the vascular architecture of tissues. In this study, all patients had malignant involvement of the pleura, of which nine were mesothelioma [42]. The authors did not find a difference in the diagnostic accuracy between NBI and white light videopleuroscopy (Fig. 13.4). We have had similar observations in 45 patients with pleural effusions of unclear etiology (unpublished data). In our cohort, 32 patients had pleural metastases, 12 had pulmonary tuberculosis, and 1 had chronic pleuritis, and all patients were followed for 12 months. Although NBI enhanced the pleural vasculature well, it was difficult to discriminate tumor neovascularization from inflammation based on vascular patterns. In patients with metastatic pleural malignancy, NBI demarcated tumor margins clearly, but there was no difference in the quality of biopsies obtained with

Fig. 13.4 Sago nodules of
tuberculous effusion

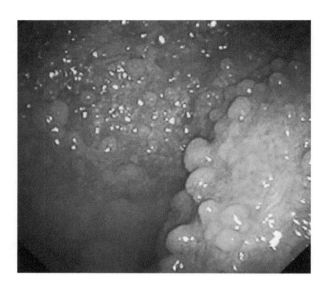

white light versus NBI. Baas and coworkers investigated if prior administration of
5-aminolaevulinic acid (ALA) before VATS could lead to the improved detection
and staging of thoracic malignancy. In this study, patients were given 5-ALA by
mouth 3–4 hours before VATS. The pleural cavity was then examined using white
light followed by fluorescence thoracoscopy (D-light Autofluorescence System,
Karl Storz, Germany). Tissue sampling of all abnormal areas was performed, and
histological diagnoses were compared against thoracoscopic findings. The fluorescence mode did not provide a superior diagnostic accuracy over white light, but led
to upstaging in 4 of 15 patients with mesothelioma due to better visualization of
visceral pleural lesions that were otherwise undetectable by white light. Several
postoperative complications were reported, but the authors concluded that fluorescence thoracoscopy using 5-ALA was feasible with minimal side effects, and it
could have potential applications in the diagnosis and staging of mesothelioma [43].

Pleuroscopy

Pleuroscopy allows inspection of the pleural cavity, guides biopsy of abnormal
pleural lesions, and removes PF and allows pleurodesis. Pooled results of 22 studies
confirm medical thoracoscopy as the procedure with the highest accuracy (93%) for
the diagnosis of pleural malignancy [37].

Historically, rigid instruments have been used [1–7, 37, 40] that require cold
(xenon) light source, camera attached to the eyepiece of the telescope, video monitor, and recorder (Fig. 13.5). The O-degree telescope is used for direct viewing,
while the oblique (30- or 50-degree) and 90-degree telescopes offer panoramic
view of the pleural cavity. A large trocar that accommodates a larger telescope with
better optics improves the quality of exploration, but compression of the intercostal

Fig. 13.5 Rigid trocars, telescopsses, and accessories

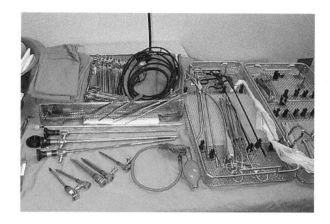

nerve during manipulation can cause discomfort if thoracoscopy is performed under local anesthesia and conscious sedation. We prefer the 7-mm trocar, direct viewing (0 degree) 4-mm or 7-mm telescope, and the 5-mm optical forceps that allow pleural biopsies without a second port. Tassi and coworkers reported excellent views of the pleural space using 3.3-mm telescope in patients with small loculated pleural effusions inaccessible to standard-sized instruments. Diagnostic yield with 3-mm biopsy forceps was comparable with conventional 5-mm biopsy forceps [40].

The flexi-rigid pleuroscope represents a major advance in the field as it allows the procedure to be performed safely in the bronchoscopy suite under local anesthesia and conscious sedation [44, 45]. The flex-rigid pleuroscope (model LTF 160, Olympus, Japan) is fashioned like the flexible bronchoscope and can be autoclaved. It consists of a handle and shaft measuring 7 mm in outer diameter, 22-cm proximal rigid portion, and 5-cm flexible distal end. The flexible tip allows two-way angulation and has a 2.8-mm working channel that accommodates biopsy forceps, needles, and electrosurgical and laser accessories (Fig. 13.6). The flex-rigid pleuroscope interfaces well with processors (CV-160, CLV-U40) and light sources (CV-240, EVIS-100 or 140, EVIS EXERA-145 or 160) made by the same manufacturer for flexible bronchoscopy or GI endoscopy [39]. Recent meta-analysis of 744 patients undergoing flex-rigid pleuroscopy demonstrates 91% sensitivity and 100% specificity for pleural malignancy [46].

Indications and Contraindications for Medical Thoracoscopy

The only absolute contraindication for pleuroscopy is the lack of pleural space due to adhesions although this can be overcome by enlarging the skin incision and digitally dissecting the lung away from the chest wall [47]. MT requires special skills and should not be undertaken without training. As the procedure is performed under conscious sedation in a spontaneously breathing patient with partial lung collapse,

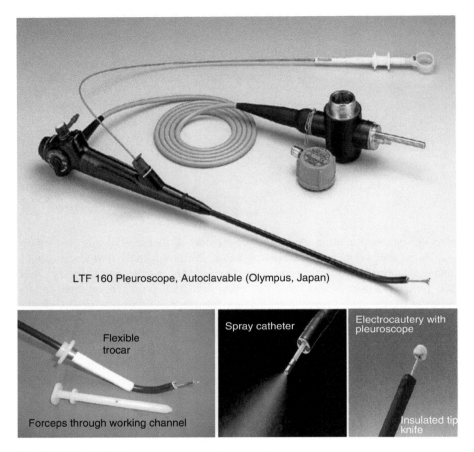

Fig. 13.6 Flex-rigid pleuroscope, trocar, and accessories

these patients must not have intolerable hypoxia unrelated to pleural effusion, an unstable cardiovascular status, bleeding diathesis, refractory cough, or allergy to the medications used.

Patient Preparation

A detailed history and physical examination together with review of CXR, CT, and US aid in the selection of appropriate entry site. The operator may remove 200 to 300 ml of fluid with angiocatheter, thoracentesis catheter, or Boutin pleural puncture needle first before opening the needle to air until stable equilibrium is achieved. Air entering the pleural cavity causes the lung to collapse away from the chest wall, thereby creating a space for trocar insertion. Conversely, the operator may choose to do the procedure directly with US, which has led to decrease in trocar access failures as well as in the number of pneumothoraces induced before pleuroscopy [48, 49].

Anesthesia

Benzodiazepines (midazolam) combined with opioids (Demerol, fentanyl, morphine) provide adequate analgesia and sedation [38, 39, 44]. Meticulous care in administering local anesthesia to the four layers (epidermis, aponeurosis, intercostal muscles, and parietal pleura at the entry site) assures patient comfort during manipulation of the thoracoscope [50]. There is a trend in recent years toward increasing utilization of propofol to enhance patient comfort if talc poudrage is planned; however, this requires monitoring by anesthesiologists in many countries and a recent study reported hypotension in 64% of patients who had propofol titrated according to comfort and 9% required corrective measures [51]. In another study, more episodes of hypoxemia (27% vs. 4%) and hypotension (82% vs. 40%) were observed in the group who received propofol compared against midazolam leading the authors to remark that propofol should not be the first choice for sedation in medical thoracoscopy [52]. We have successfully performed thoracoscopic talc poudrage for pneumothoraces and malignant effusions using benzodiazepines and opioids and anesthetizing the pleura with 250 mg of 1% lidocaine via a spray catheter prior to talc [53]. Preoperative anesthesia should be individualized according to the patient's general condition and expectations; however, physicians must be aware of potential adverse events associated with anesthetic drugs and be ready to manage them.

Technique

The patient is first placed in the lateral decubitus position with the affected side up. The patient's vital parameters, electrocardiogram (ECG), blood pressure, and oxygenation by means of pulse oximetry are monitored. The site of entry depends on the location of effusion or pneumothorax while avoiding hazardous areas such as the internal mammary artery, the axillary region with lateral thoracic artery, the infraclavicular region with the subclavian artery, and the diaphragm. A single port access located between the fourth and seventh intercostal spaces of the chest wall and along the midaxillary line is preferred for diagnostic pleuroscopy, guided pleural biopsy, and talc poudrage. A second port might be necessary to facilitate adhesiolysis, drainage of complex loculated fluid collections, lung biopsy, or sampling of pathological lesions located around the first entry site. Similarly, double port access may be necessary to evaluate the pleural space completely when the rigid telescope is used, especially if the posterior and mediastinal aspects of the hemithorax are inaccessible due to partial collapse of the lung, or when the lung parenchyma is adherent to the chest wall [4]. With the flex-rigid pleuroscope, a single port would often suffice since its nimble tip allows easy maneuverability within a limited pleural space and around adhesions. A chest tube is inserted at the end of diagnostic pleuroscopy, and the air is aspirated. The tube is removed as soon as the lung has re-expanded, and the patient may be discharged after a brief observation in a recovery area [54]. If talc pleurodesis or lung biopsy is performed, the patient is hospitalized for a period of monitoring and chest tube drainage [44, 45, 53].

Thoracoscopic-Guided Biopsy of Parietal Pleura

Biopsy of the parietal pleura should be performed over a rib to avoid the neurovascular bundle. The forceps first probes for the rib followed by grasping the abnormal pleura and stripped by tearing rather than "grab and pull" motion. The specimens are not only larger than those with Abram's or Cope needle; importantly, they are visually guided. Biopsies with the flexible forceps are limited by the size of forceps which may lack the mechanical strength in obtaining pleural specimens of sufficient depth if fibrotic pleura is encountered. This can be overcome by taking multiple biopsies (5–10) as well as several "bites" of the same area to obtain tissue of sufficient depth. Comparative studies show no difference in diagnostic yield between biopsies using flexible and rigid forceps even in mesothelioma [55, 56]. Full-thickness parietal pleural biopsies can be achieved using the insulated tip (IT) diathermic knife during flex-rigid pleuroscopy. In one study, the reported diagnostic yields were 85% with IT knife and 60% with flexible forceps. The IT knife was notably useful when smooth, thickened lesions were encountered, of which nearly half were malignant mesothelioma [57]. Cryobiopsy is another method that achieves bigger specimens and better preserved cellular architecture and tissue integrity [58] (Table 13.2).

Thoracoscopic Talc Poudrage

Chemical pleurodesis plays an integral role in the management of malignant effusions as most recur unless the primary tumor is chemosensitive. Similarly, one of the primary goals in secondary spontaneous pneumothorax management is recurrence prevention. Chemical pleurodesis can be performed via instillation of sclerosants through intercostal tubes or small-bore catheters, or via talc poudrage during thoracoscopy [59]. Chemical pleurodesis via chest drain using various agents succeeds in approximately 60% of patients with the remainder requiring further intervention. Thoracoscopic talc poudrage (Fig. 13.2) can be performed following fluid aspiration and pleural biopsy at the same sitting, and pooled data from 19 studies suggest that the efficacy of thoracoscopic talc poudrage at 1 month based on radiology is about 85% for both benign and malignant causes of effusion [37]. Various delivery devices are available such as a talc spray atomizer, a bulb syringe, or a spray catheter introduced through the working channel of the flex-rigid pleuroscope.

Complications

Mortality from MT using rigid instruments ranges between 0.09 and 0.34% [37, 60]. Talc poudrage is associated with 0.69% mortality, and a major contribution (9 deaths out of 16) was from a large randomized study conducted in the USA using

Table 13.2 Diagnostic tools for pleural disease in lung cancer

Diagnostic tool	Clinical use	Notes
Pleural imaging		
Ultrasound [14]	Ultrasonographic features indicative of malignancy include the following: Pleural thickening >1 cm, pleural nodularity and diaphragmatic thickening >7 mm	Sensitivity 73%, specificity 100%
CT-guided cutting needle biopsy	Diagnosis of malignancy in pleural-based lesions 5 mm or greater	Sensitivity 87%
Ultrasound-guided cutting needle biopsy	Diagnosis of malignancy in pleural-based lesions 20 mm or greater	Sensitivity 85.5% (100% for mesothelioma)
Tru-cut needle	Sampling of pleural nodules/masses for histopathology	Superior to Menghini-type needle
Pleural diagnosis		
Flexi-rigid pleuroscopy	Pleural cavity inspection. Direct sampling of pleural nodules/masses for histopathology	Done under local anesthesia
Autofluorescence for thoracoscopy	To detect and direct biopsies at abnormal sites not visible with conventional white light	Sensitivity 100%, specificity 75%
Fluorescence detection for thoracoscopy	To detect and direct biopsies at abnormal sites not visible with conventional white light	5-Aminolaevulinic acid taken orally before procedure
Narrow band imaging for thoracoscopy	To detect and direct biopsies at abnormal sites not visible with conventional white light	Specificity 85.3%, specificity 76.9%
Electrocautery biopsy [56]	Adjunct to flexi-rigid pleuroscopy forceps biopsy of smooth abnormal pleura	Diagnostic yield 85%
Cryobiopsy [57]	Adjunct to flexi-rigid pleuroscopy forceps biopsy	Diagnostic yield 90%
Pleural biomarkers* assayed	*From pleural fluid*	
Carcinoembryonic antigen [18]	Distinguish malignant pleural effusion from benign causes	Sensitivity 54%, specificity 94%
Carcinoembryonic antigen with Cyfra 21–1 [19]	Distinguish lung adenocarcinoma-associated malignant pleural effusion from benign causes	Sensitivity 97.6%, specificity 91.4%
Telomerase with Cyfra 21–1 [20]	Distinguish lung cancer-associated malignant pleural effusion from benign causes	Sensitivity 90%, specificity 76%
Carcinoembryonic antigen and BIRC5 mRNA [21]	Distinguish malignant pleural effusion from benign causes	Sensitivity 86.4%
Soluble mesothelin-related peptide (serum) [23–25]	Diagnosis of mesothelioma	Sensitivity 53–60%, specificity 82–89%
Vascular endothelial growth factor and endostatin [26]	Distinguish malignant pleural effusion from tuberculous pleurisy	Sensitivity 81%, specificity 97%

nongraded talc [61]. Major complications (prolonged air leak, hemorrhage, empyema, pneumonia, and port site tumor growth) occurred in 1.8%, while minor complications (subcutaneous emphysema, wound infection, fever, hypotension, and cardiac arrhythmias during the procedure) occurred in 7.3% [62].

The most serious complication of pneumothorax induction is air embolism which occurs in <0.1 percent [60]. During MT, liters of fluid can be removed with little risk of re-expansion pulmonary edema due to immediate equilibration of pressures provided by entry of air through the trocar into the pleural space. Fever may occur after talc poudrage which resolves within 48 hours, while a bronchopleural fistula may develop following thoracoscopic lung biopsy requiring chest drain and suction for longer than 3–5 days especially if biopsy is performed for interstitial lung disease. Wound infection, pneumonia, and empyema can develop from long-term drainage. In cases of mesothelioma, prophylactic radiotherapy should be carried out within 2 weeks of medical thoracoscopy to prevent tumor growth at incision sites [63].

Complications with the flex-rigid pleuroscope are rare. In fact, it has been shown to be very safe when performed by trained pulmonologists. We previously reported our safety and outcome results in 51 patients with indeterminate pleural effusions who underwent flex-rigid pleuroscopy. No morbidity or mortality was observed [44]. In a recent meta-analysis of 755 patients with indeterminate pleural effusions, no mortality was reported [46]. However, studies of complication rates involve procedures performed by specialists and may not reflect circumstances with less experienced physicians. The need for training cannot be overemphasized. Table 13.3 describes the type of patient suitable for rigid or flex-rigid pleuroscopy.

Table 13.3 Indications for rigid or semi-rigid pleuroscopy

Clinical scenario	Type of procedure
Diagnostic thoracoscopy for indeterminate, uncomplicated pleural effusion where suspicion of mesothelioma is not high	Flex-rigid pleuroscopy[a] or use of rigid telescopes under local anesthesia
Trapped lung with radiographically thickened pleura	Rigid optical biopsy forceps[a] or flex-rigid pleuroscopy with flexible forceps performing multiple bites over the same area to obtain specimens of sufficient depth or use of flexible forceps and IT knife
Mesothelioma is suspected	Rigid optical biopsy forceps[a] or flex-rigid pleuroscopy with IT knife, cryoprobe
Pleuropulmonary adhesions	Fibrous: Rigid optical biopsy forceps[a] or flex-rigid pleuroscopy with electrocautery accessories Thin, fibrinous: Flex-rigid pleuroscopy with flexible forceps
Empyema, split pleural sign, loculated pleural effusion	Rigid instruments (VATS)[a] or conversion to thoracotomy for decortication
Pneumothorax with bulla or blebs	Rigid instruments (VATS)[a] for staple bullectomy

[a]denotes procedure preferred

Conclusion

Pleuroscopy or thoracoscopy is effective when routine PF cytology fails. In institutions where pleuroscopy/thoracoscopy is available, it replaces second-attempt thoracentesis and CNB. It also offers the non-surgeon to intervene therapeutically and to break down loculations in early empyemas and talc pleurodesis for recurrent malignant effusion and pneumothorax [64]. The flex-rigid pleuroscope is a significant invention likely to replace traditional biopsy methods in the future.

References

1. McKenna RJ Jr. Thoracoscopic evaluation and treatment of pulmonary disease. Surg Clin North Am. 2002;80:1543–53.
2. Rocco G, Romano V, Accardo R, et al. Awake single-access (uniportal) videoassisted thoracoscopic surgery for peripheral pulmonary nodules in a complete ambulatory setting. Ann Thorac Surg. 2010;89:1625–7.
3. Lee P, Mathur PN, Colt HG. Advances in thoracoscopy: 100 years since Jacobaeus. Respiration. 2010;79:177–86.
4. Tassi GF, Davies RJ, Noppen M. Advanced techniques in medical thoracoscopy. Eur Respir J. 2006;28:1051–9.
5. Moisiuc FV, Colt HG. Thoracoscopy: origins revisited. Respiration. 2007;74:344–55.
6. Jacobaeus HC. Uber die Moglichkeit, die Zystoskopie bei Untersuchungen seroser Hohlungenanzuwenden. MunchMed Wschr. 1910;40:2090–2.
7. Jacobaeus HC. The practical importance of thoracoscopy in surgery of the chest. Surg Gynecol Obstet. 1922;34:289–96.
8. Hsu C. Cytologic detection of malignancy in pleural effusion: a review of 5,255 samples from 3,811 patients. Diag Cytopathol. 1987;3:8–12.
9. Renshaw AA, Dean BR, Antman KH, Sugarbaker DJ, Cibas ES. The role of cytologic evaluation of pleural fluid in the diagnosis of malignant mesothelioma. Chest. 1997;111:106–9.
10. Starr RL, Sherman ME. The value of multiple preparations in the diagnosis of malignant pleural effusions: a cost-benefit analysis. Acta Cytol. 1991;35:533–7.
11. Canto A, Ferrer G, Ramagosa V, Moya J, Bernat R. Lung cancer and pleural effusion: clinical significance and study of pleural metastatic locations. Chest. 1985;87:649–51.
12. Leung AN, Mueller NL, Miller RR. CT in differential diagnosis of diffuse pleural disease. AJR. 1990;154:487–92.
13. Traill ZC, Davies RJ, Gleeson FV. Thoracic computed tomography in patients with suspected malignant pleural effusions. Clin Radiol. 2001;56:193–6.
14. Gill RR, Umeoka S, Mamata H, Tilleman TR, Stanwell P, Woodhams R, et al. Diffusion-weighted MRI of malignant pleural mesothelioma: preliminary assessment of apparent diffusion coefficient in histologic subtypes. AJR Am J Roentgenol. 2010;195:125–30.
15. Otsuka H, Terazawa K, Morita N, Otomi Y, Yamashita K, Nishitani H. Is FDG-PET/CT useful for managing malignant pleural mesothelioma? J Med Investig. 2009;56:16–20.
16. Shim HS, Park IK, Lee CY, Chung KY. Prognostic significance of visceral pleural invasion in the forthcoming (seventh) edition of TNM classification for lung cancer. Lung Cancer. 2009;65:161–5.
17. Hersh CP, Feller-Kopman D, Wahidi M, Garland R, Herth F, Ernst A. Ultrasound guidance for medical thoracoscopy: a novel approach. Respiration. 2003;70:299–301.

18. Qureshi NR, Rahman NM, Gleeson FV. Thoracic ultrasound in the diagnosis of malignant pleural effusion. Thorax. 2009;64:139–43.
19. Chian CF, Su WL, Soh LH, Yan HC, Perng WC, Wu CP. Echogenic swirling pattern as a predictor of malignant pleural effusions in patients with malignancies. Chest. 2004;126:129–34.
20. Shi HZ, Liang QL, Jiang J, Qin XJ, Yang HB. Diagnostic value of carcinoembryonic antigen in malignant pleural effusion: a meta-analysis. Respirology. 2008;13:518–27.
21. Huang WW, Tsao SM, Lai CL, Su CC, Tseng CE. Diagnostic value of Her-2/Neu, Cyfra 21-1, and carcinoembryonic antigen levels in malignant pleural effusions of lung adenocarcinoma. Pathology. 2010;42:224–8.
22. Li H, Fu J, Xiu Y, Zhou Q. Diagnostic significance of combining telomerase activity with Cyfra21-1 level in differentiating malignant pleural effusion caused by lung cancer from benign pleural effusion. Zhongguo Fei Ai Za Zhi. 2010;13:652–4.
23. Wang T, Qian X, Wang Z, Wang L, Yu L, Ding Y, et al. Detection of cell-free birc5 Mrna in effusions and its potential diagnostic value for differentiating malignant and benign effusions. Int J Cancer. 2009;125:1921–5.
24. Pass HI, Lott D, Lonardo F, Harbut M, Liu Z, Tang N, et al. Asbestos exposure, pleural mesothelioma, and serum osteopontin levels. N Engl J Med. 2005;353:1564–73.
25. Paleari L, Rotolo N, Imperatori A, Puzone R, Sessa F, Franzi F, et al. Osteopontin is not a specific marker in malignant pleural mesothelioma. Int J Biol Markers. 2009;24:112–7.
26. Park EK, Sandrini A, Yates DH, Creaney J, Robinson BW, Thomas PS, et al. Soluble mesothelin-related protein in an asbestos-exposed population: the dust diseases board cohort study. Am J Respir Crit Care Med. 2008;178:832–7.
27. Schneider J, Hoffmann H, Dienemann H, Herth FJ, Meister M, Muley T. Diagnostic and prognostic value of soluble mesothelin-related proteins in patients with malignant pleural mesothelioma in comparison with benign asbestosis and lung cancer. J Thorac Oncol. 2008;3:1317–24.
28. Zhou WB, Bai M, Jin Y. Diagnostic value of vascular endothelial growth factor and endostatin in malignant pleural effusions. Int J Tuberc Lung Dis. 2009;13:381–6.
29. Hooper C, Lee YC, Maskell N, BTS Pleural Guideline Group. Investigation of a unilateral pleural effusion in adults: British Thoracic Society pleural disease guideline 2010. Thorax. 2010;65(Suppl 2):ii4–17.
30. Whitaker D, Shilkin KB. Diagnosis of pleural malignant mesothelioma in life: a practical approach. J Pathol. 1984;143:147–75.
31. Maskell NA, Gleeson FV, Davies RJ. Standard pleural biopsy versus CT-guided cutting-needle biopsy for diagnosis of malignant disease in pleural effusions: a randomised controlled trial. Lancet. 2003;361:1326–30.
32. Diacon AH, Schuurmans MM, Theron J, Schubert PT, Wright CA, Bolliger CT. Safety and yield of ultrasound-assisted transthoracic biopsy performed by pulmonologists. Respiration. 2004;71:519–22.
33. Tombesi P, Nielsen I, Tassinari D, Trevisani L, Abbasciano V, Sartori S. Transthoracic ultrasonography-guided core needle biopsy of pleural-based lung lesions: prospective randomized comparison between a tru-cut-type needle and a modified menghini-type needle. Ultraschall Med. 2009;30:390–5.
34. Koegelenberg CF, Bolliger CT, Theron J, Walzl G, Wright CA, Louw M, et al. Direct comparison of the diagnostic yield of ultrasound-assisted abrams and tru-cut needle biopsies for pleural tuberculosis. Thorax. 2010;65:857–62.
35. Hallifax RJ, Haris M, Corcoran JP, Leyakathalikhan S, Brown E, Srikantharaja D, Manuel A, et al. Role of CT in assessing pleural malignancy prior to thoracoscopy. Thorax. 2015;70:192–3.
36. Dixon G, de Fonseka D, Maskell N. Pleural controversies: image guided biopsy vs. thoracoscopy for undiagnosed pleural effusions? J Thorac Dis. 2015;7(6):1041–51.
37. Rahman NM, Ali NJ, Brown G, et al. Local anaesthetic thoracoscopy: British Thoracic Society pleural disease guideline 2010. Thorax. 2010;65(Suppl 2):ii54–60.

38. Lee P, Colt HG. Pleuroscopy in 2013. Clin Chest Med. 2013;34:81–91.
39. Lee P, Colt HG. Rigid and semirigid pleuroscopy: the future is bright. Respirology. 2005;10:418–25.
40. Tassi G, Marchetti G. Minithoracoscopy: a less invasive approach to thoracoscopy- minimally invasive techniques. Chest. 2003;124:1975–7.
41. Chrysanthidis MG, Janssen JP. Autofluorescence videothoracoscopy in exudative pleural effusions: preliminary results. Eur Respir J. 2005;26:989–92.
42. Ishida A, Ishikawa F, Nakamura M, Miyazu YM, Mineshita M, Kurimoto N, et al. Narrow band imaging applied to pleuroscopy for the assessment of vascular patterns of the pleura. Respiration. 2009;78:432–9.
43. Baas P, Triesscheijn M, Burgers S, van Pel R, Stewart F, Aalders M. Fluorescence detection of pleural malignancies using 5-aminolaevulinic acid. Chest. 2006;129:718–24.
44. Lee P, Hsu A, Lo C, Colt HG. Prospective evaluation of flex-rigid pleuroscopy for indeterminate pleural effusion: accuracy, safety and outcome. Respirology. 2007;12:881–6.
45. Munavvar M, Khan MA, Edwards J, et al. The autoclavable semi-rigid thoracoscope: the way forward in pleural disease? Eur Respir J. 2007;29:571–4.
46. Agarwal R, Aggarwal AN, Gupta D. Diagnostic accuracy and safety of semirigid thoracoscopy in exudative pleural effusions: a meta-analysis. Chest. 2013;144:1857–67.
47. Janssen J, Boutin C. Extended thoracoscopy: a method to be used in case of pleural adhesions. Eur Respir J. 1992;5:763–6.
48. Macha HN, Reichle G, Von Zwehl D, et al. The role of ultrasound assisted thoracoscopy in the diagnosis of pleural disease. Clinical experience in 687 cases. Eur J Cardiothorac Surg. 1993;7:19–22.
49. Medford AR, Agrawal S, Bennett JA, et al. Thoracic ultrasound prior to medical thoracoscopy improves pleural access and predicts fibrous septation. Respirology. 2010;15:804–8.
50. Migliore M, Giuliano R, Aziz T, et al. Four-step local anesthesia and sedation for thoracoscopic diagnosis and management of pleural diseases. Chest. 2002;121:2032–5.
51. Tschopp JM, Purek L, Frey JG, et al. Titrated sedation with propofol for medical thoracoscopy: a feasibility and safety study. Respiration. 2011;82:451–7.
52. Grendelmeier P, Tamm M, Jahn K, Pflimlin E, Stolz D. Propofol versus midazolam in medical thoracoscopy: a randomized, noninferiority trial. Respiration. 2014;88:126–36.
53. Lee P, Colt HG. A spray catheter technique for pleural anesthesia: a novel method for pain control before talc poudrage. Anesth Analg. 2007;104:198–200.
54. DePew ZS, Wigle D, Mullon JJ, Nichols FC, Deschamps C, Maldonado F. Feasibility and safety of outpatient medical thoracoscopy at a large tertiary medical center: a collaborative medical-surgical initiative. Chest. 2014;146:398–405.
55. Rozman A, Camlek L, Marc-Malovrh M, Triller N, Kern I. Rigid versus semi-rigid thoracoscopy for the diagnosis of pleural disease: a randomized pilot study. Respirology. 2013;18:704–10.
56. Dhooria S, Singh N, Aggarwal AN, Gupta D, Agarwal R. A randomized trial comparing the diagnostic yield of rigid and semirigid thoracoscopy in undiagnosed pleural effusions. Respir Care. 2014;59:756–64.
57. Sasada S, Kawahara K, Kusunoki Y, et al. A new electrocautery pleural biopsy technique using an insulated-tip diathermic knife during semirigid pleuroscopy. Surg Endosc. 2009;23:1901–7.
58. Thomas R, Karunarathne S, Jennings B, Morey S, Chai SM, Lee YC, Phillips MJ. Pleuroscopic cryoprobe biopsies of the pleura: a feasibility and safety study. Respirology. 2015;20:327–32.
59. Roberts ME, Neville E, Berrisford RG, BTS Pleural Disease Guideline Group, et al. Management of a malignant pleural effusion: British Thoracic Society pleural disease guideline 2010. Thorax. 2010;65(Suppl 2):ii32–40.
60. Viskum K, Enk B. Complications of thoracoscopy. Poumon-Coeur. 1981;37:25–8.

61. Dresler CM, Olak J, Herndon JE, et al. Phase III intergroup study of talc poudrage vs talc slurry sclerosis for malignant pleural effusion. Chest. 2005;127:909–15.
62. Colt HG. Thoracoscopy: a prospective study of safety and outcome. Chest. 1995;108:324–9.
63. Boutin C, Rey F, Viallat JR. Prevention of malignant seeding after invasive diagnostic procedures in patients with pleural mesothelioma. A randomized trial of local radiotherapy. Chest. 1995;108:754–8.
64. Lee P, Folch E. Thoracoscopy: advances and increasing role for interventional pulmonologists. Semin Respir Crit Care Med. 2018;39:693–703.

Chapter 14
Pneumothorax: Large-Bore Tubes Vs. Pigtail Catheter

Robert F. Browning Jr, Philip Mullenix, Matthew Middendorf, Sean McKay, and J. Francis Turner, Jr.

Background

Pneumothorax as a condition was first recognized by fifteenth-century surgeon Sabuncuoglu. He described "mihceme" or cupping therapy as a treatment technique in which an incision in the chest wall was covered with a glass and a candle was then introduced to create a vacuum for aspiration [1]. The term was officially coined by Jean Marc Itard in 1803 and later described by Rene Laennec in 1819 as "an effusion of gaseous fluid into the cavity of the pleura." Although known for many centuries, the treatment of pneumothorax was not standardized until World War II [2]. Traditionally, large-bore chest tube with surgical insertion has been the standard for pneumothorax meeting the threshold for intervention especially in the emergency room or trauma setting. Over the past several decades, there has been a shift toward more minimally invasive approaches to the treatment of pneumothorax to include percutaneous and Seldinger insertion of smaller tubes with curved (pigtail) ends (as shown in Figs. 14.1 and 14.2) which are often more comfortable for the patient and easier to place for physicians used to these techniques [3]. Despite this shift in practice and evidence for smaller treatment tubes, the variance in the

R. F. Browning Jr (✉) · M. Middendorf · S. McKay
Interventional Pulmonology, Pulmonary and Critical Care Medicine Service,
Walter Reed National Military Medical Center, Bethesda, MD, USA

P. Mullenix
Department of Cardiothoracic Surgery, Walter Reed National Military Medical Center,
Bethesda, MD, USA

J. F. Turner, Jr.
Director of Interventional Pulmonology, Director of Pulmonary Rehabilitation, Pulmonary &
Critical Care Medicine, Wyoming Medical Center, Casper, Wyoming, USA

J. F. Turner, Jr. et al. (eds.), *From Thoracic Surgery to Interventional
Pulmonology*, Respiratory Medicine,
https://doi.org/10.1007/978-3-030-80298-1_14

spectrum of tube selection for pneumothorax still exists for several important reasons that we will review in this chapter [4].

Pathophysiology

In normal subjects, the pressure within the pleural space is negative throughout the respiratory cycle during quiet respiration and is generated by both the inward elastic recoil of the lungs and the inherent outward elastic force of the chest wall. The pleural pressure is negative in comparison to atmospheric pressure, and when a communication develops between an intrapulmonary airspace (e.g., alveolus) or chest wall and the pleural space (e.g., penetrating trauma), air will flow down its pressure gradient and into the pleural space until the pressure equalizes or the communication is sealed. As the pleural space begins to fill with air and the pressure rises, it can cause a shift of the mediastinum to the contralateral side, an enlarged hemithorax, and a depressed hemidiaphragm [5]. A feared complication of pneumothorax is tension pneumothorax and should be suspected in a patient who develops sudden cardiopulmonary deterioration in the setting of a known pneumothorax, or a condition known to predispose to pneumothorax. Tension physiology is created when more air enters the pleural space during inspiration than exits during expiration causing intrapleural pressure to exceed atmospheric pressure. This scenario is usually created under positive-pressure ventilation or in the spontaneously breathing patient if a one-way valve exists [6]. Although this scenario begins as a primary lung and respiratory event, physiologically this pneumothorax creates a primarily cardiovascular stress. With decreased venous return to the heart due to the pressure from pneumothorax, there is decreased RV filling resulting in decreased RV output and LV filling (plus bowing of the septum) resulting in a loss of preload/low cardiac output in a positive feedback loop (vicious cycle) that begets more hypotension and less cardiac output. Cardiovascular collapse ensues unless the pneumothorax is decompressed (Figs. 14.1 and 14.2).

Etiology

Pneumothorax can further be subdivided into spontaneous (primary and secondary) and traumatic (iatrogenic and non-iatrogenic) causes. Primary spontaneous pneumothorax (PSP) has an incidence of 18–28/100,000 cases per annum for men and 1.2–6/100,000 for women. It occurs in patients without apparent lung disease; however, subpleural bullae are found in >90% of patients on imaging or VATS [7]. Smoking may cause small airway inflammation and early emphysema-like changes and has been associated with a 12% risk of developing pneumothorax in healthy male smokers versus 0.1% in nonsmokers [8]. PSP is more common in taller, thin males and is thought to be secondary to the increased negative pleural pressure gradient and distending forces at the lung apex which predispose to bullae formation [7]. Recurrence rates are as high as 39% for PSP and typically recur within the first month to year. After the first recurrence, the lifetime risk of another recurrence exceeds 50% if no preventive measures are taken [9].

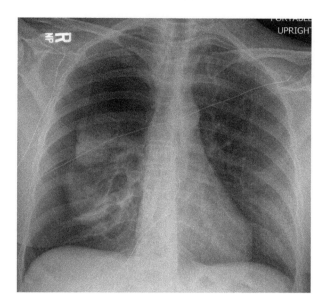

Fig. 14.1 Chest x-ray showing large right sided pneumothorax post CT guided transthoracic needle biopsy of a lung nodule

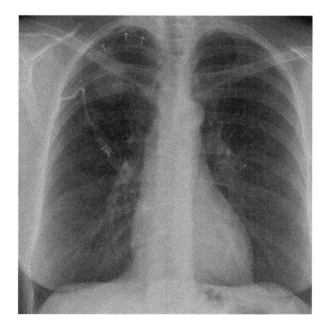

Fig. 14.2 Chest x-ray showing 10 Fr pigtail catheter placed in the anterior apical chest with near complete resolution of iatrogenic pneumothorax shown in the above figure

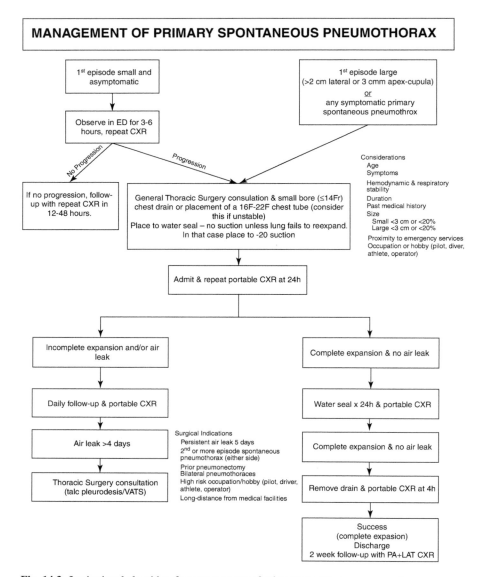

Fig. 14.3 Institutional algorithm for management of primary spontaneous pneumothorax

In general thoracic practice, video-assisted thoracoscopic surgery (VATS) is performed for any second episode or 5-day failure of the initial tube. The algorithm shown below (Fig. 14.3) highlights our institutional practice [10, 11]. In certain high-risk occupations such as pilots and divers, the first episode may be treated surgically as well.

Secondary spontaneous pneumothorax (SSP) has an incidence of 16.7/100,000 for men and 5.8/100,000 for women and is associated with underlying lung disease like COPD, cystic and interstitial lung diseases, connective tissue disease, cancers, and thoracic endometriosis in women [12]. In the eighteenth century, pulmonary tuberculosis was the most common cause of SSP in the developed world; however, currently, necrotizing bacterial pneumonias, *Pneumocystis jirovecii* pneumonia, as well as viral and fungal pneumonias are more common causes of SSP. SSP is more serious due to underlying lung disease and low pulmonary reserve and can be more difficult to manage. Recurrence rates for SSP are as high as 45% even if measures are taken to prevent recurrence. [10]

Traumatic pneumothorax can result from either penetrating or non-penetrating chest trauma in which air enters the pleural space directly through the chest wall or the visceral pleura through the tracheobronchial tree. Non-iatrogenic causes can include penetrating trauma (stab, gunshot wounds, etc.), blunt trauma such as rib fracture, or pulmonary barotraumas as seen in air travel and scuba diving. At altitude, air trapped in pleural blebs is exposed to lower atmospheric pressure and may expand causing rupture. Divers breathe compressed air at depth that re-expands on ascent and may cause barotrauma [13]. Transthoracic needle aspiration is the most common iatrogenic cause with an incidence of 25% and increases if the patient has COPD [14]. Other less common causes are mechanical ventilation, central venous cannulation, thoracentesis, and transbronchial lung biopsies. [14]

Pneumothorax Size and Intervention Considerations

CT scanning is considered the gold standard in the detection and size determination of pneumothorax and is helpful in identifying underlying causes for pneumothorax like bullae or emphysema. The 2010 British Thoracic Society guidelines use a cutoff of >2 cm between the lung margin and the inner chest wall at the level of the hilum in distinguishing between small and large pneumothoraces [7]. A 2 cm radiographic pneumothorax equates to an approximately 50% pneumothorax by lung volume and is used as the cutoff for intervention in a symptomatic patient. Two cm is a compromise between reducing the risk of needle trauma for intervention on a smaller pneumothorax and the significant length of time it may take for a larger pneumothorax to spontaneously resolve [15]. However, size of the pneumothorax is less important than symptoms and clinical status when determining an intervention. Patients with preexisting lung disease tolerate pneumothorax less well, and an effort should be made to evaluate for suspected primary spontaneous pneumothorax (PSP) versus secondary spontaneous pneumothorax (SSP) as this will influence management. Patients with small PSP without breathlessness and select asymptomatic patients with large PSP may be managed by observation alone. All patients with SSP should be admitted to the hospital for observation and most will need a small-bore chest drain. Regardless of the classification, any patient with significant breathlessness, bilateral pneumothoraces, or hemodynamic instability should undergo an intervention. Needle aspiration has shown similar initial success rates to large-bore chest drains in PSP (7); however, from a practical and inhospital management perspective, we generally employ small-bore chest drains in the management of pneumothorax if an intervention is warranted. All admitted patients should receive high-flow oxygen to correct hypoxia and aid in the resolution of pneumothorax [16].

In many trauma centers and within the military, traumatic pneumothoraces generally are treated with larger bore chest tube (concomitant injuries, possible need for air evacuation, possible development of hemothorax, presence of rib injuries, control of pleural space) because the patient may be on a ventilator for head injury, or about to go under general anesthesia for exploratory laparotomy or other surgeries. Smaller tubes have a risk of clogging with clot or debris and are often not trusted to maintain patency throughout the emergent surgeries. In the military and trauma setting, it is standard to place larger chest tubes even if the patient has no "symptoms." In our institutional practice, traumatic pneumothoraces that are small enough that they can only be visualized by CT scan only do not necessarily get chest tubes unless there is some other indication to place one (i.e., hemothorax, pleural effusion, etc.). In a combat environment, the chest tube in trauma threshold is even lower. Physical examination is relatively insensitive for the detection of a small pneumothorax generally, and nearly impossible in that noisy setting. Chest radiography in a trauma setting may similarly miss a small pneumothorax (and is not universally available). Even a small/clinically occult pneumothorax may become clinically significant during the medical evacuation flight. A chest tube is often placed for any patient pending air evacuation if there is a clinical suspicion that a pneumothorax may be present. If injury mechanism and/or physical examination suggests the possibility of a pneumothorax, a chest tube is generally placed because the potential negative consequences of symptomatic or tension pneumothorax during transport are significant.

Options for Pneumothorax Intervention Tube Selection

Medical chest tube catheter sizes are measured by French gauge (Fr). The measurement describes the outer diameter of the catheter. One Fr is equal to 1/3 mm, so a 3 Fr catheter has an outer circumference of 1 mm [17]. The typical options for chest tube size ranges from 6 Fr to 40 Fr size catheters. The definition of small versus large-bore chest tubes varies among studies, but generally accepted classification would include sizes 8 Fr–14 Fr as small bore and 28 Fr to 40 Fr as large bore with 16 Fr to 20 Fr considered small or large depending on the study [18].

In addition to tube size, the other major selection option is the choice between a straight tube and a "pigtail" or curved distal tip catheter (Fig. 14.4). The straight chest tubes tend to be the larger bore chest tubes (although not necessarily). These tubes are usually stiffer often due to their larger gauge. The curved pigtail catheters are straight when inserted with some type of inner stylet/trocar or cannula that allows for direction and easy insertion through the chest wall and then when in the

Fig. 14.4 Large bore 28 Fr straight chest tube (left) and small bore 10 Fr locking pigtail catheter (right)

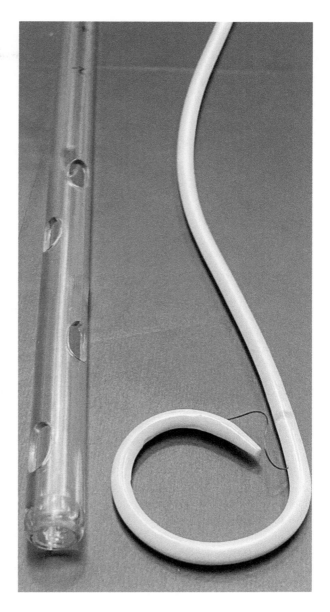

pleural space can be removed to regain the soft curved distal tip. This curve at the end can be "locked" or "unlocked." A locking catheter has an inner string attached to the distal tip that when pulled taught will secure the distal ring closed to keep the circular "pigtail" shape of the distal tip and prevent inadvertent migration out of the pleural space [19] (Fig. 14.5). Practically, the largest pigtail catheter is a 14 Fr catheter, so all pigtail chest tubes are small-bore tubes.

Fig. 14.5 Pleuroscopic image of 10 Fr locking pigtail catheter withdrawn to the chest wall. Note all fenestrations remain within the chest cavity and are prevented from migration outside the pleural space due to the ring formed by the pigtail and locked with the inner string

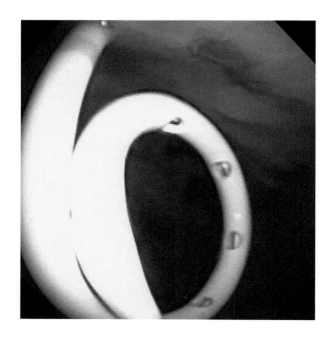

Insertion of the larger bore straight tube is most commonly performed using a surgical approach with scalpel and dissection through the chest wall. There are some commercially available straight tubes that can be inserted through a percutaneous approach and Seldinger technique with serial dilations to insert the tube, but the larger sizes require significant dilations, so more often these are only used with smaller bore straight tubes. The pigtail catheters are usually inserted using a guidewire or trocar. If a guidewire is used, dilators may be used in conjunction if the 10 Fr to 14 Fr catheters are placed.

The evidence for selecting the tube size for treatment of pneumothorax is limited. Extrapolation from similar literature with pleural effusions is reasonable as any pleural fluid will have a higher viscosity than the gas found in a pneumothorax. A 2018 meta-analysis of large (>14 Fr)-bore versus small (< or equal to 14 Fr)-bore chest tubes in treatment of malignant pleural effusion showed no difference in efficacy of pleurodesis and no difference in complications [20]. There is some evidence available specific to pneumothorax. Meta-analysis of large-bore chest tube versus small-bore pigtail catheters for treatment of pneumothorax by Chang and colleagues [2] published in 2018 found only two randomized controlled trials with a total of 62 patients enrolled with all other studies listed as retrospective cohorts. Conclusions of this meta-analysis found drainage duration and hospital stay were reduced with the pigtail catheter use, and in secondary pneumothorax, the complication rate was lower [2]. One of the studies supporting the efficacy of small-bore versus large-bore chest tubes was published in 2012 and showed in a cohort of 238 patients with pneumothorax no difference in efficacy of small vs. large chest tubes although in this study small size was defined as a straight 28–32 Fr versus large size as 36–40 Fr and was performed in a trauma setting. [21] More recently in 2020, a randomized controlled trial by Baumen et al. with 43 patients comparing 14 Fr pigtail catheter to 28–32 Fr chest tube in trauma patients with hemothorax and hemopneumothorax, the smaller pigtail catheters were found to be equally effective as the larger chest tubes demonstrating no clinical significance of the larger inner tube diameter even with fluid as viscous as blood is limited [22]. Despite common practice to place the tip of the tube or catheter in an apical anterior location, limited evidence that we have does not support this. In a 2017 paper from Riber et al., the retrospective review of 134 identified primary spontaneous pneumothorax cases treated with

Fig. 14.6 Chest x-ray showing large right sided hydropneumothorax

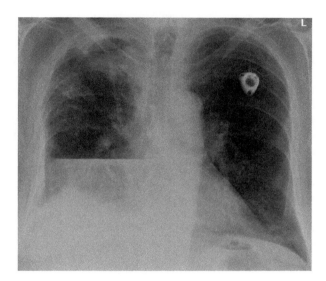

Fig. 14.7 Chest x-ray showing near complete resolution of hydropneumothorax with a basilar placed 12 Fr pigtail catheter

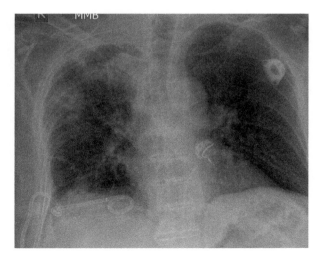

either a pigtail catheter (12–16 Fr) or a surgical chest tube (21–24 Fr) showed no difference in the location of the tube apical versus basal tip placement but did show a longer length of stay and increased patient discomfort in the surgical chest tube cohort [23]. In some cases, insertion in the basal chest is more easily performed when inserting into the fluid portion of a hydropneumothorax and is still effective in treating both the effusion (Figs. 14.6 and 14.7).

Decreased pain with smaller chest tube size is intuitive in theory, but the TIME1 study which is the largest study to date specifically compares pain control in 12 Fr versus 14 Fr chest tubes in malignant pleural effusions, and pain was statistically less in the 12 Fr group, but the difference did not meet the clinically significant level [24]. This study was in patients with malignant disease attempting to achieve pleurodesis which may confound the pain assessments though.

Understanding the etiology and extent of the air leak in a patient with pneumo-thorax can help guide the selection. If we use the analogy of a sink and drain with the pleural space being the sink and the drain being the tube you select to place into the space, it is simply understood that if the rate of air leak (faucet pouring into the sink) exceeds the capability of the tube to drain the contents, the sink will overflow. In the case of the closed pleural space, tension physiology will occur. Therefore, we must understand the degree and etiology of the air leak to choose the tube size and type appropriately. For a large air leak either from a large defect or from increased airflow from positive-pressure ventilation and possibly significant subcutaneous emphysema, a larger tube or additional tubes will be needed to keep up with the rate of accumulation in the chest (Figs. 14.8 and 14.9).

Additional considerations for a larger chest tube include the presence of a fluid or other debris in the pleural space that might occlude or limit the flow through the selected tube. Clot, tumor, and fibrinous debris can all partially or completely clog a tube and allow the rate of pneumothorax accumulation to outpace the rate of gas removal and tip the scales toward tension physiology and/or lung collapse. For this

Fig. 14.8 Chest x-ray showing extensive subcutaneous emphysema in a ventilated patient with a right pneumothorax and an apically placed right sided 14 Fr pigtail catheter

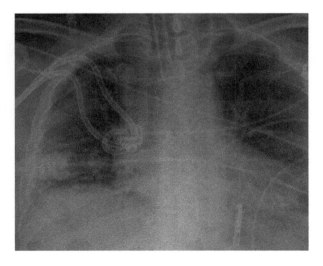

Fig. 14.9 Chest x-ray showing a second right sided 14 Fr pigtail catheter in the same patient shown in Fig. 14.8 with reduced subcutaneous emphysema and improved right sided lung volume

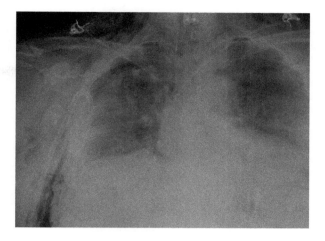

reason, a large-bore tube may better at confident evacuation of the space. So large-bore tube just to be safe is one approach, but the limited data does not support this, and practically speaking, a large tube can be more painful for the patient at insertion and while it is in place (20). For complicated pleural spaces with adhesions and loculations, the lung may be injured during insertion, and if not needed, smaller tubes are more comfortable for the patient and can work just as well. While comfort is increased with a small-bore chest tube or pigtail catheter, the smaller flexible tubing is more likely to experience kinking which will obstruct airflow and fluid drainage from the pleural space [20]. Clogging with fibrinous debris in the lumen of a small-bore chest tube may be managed with periodic flushing with sterile saline (every 6–12 hours) or with some thrombolytic dosing [25].

The traditional straight large-bore chest tube does have advantages. Due to the larger size, it has more rigidity and stiffness than a smaller tube especially the pigtail design. This can be helpful in directing the tube after insertion to a more apical and anterior position (usually the most common place for pneumothorax to accumulate in the chest in a patient that is upright or supine). This advantage is not always reliable though as it is often placed or migrates into the fissure or posteriorly. This migration may be true of any tube in the lung that is not fixed in a loculated space. This is why using the locked pigtail and inserting at a very apical and anterior position on the chest can allow the tube to be pulled back if it migrates to a low or posterior position without the risk of exposing the fenestrations outside the chest wall. In patients with pneumothorax and large air leak (i.e., on mechanical ventilation or a large bronchopleural fistula), multiple tubes or larger tubes may be required to evacuate pneumothorax [26]. For very rapidly reaccumulating pneumothoraces, multiple large-bore chest tubes may be required to prevent tension physiology. As noted above in combat and trauma, the added confidence in patency of a large-bore chest tube is often preferred. From the thoracic surgical perspective, large-bore chest tubes are the standard post-surgery to control the fluid, perhaps a lot of air, and because it is durable and will not kink (Fig. 14.10).

Fig. 14.10 Chest x-ray showing standard institutional post op chest tube management with a 28 Fr straight chest tube extending from the basilar lateral chest to the apex to remove air from the pleural space and a lower 24 Fr fluted flexible Blakemore drain placed on the diaphragm to remove residual fluid

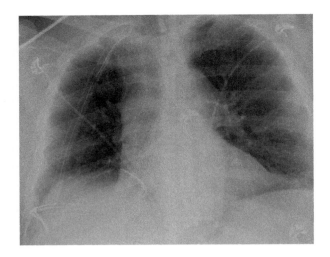

This provides confidence for control of space during postop rehabilitation. Besides these limited scenarios, both the evidence, guidelines, and changing practice patterns favor small-bore or pigtail catheter over the large-bore chest tubes. Even in complicated fluid/air collections like empyema or hydropenumo−/pyo-pneumothorax, the small-bore image-guided tubes (even if it is multiple pigtails for multiple collections) are preferred.

In practice, pneumothorax tube selection can be simplified using the guiding principles of choosing the smallest tube size with greatest patient comfort that has a reasonable likelihood of success in treating pneumothorax in the face of any complicating factors including etiology, combined effusion, hemothorax, trauma, positive-pressure ventilation, etc. In some cases, success will not be full re-expansion of the lung especially when there is abnormal lung parenchyma and/or pleura. A stable or loculated pneumothorax may be the best obtainable outcome in some patients, but ideally full pleural apposition for as much of the lung surface area as possible is the goal of any interventions.

References

1. Kaya SO, Karatepe M, Tok T, Onem G, Dursunoglu N, Goksin I. Were pneumothorax and its management known in 15th-century anatolia? Tex Heart Inst J. 2009;36(2):152–3.
2. De L'Auscultation Médiate. Ou Traité du diagnostic des maladies des Poumons et du Cœur, fondé principalement Sur ce nouveau Moyen d'Exploration. Edinb Med Surg J. 1822;18(72):447–74.
3. Martin K, Emil S, Zavalkoff S, Lo A, Ganey M, Baird R, Gaudreault J, Mandel R, Perreault T, Pharand A. Transitioning from stiff chest tubes to soft pleural catheters: prospective assessment of a practice change. Eur J Pediatr Surg. 2013;23(5):389–93. https://doi.org/10.1055/s-0033-1333641. Epub 2013 Feb 26. PMID: 23444073.
4. Havelock T, Teoh R, Laws D, Gleeson F, BTS Pleural Disease Guideline Group. Pleural procedures and thoracic ultrasound: British Thoracic Society pleural disease guideline 2010. Thorax. 2010;65(Suppl 2):ii61–76. https://doi.org/10.1136/thx.2010.137026. PMID: 20696688.b.

5. Light RW. Pleural diseases. 6th ed. Baltimore: Lippincott Williams & Wilkins; 2013.
6. Leigh-Smith S, Harris T. Tension pneumothorax--time for a re-think? Emerg Med J. 2005;22(1):8–16. https://doi.org/10.1136/emj.2003.010421. PMID: 15611534; PMCID: PMC1726546.
7. MacDuff A, Arnold A, Harvey J, BTS Pleural Disease Guideline Group. Management of spontaneous pneumothorax: British Thoracic Society pleural disease guideline 2010. Thorax. 2010;65(Suppl 2):ii18–31. https://doi.org/10.1136/thx.2010.136986.
8. Bense L, Eklund G, Wiman LG. Smoking and the increased risk of contracting spontaneous pneumothorax. Chest. 1987;92(6):1009–12. https://doi.org/10.1378/chest.92.6.1009.
9. Murray M, Jay A, Nadel (Hon), DLaw (Hon). Murray & Nadel's textbook of respiratory medicine Vol. 2. 6th ed. Philadelphia: Elsevier Saunders; 2015. p. 1439–66.
10. Baumann MH, et al. Management of spontaneous pneumothorax; an American College of Chest Physicians Delphi consensus statement. Chest. 2001;119:590–602.
11. Brunelli A, et al. Consensus definitions to promote and evidence-based approach to management of the pleural space. A collaborative proposal by ESTS, AATS, STS, and GTSC. Eur J Cardiothorac Surg. 2011;40:291–7.
12. Sahn SA, Heffner JE. Spontaneous pneumothorax. N Engl J Med. 2000;342(12):868–74.
13. Sharma A, Jindal P. Principles of diagnosis and management of traumatic pneumothorax. J Emerg Trauma Shock. 2008;1(1):34–41.
14. Vitulo P, Dore R, Cerveri I, Tinelli C, Cremaschi P. The role of functional respiratory tests in predicting pneumothorax during lung needle biopsy. Chest. 1996;109(3):612–5.
15. Baumann MH, Strange C, Heffner JE, et al. Management of spontaneous pneumothorax: an American College of Chest Physicians Delphi consensus statement. Chest. 2001;119(2):590–602.
16. Northfield TC. Oxygen therapy for spontaneous pneumothorax. Br Med J. 1971;4(5779):86–8.
17. Iserson KV. J.-F.-B. Charrière: the man behind the "French" gauge. J Emerg Med. 1987;5(6):545–8. https://doi.org/10.1016/0736-4679(87)90218-6. PMID: 3323304.
18. Chang SH, Kang YN, Chiu HY, Chiu YH. A systematic review and meta-analysis comparing pigtail catheter and chest tube as the initial treatment for pneumothorax. Chest. 2018;153(5):1201–12. https://doi.org/10.1016/j.chest.2018.01.048. Epub 2018 Feb 13. PMID: 29452099.
19. Porcel JM. Chest tube drainage of the pleural space: a concise review for pulmonologists. Tuberc Respir Dis (Seoul). 2018;81(2):106–15. https://doi.org/10.4046/trd.2017.0107. Epub 2018 Jan 24. PMID: 29372629; PMCID: PMC5874139.
20. Thethi I, Ramirez S, Shen W, Zhang D, Mohamad M, Kaphle U, Kheir F. Effect of chest tube size on pleurodesis efficacy in malignant pleural effusion: a meta-analysis of randomized controlled trials. J Thorac Dis. 2018;10(1):355–62. https://doi.org/10.21037/jtd.2017.11.134. PMID: 29600067; PMCID: PMC5863112.
21. Inaba K, Lustenberger T, Recinos G, Georgiou C, Velmahos GC, Brown C, Salim A, Demetriades D, Rhee P. Does size matter? A prospective analysis of 28-32 versus 36-40 French chest tube size in trauma. J Trauma Acute Care Surg. 2012;72(2):422–7. https://doi.org/10.1097/TA.0b013e3182452444. PMID: 22327984.
22. Bauman ZM, Kulvatunyou N, Joseph B, Gries L, O'Keeffe T, Tang AL, Rhee P. Randomized clinical trial of 14-French (14F) pigtail catheters versus 28-32F chest tubes in the management of patients with traumatic hemothorax and hemopneumothorax. World J Surg. 2021;45(3):880–6. https://doi.org/10.1007/s00268-020-05852-0. Epub 2021 Jan 7. PMID: 33415448; PMCID: PMC7790482.
23. Riber SS, Riber LP, Olesen WH, Licht PB. The influence of chest tube size and position in primary spontaneous pneumothorax. J Thorac Dis. 2017;9(2):327–32. https://doi.org/10.21037/jtd.2017.02.18. PMID: 28275481; PMCID: PMC5334075.
24. Rahman NM, Pepperell J, Rehal S, Saba T, Tang A, Ali N, West A, Hettiarachchi G, Mukherjee D, Samuel J, Bentley A, Dowson L, Miles J, Ryan CF, Yoneda KY, Chauhan A, Corcoran JP, Psallidas I, Wrightson JM, Hallifax R, Davies HE, Lee YC, Dobson M, Hedley EL, Seaton D, Russell N, Chapman M, McFadyen BM, Shaw RA, Davies RJ, Maskell NA, Nunn AJ, Miller RF. Effect of opioids vs NSAIDs and larger vs smaller chest tube size on pain control

and pleurodesis efficacy among patients with malignant pleural effusion: the TIME1 randomized clinical trial. JAMA. 2015;314(24):2641–53. https://doi.org/10.1001/jama.2015.16840. Erratum in: JAMA. 2016 Feb 16;315(7):707. Erratum in: JAMA. 2016 Apr 19;315(15):1661.

25. Bremer W, Ray CE Jr. A primer on the management of pleural effusions. Semin Intervent Radiol. 2018;35(5):486–91. https://doi.org/10.1055/s-0038-1676361. Epub 2019 Feb 5. PMID: 30728665; PMCID: PMC6363553.

26. Lin YC, Tu CY, Liang SJ, et al. Pigtail catheter for the management of pneumothorax in mechanically ventilated patients. Am J EmergMed. 2010;28:466–71.

Chapter 15
Pleurodesis: From Thoracic Surgery to Interventional Pulmonology

Maher Tabba and Kazuhiro Yasufuku

History

The concept of creating an attachment of the pleural layer to the chest wall after open thoracic surgery or acute chest trauma which is complicated by pneumothorax evolved after observing acute cardiopulmonary decompensation and increased mortality in animal experiments and patients. Several physicians contributed to the extensive work, mostly done in the 1800s, to understand the pathophysiology of this phenomenon. Quenu and Longuet are French physicians who presented a summary of all the works done in this area throughout the nineteenth century and adopted several methods to prevent this complication: (1) provoke adhesions by the application of irritants, (2) adhesions obtained by acupuncture or by trocars allowed to remain in situ, and (3) adhesions or, secondarily, after the pleura has been opened in order to anchor the lung to the chest wall obtained by suturing the pleural surfaces as a preliminary to operations. Multiple agents were utilized for this purpose such as aseptic foreign bodies in the pleura, ignipuncture with the thermo-cautery, electrolysis, and harpooning and transfixing the pleura and lung subcutaneously [2]. These procedures did not lead to a good outcome. Samuel Robinson (1914), an American thoracic surgeon, introduced pleurodesis as an important first step in a two-stage lobectomy for patients with bronchiectasis in the early twentieth century

M. Tabba (✉)
Division of Pulmonary and Critical Care and Sleep Medicine, Tufts Medical Center,
Boston, MA, USA
e-mail: MTabba@tuftsmedicalcenter.org

K. Yasufuku
Division of Thoracic Surgery, Toronto General Hospital, University Health Network,
University of Toronto, Toronto, ON, Canada
e-mail: kazuhiro.yasufuku@uhn.ca

to avoid pneumothorax after resecting the diseased lobe. The technique was modified by a Canadian surgeon, Norman Bethune (1935), who described the use of "pleural poudrage" with iodized talc for an improved outcome [3]. Significant changes took place post World War II with more attention devoted to patients with tuberculosis and the emergence of antibiotics [4].

The first actual pleurodesis was first performed more than 100 years ago by Lucius Spengler in 1901, when he described the use of the hypertonic solution of glucose with an unsuccessful result. In 1906, he described the use of 0.5% solution of silver nitrate in treating spontaneous pneumothorax [5–7]. Over time, the development of this procedure focused on finding the proper agent and achieved a higher success rate of pleurodesis. In 1939, two groups, Chandler at London Chest Hospital and Hennell and Steinberg at Mount Sinai Hospital in New York, described the use of oil of gomenol in olive oil in pleurodesis and reported good results [8–10]. Mechanical abrasion was first performed in 1941 by an American surgeon, Edward Delos Churchill [11]. Cer Movitt and others (1947) reviewed the value of several elements in pleurodesis, including blood, guaiacol, iodoform, and lipiodol, but none of them gave satisfactory results [12]. Brock (1948) described a series of patients with pneumothorax who underwent pleurodesis by using silver nitrate solution [13].

In the past century, multiple agents have been used in pleurodesis including talc, antibiotics, chemotherapy agents, radioactive materials, auto blood, cytokines, and bacteria and its products [14].

Indications

The two major indications for pleurodesis are recurrent and symptomatic pleural effusion (malignant or benign) and recurrent pneumothorax. The objective of the former is to alleviate the respiratory symptom (dyspnea), and the objective of the latter is to prevent the condition from relapsing.

Techniques

Pleurodesis can be achieved by many methods:

1. *Video-Assisted Thoracoscopy (VAT):* refers to a thoracic procedure performed in the operating room, under general anesthesia, and required single lung ventilation. Multiple instruments are needed for this procedure (Fig. 15.1). Three chest wall entry points are necessary to access the thoracic cavity. A VAT procedure helps in achieving a full diagnostic evaluation of the pleural cavity, obtaining parietal, visceral, or lung parenchymal biopsy, performing chemical or mechanical pleurodesis, and carrying out decortication and resection (wedge, lobectomy, or pneumonectomy) [15–17].

Fig. 15.1 Equipment
necessary for surgical
thoracotomy and video-
assisted thoracoscopy

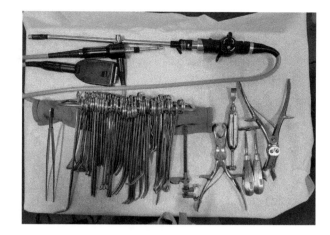

Fig. 15.2 Medical
thoracoscopy (MT) is
performed in endoscopy
suite

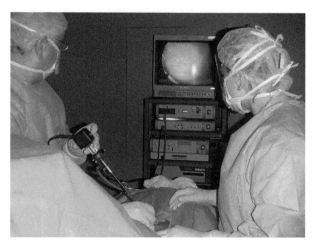

2. *Medical Pleuroscopy or Thoracoscopy (MT):* refers to a thoracoscopic procedure performed in the endoscopy suite or operating room. The procedure is routinely done under conscious sedation with local anesthetics (Fig. 15.2). Intubation
   is not required except in special circumstances related to the patient's condition.
   The equipment is usually simple and consists of rigid or semi-rigid pleuroscope,
   trocar, pleural biopsy forceps, and suction catheter. The procedure helps in performing diagnostic evaluation of the pleural cavity, especially in patients with
   exudative pleural effusion of unknown etiology, obtaining parietal pleural biopsy,
   accomplishing localized or complete pleurodesis, and guiding the placement of
   the indwelling pleural catheter or chest tube.
3. *Indwelling Pleural Catheter:* refers to a placement of 15.5 Fr and 66 cm long
   silicone rubber catheter with fenestrations along the proximal 24 cm. The distal
   end is provided with a valve to prevent the fluid or air from passing in either

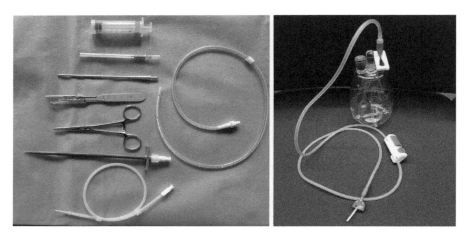

Fig. 15.3 Indwelling pleural catheter with vacuum bottle draining system

direction through the catheter, unless the catheter is attached to a comparable drainage line. The catheter is placed subcutaneously with the proximal end inserted inside the pleural cavity and the distal end kept externally, coiled and covered with a layer of gauze (Fig. 15.3). The pleural fluid is drained by inserting the access tip of the drainage line into the valve of the catheter, and then draining the fluid via an external tube into vacuum bottles. It received FDA approval in 1997 for recurrent and symptomatic malignant pleural effusion. It can be placed under conscious sedation and/or just local anesthesia.

4. *Chest Tube Slurry:* refers to administrating the sclerosing agent through the chest tube after optimizing the pleural fluid drainage (Fig. 15.4).

Pleurodesis Agents

An ideal sclerosing agent should have multiple important features including high molecular weight, steep dose-response curve, and few side effects [18]. There are multiple agents that have been used for pleurodesis for over ten decades, including biological irritants (autologic blood, dry killed *Corynebacterium parvum*, and OK-432) [19–22], chemical irritants such as cytostatic agents (bleomycin, mitoxantrone, nitrogen mustard, mitomycin C, and doxorubicin) [23–29], antiseptics (silver nitrate and iodopovidone) [30, 31], antibiotics (tetracycline and its derivative) [32–35], quinacrine [36], transforming growth factor-β (TGF-β) [37], radioactive colloidal gold [38], hypertonic glucose [39], essential oils, mineral (talc) [40, 41], thermal irritant (Nd-YAG laser or electrocautery) [42], mechanical (rough gauze) [43], or by placing a special draining indwelling tunneled catheter [44].

The choice of a sclerosing agent will be determined by the efficacy or success rate of the agent, accessibility, safety, ease of administration, number of administrations

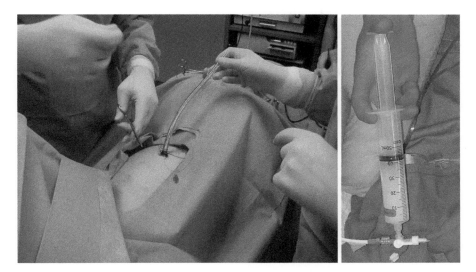

Fig. 15.4 Talc slurry pleurodesis is performed after inserting the chest tube and injecting the talc directly to the pleural cavity

to achieve complete and adequate anticipated response, and cost. Despite the evaluation of a wide variety of agents over a century, there is still no ideal sclerosing agent that exists to date.

Types of Pleurodesis Outcome

Defining the degree of successful pleurodesis varies in the literature. Multiple criteria were used to define this success including the degree of the clinical improvement, the amount of radiographic resolution of the pleural fluid, and the need for repeated thoracentesis within a variable period of time. In general, the success of a pleurodesis outcome has been categorized into three levels: (1) **Complete**, when the symptoms associated with the effusion and the radiographic signs of pleural effusion are resolved on the long term without recurrence; (2) **Partial**, when there is significant improvement in the symptoms without complete resolution accompanied by more than 50% decrease in the amount of the pleural fluid radiographically; and (3) **Failure**, when there is neither clinical improvement nor radiographic changes in the amount of pleural effusion [45].

In general, a successful pleurodesis should not be measured only by the resolving amount of pleural fluid but by no further effusion-related drainage procedure [46], symptomatic relief of dyspnea, improving the quality of life, and minimizing hospital admissions [47].

Mechanisms of Pleurodesis

Multiple mechanisms are involved in the pleurodesis process including stimulation of inflammatory reaction on the level of cytokines, disturbing the balance in the intrapleural coagulation cascade on the one hand and the fibrinogenesis and fibrinolysis on the other hand, and impeding intrapleural angiogenesis and angiostasis pathways [48].

The sclerosing agent typically stimulates the mesothelial cells to release a variety of mediators that stimulate multiple inflammatory pathways. These are interleukin-8 (IL-8), monocyte chemoattractant protein-1 (MCP-1), growth factors, vascular endothelial growth factor (VEGF), platelet-derived growth factor (PDGF), basic fibroblast growth factor (bFGF), transforming growth factor-β (TGF-β), and others [49, 50].

There is constant balance between the fibrinogenesis and fibrinolysis process in the pleura due to the continuous mesothelial cell substance release of tissue plasminogen activator (tPA) (anticoagulant factor) and plasminogen activator inhibitor-1 (PAI-1) (anticoagulant factors). Damaging the mesothelial cell will lead to the disruption of this balance and generates fibrosis [51]. Pleurodesis also favors proliferation of fibroblasts, collagen, and extracellular matrix component [52]. Finally, there is evidence that the vascular regulatory pathways are disrupted by the pleurodesis [53, 54].

In summary, all sclerosing agents lead to unspecific organizing fibrotic pleuritis which leads to.

pleural fibrosis and contributes to the pleurodesis.

Talc

Talc has been used in pleurodesis for over eight decades and considered the most used agent for that purpose (Fig. 15.5). It showed to be the most effective sclerosant available with success that can reach up to 70–100% and is associated with less pleural effusion recurrence [55]. It is also more effective than pleurectomy or mechanical pleural abrasion [56].

During preparation for medical use, the talc should be "graded" (processed into powder) and "calibrated" (filtered to remove small particles). Historically, talc was started to be purified after 1970 to remove asbestos particles. The mean particle size used in the United States is 10.8 μm, as compared to >30 μm in France and Taiwan [57]. Developing systemic inflammatory response (SIR) following intrapleural talc administration is a known side effect of talc pleurodesis. It may rarely progress to acute respiratory distress syndrome (ARDS). This response is typically related to using smaller particle size and higher talc dose during pleurodesis. The incidence of this side effect ranged from 0 to 15% of the patients undergoing talc pleurodesis

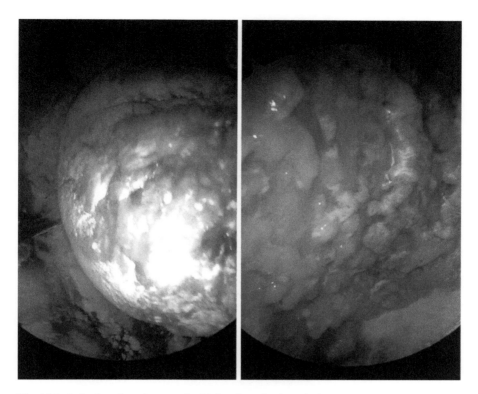

Fig. 15.5   *Left:* pleural carcinomatosis; *Right:* after talc pleurodesis

[58–60]. The most acceptable mechanism is the change in alveolar-capillary membrane permeability, dissemination of talc particles, and fast lymphatic absorption [61, 62]. Talc particles were found in the lung and almost all organs of affected patients [63, 64]. In one large study including patients with MPE, using large particle talc (MPS 24.5 μm) led to high level of efficacy and safety with zero incidence of ARDS [65].

The dose of the talc that appears to provide effective pleurodesis with low risk of ARDS is generally agreed among experts to be not more than 5 grams, instilled unilaterally, in a 70 kg adult, and in agreement with the American Thoracic Society 2000 consensus recommendations [66].

Talc can be delivered directly to the pleural cavity during thoracoscopy (Fig. 15.6) and can also be administrated through chest tube (slurry pleurodesis) or through the IPC (Figs. 15.2 and 15.7). The latter may achieve symptomatic improvement in 90% and pleurodesis in 42–60% of the patients [67]' [68]. A randomized study in patients with malignant pleural effusion showed a higher rate of successful pleurodesis in patients with IPC who received outpatient talc instillation 2 weeks later compared to placebo instillation [69].

Fig. 15.6 Talc delivery
system

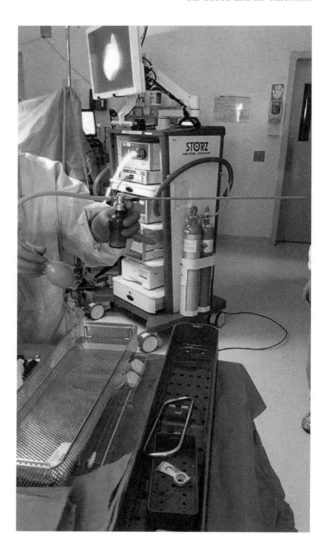

Fig. 15.7 Talc pleurodesis
followed by indwelling
pleural catheter placement

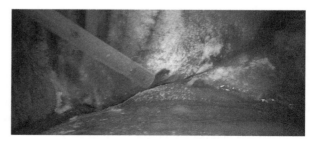

Finally, despite the fact that there are suggestions in the literature to link talc with female genital malignancies, there is no clear correlation to connect intrapleural talc instillation to mesothelioma, or any intra- or extrathoracic malignancy [70].

Indications for Pleurodesis

A-Malignant Pleural Effusion

Introduction

Malignant pleural effusion (MPE) is the most common indication to perform pleurodesis. Approximately >40,000 in the UK [71], >150,000 in the USA, and more than one million worldwide [72] patients have been affected annually. About 15% of patients with malignancy will initially present with MPE and 46% will develop MPE during the disease process [73]. Malignancy of the lung, breast, and lymphoma consists of 75% of the total MPEs [74]. The incidence of MPE in lung cancer patients varies from 7 to 23% [75]. Paramalignant pleural effusion might also occur in patients with malignancy but without pleural involvement confirmed with negative cytology or nondiagnostic thoracoscopy for cancer. It results from the pleural lymphatic obstruction from the mediastinal lymphadenopathy, lung atelectasis or collapse from endobronchial obstruction, trapped lung, pulmonary embolism, hypoalbuminemia, congestive heart failure, pericardial effusion, ascites, and others [76]. Almost half of the pleural effusions resulting from cancer are paramalignant effusion with lung and breast cancers as the leading etiologies [77]. Developing MPE reduced the life expectancy significantly in cancer patients and represents advanced disease stage [78]. The median survival time ranged between 3 and 12 months and it depends on the type of cancer. The shortest is lung cancer at about 3–4 months, breast cancer and cancer of unknown primary is intermediate with about 5–6 months, and the longest is ovarian cancer at around 15 months [79–82].

Multiple prognostic scores were validated to predict survival in patients with MPE. The most useful scores are:

(a) LENT (pleural fluid lactate dehydrogenase, Eastern Cooperative Oncology Group performance score, neutrophil-to-lymphocyte ratio, and tumor type). This is a risk stratification score which classified patients to low, intermediate, and high mortality risk and correlate with median survival of 319 days, 130 days, and 44 days, respectively [83].

(b) PROMISE score (hemoglobin, CRP, WBC, ECOG performance status, cancer type, pleural fluid TIMP1 concentration, prior chemo-/radiotherapy) is also a risk stratification system evaluating 17 biomarker candidates for survival and seven for pleurodesis [84].

Treatment consists of observation, frequent therapeutic aspiration, chest tube drainage, indwelling pleural catheter (IPC), pleurodesis, and combination of these therapeutic modalities [85].

Pleurodesis for MPE

1. Video-Assisted Thoracoscopy (VAT) for Pleurodesis.

For different reasons, not all patients with MPE are candidates for VAT pleurodesis. Poor respiratory condition with significant hypoxemia and hypercapnia, advanced cardiovascular diseases, and malnutrition are among the major conditions that put the patients at high risk for administrating anesthesia or undergoing surgical intervention. Thoracotomy and more popular VAT are very useful in performing direct evaluation of the pleural cavity, obtaining pleural biopsies, carrying out decortication and detaching the pleural adhesions to release the trapped portion of the lung, accomplishing poudrage pleurodesis, and placing chest tube or IPC under direct visualization. The success rate in achieving pleurodesis is over 90% for the patients. Among the failed cases, 29.5% were found to have trapped lung [86–89].

2. Medical Thoracoscopy (MT).

Medical pleuroscopy was described by a Swedish physician, Hans Christian Jacobaeus, who explored the pleural cavity of patients with TB and cutting adhesions using a cystoscope in 1910 [90]. This procedure has gained more popularity in the last two or three decades. The development of flexible bronchoscopy in the late 1960s encouraged using similar equipment for medical thoracoscopy [91]. The semiflexible thoracoscope was invented in 1998 which gave the operators better equipment to perform medical thoracoscopy and obtain pleural biopsy [92].

Compared with VAT procedure, MT requires simpler setup, less equipment, and limited working space. The procedure is typically more tolerated by the patients. Usually, there is no need for intubation or general anesthesia to perform the procedure and the recovery is quicker. The procedure is associated with fewer complications and it is more cost-effective. Technology development and inventing the semirigid pleuroscope helps in improving the procedural maneuvering to optimize the benefit of the procedure and increase the flexibility to inspect the entire pleura and improve the sampling capability [93]. The narrowband imaging device was added to the pleuroscope to add further ability to enhance blood vessels and distinguish benign from malignant or abnormal pleural surface [94]. Autofluorescence device was also added to the pleuroscope to increase the yield of detecting malignant pleural lesions [95].

Overall, the diagnostic yield of MT is 95% in patients with malignant pleural disease, with approximately 90% successful pleurodesis for patients with MPE and 95% for pneumothorax [96–99].

The increasing number of specialized pulmonologists in performing MT and the growing number of interventional pulmonology fellowship training programs help in promoting the utilization of this procedure and expanding the indications.

3. Chest Tube Slurry.

   It is performed by inserting the chest tube to drain the pleural effusion and then administrating the sclerosing agent. In meta-analysis to evaluate the efficacy and safety of chest tube size in the management of MPE, chest tubes <14Fr versus chest tube >14 Fr have similar successful pleurodesis of 73.8% vs. 82.0% and complication rate of 13.0% vs. 10.5%, respectively [100].

Poudrage Vs. Slurry Talc Pleurodesis

There are two methods to apply sclerosing agent on the pleura when performing pleurodesis: poudrage (direct application of the sclerosing agent on the pleural and the surface of the lung) or slurry (when the sclerosing agent is injected into the chest tube or indwelling pleural catheter). The success of either of these strategies over the other has been debatable. In studying 482 patients, both methods showed similar success during 30-day outcome [101]. In another study, 109 patients showed talc poudrage is more effective than talc slurry on the short term (87.5% vs. 73%) and long term (82% vs. 62%) follow-up [102]. In reviewing the randomized controlled trials published between 1980 and 2014 and comparing the two strategies, there was no difference in success rates of pleurodesis based on patient-centered outcomes between talc poudrage and talc slurry treatments. Respiratory complications are more common with talc poudrage via thoracoscopy [103].

The TAPPS (evaluating the efficacy of thoracoscopy and talc poudrage versus pleurodesis using talc slurry) trial studied 330 adults with a confirmed diagnosis of MPE found no significant difference in 90-day pleurodesis failure (the primary outcome) between poudrage and slurry, 22% vs. 24%, respectively. There was also no differences in the secondary outcomes which include 90-day hospital stay, all-cause mortality at 180 days, and cost-effectiveness [104]. In another randomized clinical trial studying 53 patients, they found no significant difference in hospital stay, chest tube drainage duration, analgesic requirement, or recurrence rates of effusion [105].

Mechanical Pleurodesis

Mechanical pleurodesis, which is performed with thoracotomy or thoracoscopy, involves mechanical irritation of the pleura or removal of parietal pleura. The mechanical irritation can be performed by using Nd:YAG laser, electrocautery, argon beam coagulation (APC), or rough gauze. All these techniques lead to the damage of the mesothelial layer and create pleurodesis. Recent studies showed the mesothelial cells inhibit the biological cascade of fibrinogenesis. Mechanical irritation of the pleura has been used mostly in patients with pneumothorax rather than with MPE (Figs. 15.8 and 15.9). The success rate is very good with low recurrence [106]. Mechanical and chemical thoracoscopic pleurodesis have an equal success rate >90% with the former having less perioperative complications and less chest tube drainage days [107].

Pleurectomy is used to be performed on patients with MPE when there is failure to control the effusion by tube drainage and instillation of chemical or radioactive agents, presence of trapped lung, and presence of malignant effusion at the time of thoracotomy for resection of an intrathoracic tumor [108]. The procedure is performed by VAT. It is usually successful in controlling the effusion but has high rate of morbidity and mortality, 10–19% [109–111]. The major complications of this procedure are empyema, bleeding, and cardiorespiratory failure. It was described more in the literature in patients with mesothelioma.

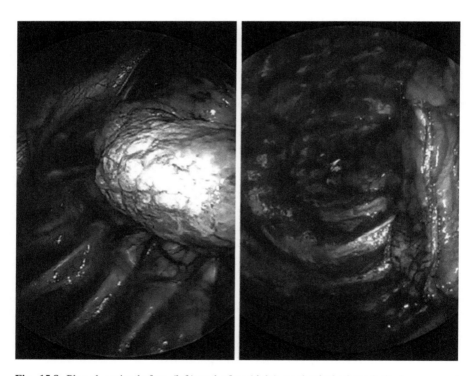

Fig. 15.8 Pleural cavity before (left) and after (right) mechanical pleurodesis for recurrent pneumothorax

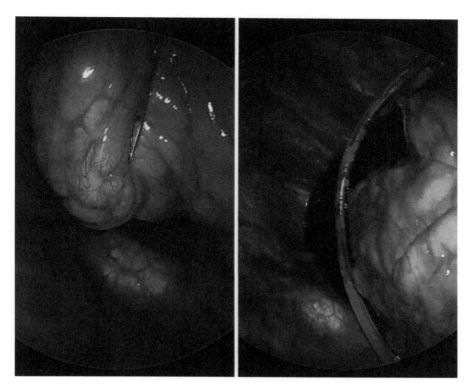

Fig. 15.9 Pleural cavity before (left) and after (right) mechanical pleurodesis followed by doxy-cycline application for recurrent pneumothorax

Pleuroperitoneal Pump

A pleuroperitoneal shunt is a subcutaneous pumping chamber which is inserted by VAT procedure with one end into the chest cavity and the other into the abdomen. The procedure has been suggested for patients with MPE with trapped lung when the pleural drainage or pleurodesis failed in expanding the lung [112–114]. The presence of ascites precludes insertion of these shunts. Draining the pleural fluid into the peritoneal cavity required several hundred manual pumps daily. Dyspnea is relived in the majority of the patients >95%. The complications rate is about 15% including catheter clotting, skin erosion, infection, catheter break, and malignancy seeding along the tract. The procedure became less popular because of the need for frequent fluid pumping and the catheter malfunction.

4. IPC for Malignant Pleural Effusion.

The major advantages of IPC placement in patient with malignant pleural effusion are symptomatic relief such as dyspnea or chest pain, shorter hospital stay, and improved quality of life [115]. IPC has been an easy and more practical procedure to perform and currently is considered the first-line therapy for patients with MPE to control the respiratory symptoms, create spontaneous pleurodesis, and prevent further fluid accumulation.

Despite the fact that pleurodesis is an indicator for cytology confirmed malignant effusion, it has been performed in patients with cytology-negative pleural effusion [116]. Evaluating patient for pleurodesis should include a trial of therapeutic thoracentesis, survival of more than 1–3 month(s), type of malignancy not responsive to chemotherapy, sufficient expandability of the lung, and adequate functional status unless it is performed for palliation purpose [117]. Performing large volume thoracentesis to evaluate for symptomatic relief and lung expandability is recommended as an initial step of the evaluation [118, 119]. Using pleural manometry to assess for this purpose does not usually have any advantage over the clinical symptomatic evaluation such as improvement in dyspnea or radiographic appearance before and after the thoracentesis [120]. IPC achieves spontaneous pleurodesis in 50–70% of the patients [121, 122]. Comparing patients who are being treated with chemotherapy versus no chemotherapy, there is no statistical significance in achieving spontaneous pleurodesis [123].

The mechanisms of pleurodesis in IPC are poorly understood. Most of the suggested mechanisms for autopleurodesis are due to inflammatory reactions produced by the presence of the foreign body (the catheter) in the pleural cavity and frequent fluid suctioning, which increase the probability for the catheter to rub the pleura on dry cavity [124, 125].

There are multiple factors that influence the success of IPC placement in achieving spontaneous pleurodesis include breast and gynecological malignancy, absence of the chest wall radiation, positive cytology, and non-trapped lung [126]. Also, daily drainage of pleural fluid is associated with a higher rate of autopleurodesis and a faster time to liberate the patient from the catheter [127]. There are multiple series that report the use of the IPC in patients with malignant pleural effusion and trapped lung with adequate symptomatic relief and satisfactory quality of life by applying high drainage frequency [128–131].

The IPC can also be used to install sclerosing agent such as talc to achieve a higher pleurodesis rate of 92% [132]. The rapid pleurodesis protocol was carried out by placing IPC in patients with MPE following medical pleuroscopy, and talc pleurodesis has achieved pleurodesis in 92% and within a short period of time (7.54 days) [133].

Complications are minimal and include pain, dislodgment, bleeding, infection, and mechanical failure [134]. IPC pleurodesis should not be considered in an asymptomatic patient, in patient with a small amount of pleural effusion, or in patients with chemotherapy- or radiation therapy-responsive tumor [135–137]. When there is no improvement in the patient's dyspnea despite large volume thoracentesis, the focus should be shifted to possible other consequences related to the malignancy such as lymphangitis carcinomatosis, endobronchial obstruction, trapped lung or concomitant medical conditions such as COPD, CHF, thromboembolic disease, malnutrition, general deconditioning, or others [138].

Silver Nitrate-Coated Indwelling Pleural Catheter (SNCIPC)

Drug-eluting indwelling pleural catheter with silver nitrate (sclerosing agent) has been studied and showed higher successful pleurodesis results [139]. The clinical trial SWIFT (Safety and Effectiveness of a New Pleural Catheter for Symptomatic, Recurrent, MPEs Versus Approved Pleural Catheter) is intended to assess the effectiveness of SNCIPC on the rate of autopleurodesis compared with uncoated IPCs [140].

Prediction of Successful Pleurodesis

Pleurodesis failure may be due to incomplete drainage of the pleural fluid, nonhomogeneous distribution of sclerosing agents in the pleural cavity, or trapped lung. The characteristics of the MPE may also predict pleurodesis failure. Multiple studies have shown that the low PH of the pleural fluid (<7.28) is typically predictive of pleurodesis failure, extensive pleural tumor burden, and short survival [141]. In other studies, female gender, good Karnofsky performance status, low pH, elevated cholesterol, and elevated adenosine deaminase level showed a significant association with the probability of pleurodesis success [142]. The meta-analyses of 34 studies involving 4626 patients have shown that pleurodesis success is associated with increased pleural fluid pH, smaller pleural effusion, full lung expandability, shorter duration of tube drainage, higher pleural fluid glucose, lower LDH, and lower pleural tumor burden [143].

In reviewing 155 patients with a 78% success rate from pleurodesis, the following factors were associated with incomplete and unsuccessful procedure: the presence of purulent adhesion, extensive spread of pleural lesions, systemic corticosteroid, and prolonged time period between the clinical diagnoses of the malignant pleural effusion and undergoing the pleurodesis [144].

Using transthoracic ultrasound in evaluating the pleural-lung interaction (sliding sign and pleural adherence score) has been found very useful when performing the pleurodesis and evaluating the success of the procedure. The pleural adherence score is calculated by adding together lung sliding scores (0 = present, 1 = questionable, 2 = absent) from nine lung zones within the treated hemithorax. A 24-hour score of 10 or more after the procedure has a sensitivity and specificity of 82% and 92% retrospectively for predicting pleurodesis success at 1 month [145, 146].

B-Pleurodesis in Refractory Benign (BPE) or Nonmalignant Pleural Effusion

IPC was used in reliving symptomatic large pleural effusion in nonmalignant pleural effusions. In a single-center retrospective observational study evaluating 54 patients with BPE, the most common etiology is CHF, liver disease complicated with cirrhosis, and renal failure. Other conditions leading to symptomatic pleural effusion were also included. In general there is symptomatic relief in >90% of the patients and pleurodesis was achieved in about 45%. Complications were 24% (CHF 16% and liver disease 37%) [147]. In another retrospective study comparing talc pleurodesis and IPC placement vs. IPC only, there was higher pleurodesis rate achieved in the former (80%) compared with the latter (25%). This success was associated with decrease hospitalization [148].

In a large clinical trial studying the IPC placement in patients with hepatic hydrothorax, pleurodesis was achieved in 28%, and median time for pleurodesis was 55 days. Complication rates were about 10% and 2.5% died secondary to catheter-related sepsis [149] .

Finally, in a systemic review and meta-analysis of 325 patients with recurrent benign pleural effusion including patients with CHF, liver cirrhosis, renal disease, yellow nail syndrome, chylothorax, empyema, and others, spontaneous pleurodesis was achieved in 42% of cardiac patients. In noncardiac patients, spontaneous pleurodesis was achieved in 61%. The analysis showed that IPC led to less hospital stays and admissions [150].

C-Pneumothorax

Pneumothorax refers to the presence of air in the pleural space. Primary spontaneous pneumothorax (PSP) occurs in patients with no underlying pulmonary disease. On the other hand, secondary spontaneous pneumothorax (SSP) occurs in patients with chronic lung condition. The incidence and the recurrence of SSP have been on the rise in the last 50 years [151, 152]. Risk factors associated with the recurrence include pulmonary fibrosis, emphysema, and advanced age [153, 154]. SSP is also associated with higher mortality than PSP [155].

The size and stage of pneumothorax are defined by the radiographic (preferably CT scan of the chest) and thoracoscopic appearance of the pleural cavity, respectively. In 1981, Vanderschueren defined four stages of pneumothorax based upon direct visualization of the pleural space: Stage I, lung endoscopically normal; Stage II, pleuro-pulmonary adhesions; Stage III, small bullae and blebs <2 cm in diameter; and Stage IV, large bullae >2 cm in diameter [156]. The risk of recurrence of ipsilateral or contralateral pneumothorax was significantly related to the presence of blebs or bullae, or both, on the high-resolution CT scan of the chest [157].

The British Thoracic Society (BTS) and the American College of Chest Physicians (ACCP) have published guidelines regarding the management of spontaneous and secondary pneumothorax [158, 159]. The goals of the treatment are to evacuate the air from the pleural cavity, repair the defect, and prevent recurrence by inducing pleurodesis. All patients should be admitted and provided with high oxygen supplement. A small size chest tube (<14Fr) should be inserted first. In comparing a variety of treatment methods, chest drainage with pleurodesis has much lower recurrence rate than chest drainage alone [160]. Thoracic surgical intervention to evaluate the pleural cavity and perform pleurodesis is the procedure of choice [161]. It allows for performing bullectomy, apical pleurectomy, or mechanical abrasion, and can be converted over to open thoracotomy if needed.

Overall, the surgical intervention to treat pneumothorax is controversial due to the lack of good prospective trials comparing various methods. The recent recommendations from the BTS suggest that a surgical opinion should be obtained for a second ipsilateral pneumothorax, first contralateral pneumothorax, synchronous bilateral spontaneous pneumothorax, persistent air leak (despite 5–7 days of chest tube drainage), failure of lung re-expansion, spontaneous hemothorax, pregnancy, and professionals at risk (e.g., pilots, divers) [162]. The ACCP guidelines recommend either surgical or medical pleurodesis is adequate [163].

Despite the fact that open thoracotomy provides less recurrence compared with VAT, the latter carries less complications such as operative and hospitalization time, bleeding, and chest pain [164]. In patients with Vanderschueren's stage III or IV blebs/bullae, VATS is the preferred modality of treatment over medical thoracoscopy because it allows for the ability to perform further surgical intervention such as bullectomy or apical pleurectomy if needed.

Contraindications

There are no absolute contraindications to perform thoracoscopy, IPC placement, or pleurodesis. There are multiple factors that should be taken into consideration to identify high-risk patients for the procedure and for the potential to develop serious complications. These factors are inability to tolerate the procedure, persistent and uncorrectable coagulopathy, inability of the lung to expand (trapped lung), complicated pleural cavity with multiple loculation, unstable respiratory status secondary to advanced pulmonary diseases such as interstitial lung disease, tracheal disease with inability to tolerate intubations, severe refractory cough, severe hypoxemia and hypercapnia, advanced cardiovascular disease, fever, cellulitis of the chest, and allergy to the medications used in the procedure [165–167].

Complications

IPC complication rate is less than 5% [168]. These include cellulitis, empyema, loculation, chest pain, and catheter blockage [169]. IPC fracture has been as high as 10% [170]. Catheter-related metastasis has been described and reported as high as 10% and occurs especially in patients with mesothelioma and adenocarcinoma. It can be recognized clinically as development of subcutaneous nodule near the IPC insertion site [171].

The complication rate in MT is 2–5% and the mortality rate is <0.1% [172]. There are multiple potential complications resulting from performing pleurodesis including chest pain, skin infection, empyema, subcutaneous emphysema, air leakage, persistent pneumothorax, bleeding, pulmonary embolism, oversedation, acute respiratory distress, and neoplastic invasion of the thoracoscopy tract [173].

Comparing video-assisted thoracoscopic surgery (VATS) and standard thoracostomy, complications were noticed in 3.3% of patients who underwent VAT pleurodesis vs. 15.0% in standard thoracostomy [174].

Cost

The coast of treating patient with MPE in order from the less to the most expensive procedure is repeated thoracentesis, IPC, bedside pleurodesis, and thoracoscopy. When measuring the incremental cost-effectiveness ratio (ICER) (estimated as the cost per quality-adjusted life-year gained over the patient's remaining lifetime), IPC is the preferred treatment for patients with malignant pleural effusion and limited survival. Bedside pleurodesis is the most cost-effective treatment for patients with more prolonged expected survival [175]. In primary spontaneous pneumothorax, thoracoscopic talc pleurodesis under local anesthesia is more cost-effective and superior to conservative treatment by inserting a chest tube and allowing for drainage [176, 177].

Future

Pleurodesis has been playing an important role in treating patients with MPE regardless of the methods of application of the sclerosing agent (chest tube, IPC, or thoracoscopy). Many concomitant conditions may contribute to the etiology of the pleural effusion in patients with malignancy besides cancer such as congestive heart failure, malnutrition, hypoalbuminemia, pulmonary atelectasis, trap lung, thromboembolic disease, or others. Careful evaluation and optimizing the management of the reversible elements of the pleural effusion is crucial before proceeding with further chest drainage and pleurodesis.

The management plan for MPE should be customized according to the clinical condition of the patient, factors predicting outcome, and available therapeutic interventions. IPC is the most practical intervention in treating patients with MPE. It proves its efficacy and low complication rates. It can be managed mostly in the outpatient setting. Medical thoracoscopy (MT) is a highly effective modality in performing pleurodesis. It can be done for diagnostic and therapeutic purpose at the same time. Over the past two decades, it has gained a great deal of attention and popularity compared with VAT especially after the growth of interventional pulmonology field [178], increase in educational courses, advancement in technology to develop better operating equipment, and widespread use of ultrasonography which facilitates a safer procedure [179–181]. It also allows more physicians to provide this service in areas where there is no sufficient number of thoracic surgeons to provide the necessary procedures. Finally, the cost of the infrastructure (procedure location, equipment, and supporting staff) for MT is much more affordable than the VAT.

Acknowledgments I would like to acknowledge and thank the following physicians for providing pictures included in this chapter: John Beamis, MD; Antonio Lassaletta, MD; Adnan Majid, MD; Erik Folch, MD; Anjan Devaraj, MD; and Daniel Ospina Delgado.

References

1. Light RW. Pleural effusions related to metastatic malignancies. In: Light RW, Light RW, Pleural diseases. 4th. Philadelphia: Lippincott, Williams and Wilkins; 2001. p. 121–124.
2. Matas RI. On the Management of Acute Traumatic Pneumothorax. Ann Surg. 1899;29(4):409.
3. Bethune N. Pleural poudrage: new technique for deliberate production of pleural adhesions as preliminary to lobectomy. J Thorac Surg. 1935;4(1):251–61.
4. Astoul P, Tassi G, Tschopp JM. Thoracoscopy for pulmonologists. Berlin: Springer; 2016. p. 12–3.
5. Spengler L. Zur chirurgie des pneumothorax. Laupp; 1906.
6. Hennell H, Steinberg MF. Tense pneumothorax: treatment of chronic and recurrent forms by induction of chemical pleuritis. Arch Intern Med. 1939;63(4):648–63.
7. Maxwell J. The production of pleural adhesions by kaolin injection. Thorax. 1954;9(1):10.
8. Hetherington LH, Spencer GE. Treatment of recurrent spontaneous pneumothorax with Gomenol. Dis Chest. 1947;13(6):652–7.
9. Chandler FG. Valvular pneumothorax treated by mechanical valve and obliterative pleurisy. Lancet. 1939;234(6055):638–40.
10. Hennell H, Steinberg MF. Tense pneumothorax: treatment of chronic and recurrent forms by induction of chemical pleuritis. Arch Intern Med. 1939;63(4):648–63.
11. Tyson MD, Crandall WB. The surgical treatment of recurrent idiopathic spontaneous pneumothorax. J Thorac Surg. 1941;10:566–70.
12. Movitt CE, Smith JV, Elosser L. Treatment of spontaneous pneumothorax. Chest J. 1947;13(3):221–36.
13. Brock RC. Recurrent and chronic spontaneous pneumothorax. Thorax. 1948;3(2):88–111.
14. Mierzejewski M, Korczynski P, Krenke R, Janssen JP. Chemical pleurodesis—a review of mechanisms involved in pleural space obliteration. Respir Res. 2019;20(1):1–6.
15. Colt HG. Thoracoscopy: window to the pleural space. Chest. 1999;116(5):1409–15.

16. Moisiuc FV, Colt HG. Thoracoscopy: origins revisited. Respiration. 2007;74(3):344–55.
17. McKenna RJ Jr. Thoracoscopic evaluation and treatment of pulmonary disease. Surg Clin North Am. 2002;80:1543–53.
18. Roberts ME, Neville E, Berrisford RG, Antunes G, Ali NJ. Management of a malignant pleural effusion: British Thoracic Society pleural disease guideline 2010. Thorax. 2010;65(Suppl 2):ii32–40.
19. Keeratichananont W, Limthon T, Keeratichananont S. Efficacy and safety profile of autologous blood versus tetracycline pleurodesis for malignant pleural effusion. Ther Adv Respir Dis. 2015;9(2):42–8.
20. Rahman NM, Davies HE, Salzberg M, Truog P, Midgely R, Kerr D, Clelland C, Hedley EL, Lee YG, Davies RJ. Use of lipoteichoic acid-T for pleurodesis in malignant pleural effusion: a phase I toxicity and dose-escalation study. Lancet Oncol. 2008;9(10):946–52.
21. Felletti RA, Ravazzoni CE. Intrapleural Corynebacterium parvum for malignant pleural effusions. Thorax. 1983;38(1):22–4.
22. Antony VB, Nasreen N, Mohammed KA, Sriram PS, Frank W, Schoenfeld N, Loddenkemper R. Talc pleurodesis: basic fibroblast growth factor mediates pleural fibrosis. Chest. 2004;126(5):1522–8.
23. Luhr KT, Yang PC, Kuo SH, Chang DB, Yu CJ, Lee LN. Comparison of OK-432 and mitomycin C pleurodesis for malignant pleural effusion caused by lung cancer. A Randomized Trial Cancer. 1992;69(3):674–9.
24. Lynch T, Kalish L, Mentzer S, Decamp M, Strauss G, Sugarbaker D. Optimal therapy of malignant pleural effusions. Int J Oncol. 1995;8(1):183–90.
25. Marchi E, Vargas FS, Teixeira LR, Fagundes DJ, Silva LM, Carmo AO, Light RW. Comparison of nitrogen mustard, cytarabine and dacarbazine as pleural sclerosing agents in rabbits. Eur Respir J. 1997;10(3):598–602.
26. Kishi K, Homma S, Sakamoto S, Kawabata M, Tsuboi E, Nakata K, Yoshimura K. Efficacious pleurodesis with OK-432 and doxorubicin against malignant pleural effusions. Eur Respir J. 2004;24(2):263–6.
27. Jones JM, Olman EA, Egorin MJ, Aisner J. A case report and description of the pharmacokinetic behavior of intrapleurally instilled etoposide. Cancer Chemother Pharmacol. 1985;14(2):172–4.
28. Barbetakis N, Antoniadis T, Tsilikas C. Results of chemical pleurodesis with mitoxantrone in malignant pleural effusion from breast cancer. World J Surg Oncol. 2004;2(1):16.
29. Mark JB, Goldenberg IS, Montague AC. Intrapleural mechlorethamine hydrochloride therapy for malignant pleural effusion. JAMA. 1964;187(11):858–60.
30. Bucknor A, Harrison-Phipps K, Davies T, Toufektzian L. Is silver nitrate an effective means of pleurodesis? Interact Cardiovasc Thorac Surg. 2015;21(4):521–5.
31. Caglayan B, Torun E, Turan D, Fidan A, Gemici C, Sarac G, Salepci B, Kiral N. Efficacy of iodopovidone pleurodesis and comparison of small-bore catheter versus large-bore chest tube. Ann Surg Oncol. 2008;15(9):2594–9.
32. Tabatabaei SA, Hashemi SM, Kamali A. Silver nitrate versus tetracycline in pleurodesis for malignant pleural effusions; a prospective randomized trial. Adv Biomed Res. 2015;4.
33. Balassoulis G, Sichletidis L, Spyratos D, Chloros D, Zarogoulidis K, Kontakiotis T, Bagalas V, Porpodis K, Manika K, Patakas D. Efficacy and safety of erythromycin as sclerosing agent in patients with recurrent malignant pleural effusion. Am J Clin Oncol. 2008;31(4):384–9.
34. Chen JS, Chan WK, Yang PC. Intrapleural minocycline pleurodesis for the treatment of primary spontaneous pneumothorax. Curr Opin Pulm Med. 2014;20(4):371–6.
35. Salomaa ER, Pulkki K, Helenius H. Pleurodesis with doxycycline or Corynebacterium parvum in malignant pleural effusion. Acta Oncol. 1995;34(1):117–21.
36. Mierzejewski M, Korczynski P, Krenke R, Janssen JP. Chemical pleurodesis–a review of mechanisms involved in pleural space obliteration. Respir Res. 2019;20(1):1–6.
37. Light RW, Lane K, Cheng DS, Rogers J. A single intrapleural injection of transforming growth factor beta (tgf [beta]) induces an excellent pleurodesis in rabbits. Chest. 1999;116(4):269S.

38. Botsford TW. Experiences with radioactive colloidal gold in the treatment of pleural effusion caused by metastatic cancer of the breast. N Engl J Med. 1964;270(11):552–5.
39. Lai Y, Zheng X, Yuan Y, Xie TP, Zhao YF, Zhu ZJ, Hu Y. A modified pleurodesis in treating postoperative chylothorax. Ann Translat Med. 2019;7(20).
40. Feller-Kopman DJ, Reddy CB, DeCamp MM, Diekemper RL, Gould MK, Henry T, Iyer NP, Lee YG, Lewis SZ, Maskell NA, Rahman NM. Management of malignant pleural effusions. An official ATS/STS/STR clinical practice guideline. Am J Respir Crit Care Med. 2018;198(7):839–49.
41. Weissberg D, Ben-Zeev I. Talc pleurodesis: experience with 360 patients. J Thorac Cardiovasc Surg. 1993;106(4):689–95.
42. Torre M, Grassi M, Nerli FP, Maioli M, Belloni PA. Nd-YAG laser Pleurodesis via Thoracoscopy: Nd-YAG laser Pleurodesis via Thoracoscopy. Chest. 1994;106(2):338–41.
43. Youmans CR Jr, Williams RD, McMinn MR, Derrick JR. Surgical management of spontaneous pneumothorax by bleb ligation and pleural dry sponge abrasion. Am J Surg. 1970;120(5):644–8.
44. Tremblay A, Michaud G. Single-center experience with 250 tunnelled pleural catheter insertions for malignant pleural effusion. Chest. 2006;129(2):362–8.
45. Rafei H, Jabak S, Mina A, Tfayli A. Pleurodesis in malignant pleural effusions: outcome and predictors of success. Integr Cancer Sci Therap. 2015;2:216–21.
46. Suzuki K, Servais EL, Rizk NP, Solomon SB, Sima CS, Park BJ, Kachala SS, Zlobinsky M, Rusch VW, Adusumilli PS. Palliation and pleurodesis in malignant pleural effusion: the role for tunneled pleural catheters. J Thorac Oncol. 2011;6(4):762–7.
47. Lee YG, Fysh ET. Indwelling pleural catheter: changing the paradigm of malignant effusion management. J Thorac Oncol. 2011;6(4):655–7.
48. Mierzejewski M, Korczynski P, Krenke R, Janssen JP. Chemical pleurodesis–a review of mechanisms involved in pleural space obliteration. Respir Res. 2019;20(1):1–6.
49. Schwarz Y, Star A. Role of talc modulation on cytokine activation in cancer patients undergoing pleurodesis. Pulmonary Med. 2012;1:2012.
50. Idell S, Zwieb C, Kumar A, Koenig KB, Johnson AR. Pathways of fibrin turnover of human pleural mesothelial cells in vitro. Am J Respir Cell Mol Biol. 1992;7(4):414–26.
51. Light RW. Pleural diseases, vol. 50. 5th ed. Lippincott Williams & Wilkins; 2007.
52. Hurewitz AN, Lidonicci K, Wu CL, Reim D, Zucker S. Histologic changes of doxycycline pleurodesis in rabbits: effect of concentration and pH. Chest. 1994;106(4):1241–5.
53. Felbor U, Dreier L, Bryant RA, Ploegh HL, Olsen BR, Mothes W. Secreted cathepsin L generates endostatin from collagen XVIII. EMBO J. 2000;19(6):1187–94.
54. Shichiri M, Hirata Y. Antiangiogenesis signals by endostatin. FASEB J. 2001;15(6):1044–53.
55. Roberts ME, Neville E, Berrisford RG, Antunes G, Ali NJ. Management of a malignant pleural effusion: British Thoracic Society pleural disease guideline 2010. Thorax. 2010;65(Suppl 2):ii32–40.
56. Sepehripour AH, Nasir A, Shah R. Does mechanical pleurodesis result in better outcomes than chemical pleurodesis for recurrent primary spontaneous pneumothorax? Interact Cardiovasc Thorac Surg. 2012;14(3):307–11.
57. Ferrer J, Villarino MA, Tura JM, Traveria A, Light RW. Talc preparations used for pleurodesis vary markedly from one preparation to another. Chest. 2001;119(6):1901–5.
58. Shinno Y, Kage H, Chino H, Inaba A, Arakawa S, Noguchi S, Amano Y, Yamauchi Y, Tanaka G, Nagase T. Old age and underlying interstitial abnormalities are risk factors for development of ARDS after pleurodesis using limited amount of large particle size talc. Respirology. 2018;23(1):55–9.
59. Rehse DH, Aye RW, Florence MG. Respiratory failure following talc pleurodesis. Am J Surg. 1999;177(5):437–40.
60. Cardillo G, Facciolo F, Carbone L, Regal M, Corzani F, Ricci A, Di Martino M, Martelli M. Long-term follow-up of video-assisted talc pleurodesis in malignant recurrent pleural effusions. Eur J Cardiothorac Surg. 2002;21(2):302–6.

61. Baiu I, Yevudza E, Shrager JB. Talc pleurodesis: a medical, medicolegal, and socioeconomic review. Ann Thorac Surg. 2020;109(4):1294–301.
62. Shinno Y, Kage H, Chino H, Inaba A, Arakawa S, Noguchi S, Amano Y, Yamauchi Y, Tanaka G, Nagase T. Old age and underlying interstitial abnormalities are risk factors for development of ARDS after pleurodesis using limited amount of large particle size talc. Respirology. 2018;23(1):55–9.
63. Bouchama A, Chastre J, Gaudichet A, Soler P, Gibert C. Acute pneumonitis with bilateral pleural effusion after talc pleurodesis. Chest. 1984;86(5):795–7.
64. Milanez Campos JR, WEREBE C, Vargas FS, Jatene FB, Light RW. Respiratory failure due to insufflated talc. Lancet (British edition). 1997;349(9047):251–2.
65. Janssen JP, Collier G, Astoul P, Tassi GF, Noppen M, Rodriguez-Panadero F, Loddenkemper R, Herth FJ, Gasparini S, Marquette CH, Becke B. Safety of pleurodesis with talc poudrage in malignant pleural effusion: a prospective cohort study. Lancet. 2007;369(9572):1535–9.
66. THIS OFFICIAL STATEMENT OF THE AMERICAN THORACIC SOCIETY WAS ADOPTED BY THE ATS BOARD OF DIRECTORS. Management of malignant pleural effusions. Am J Respira Crit Care Med. 2000;162(5):1987–2001.
67. Myers R, Michaud G. Tunneled pleural catheters. Clin Chest Med. 2013;34(1):73–80.
68. Van Meter ME, McKee KY, Kohlwes RJ. Efficacy and safety of tunneled pleural catheters in adults with malignant pleural effusions: a systematic review. J Gen Intern Med. 2011;26(1):70–6.
69. Bhatnagar R, Keenan EK, Morley AJ, Kahan BC, Stanton AE, Haris M, Harrison RN, Mustafa RA, Bishop LJ, Ahmed L, West A. Outpatient talc administration by indwelling pleural catheter for malignant effusion. N Engl J Med. 2018;378(14):1313–22.
70. Baiu I, Yevudza E, Shrager JB. Talc pleurodesis: a medical, medicolegal, and socioeconomic review. Ann Thorac Surg. 2020;109(4):1294–301.
71. Egan AM, McPhillips D, Sarkar S, Breen DP. Malignant pleural effusion. QJM. 2013:hct245.
72. Penz ED, Mishra EK, Davies HE, Manns BJ, Miller RF, Rahman NM. Comparing cost of indwelling pleural catheter vs talc pleurodesis for malignant pleural effusion. Chest J. 2014;146(4):991–1000.
73. Antony VB, Loddenkemper R, Astoul P, BOUTIN C, GOLDSTRAW P. Management of malignant pleural effusions. Am J Respir Crit Care Med. 2000;162(5):1987–2001.
74. Light RW. Approach to the patient. In: Light RW, Light RW, editors. Pleural diseases. 5th ed. Philadelphia: Lippincott, Williams and Wilkins; 2011. p. 111–2.
75. Froudarakis ME. Pleural effusion in lung cancer: more questions than answers. Respiration. 2012;83(5):367–76.
76. Gonlugur TE, Gonlugur U. Transudates in malignancy: still a role for pleural fluid. Ann Acad Med Singap. 2008;37(9):760–3.
77. Gurung P, Goldblatt MR, Huggins JT, Doelken P, Sahn SA. Pleural fluid characteristics of paramalignant effusion. Chest J. 2009;(4_MeetingAbstracts):136, 44S–c.
78. Chernow B, Sahn SA. Carcinomatous involvement of the pleura: an analysis of 96 patients. Am J Med. 1977;63(5):695–702.
79. Abbruzzese JL, Abbruzzese MC, Hess KR, Raber MN, Lenzi R, Frost P. Unknown primary carcinoma: natural history and prognostic factors in 657 consecutive patients. J Clin Oncol. 1994;12(6):1272–80.
80. Van de Molengraft FJ, Vooijs GP. Survival of patients with malignancy-associated effusions. Acta Cytol. 1988;33(6):911–6.
81. Sears D, Hajdu SI. The cytologic diagnosis of malignant neoplasms in pleural and peritoneal effusions. Acta Cytol. 1986;31(2):85–97.
82. Bonnefoi H, Smith IE. How should cancer presenting as a malignant pleural effusion be managed? Br J Cancer. 1996;74(5):832.
83. Clive AO, Kahan BC, Hooper CE, Bhatnagar R, Morley AJ, Zahan-Evans N, Bintcliffe OJ, Boshuizen RC, Fysh ET, Tobin CL, Medford AR. Predicting survival in malignant

pleural effusion: development and validation of the LENT prognostic score. Thorax. 2014;69(12):1098–104.

84. Psallidas I, Kanellakis NI, Gerry S, Thézénas ML, Charles PD, Samsonova A, Schiller HB, Fischer R, Asciak R, Hallifax RJ, Mercer R. Development and validation of response markers to predict survival and pleurodesis success in patients with malignant pleural effusion (PROMISE): a multicohort analysis. Lancet Oncol. 2018;19(7):930–9.

85. Roberts ME, Neville E, Berrisford RG, Antunes G, Ali NJ. Management of a malignant pleural effusion: British Thoracic Society pleural disease guideline 2010. Thorax. 2010;65(Suppl 2):ii32–40.

86. Fitzgerald DB, Koegelenberg CF, Yasufuku K, Lee YG. Surgical and non-surgical management of malignant pleural effusions. Expert Rev Respir Med. 2018;12(1):15–26.

87. Cardillo G, Facciolo F, Carbone L, Regal M, Corzani F, Ricci A, Di Martino M, Martelli M. Long-term follow-up of video-assisted talc pleurodesis in malignant recurrent pleural effusions. Eur J Cardiothorac Surg. 2002;21(2):302–6.

88. de Campos JR, Cardoso P, Vargas FS, de Campos WE, Teixeira LR, Jatene FB, Light RW. Thoracoscopy talc poudrage: a 15-year experience. Chest. 2001;119(3):801–6.

89. Alihodzic-Pasalic A, Maric V, Hadzismailovic A, Pilav A, Grbic K. Comparison of efficiency of pleurodesis between video assisted thoracoscopic surgery (VATS) and standard thoracostomy. Acta Informatica Medica. 2018;26(3):185.

90. Tassi GF, Tschopp JM. The centenary of medical thoracoscopy.

91. Senno A, Moallem S, Quijano ER, Adeyemo A, Clauss RH. Thoracoscopy with the fiberoptic bronchoscope: a simple method in diagnosing pleuropulmonary diseases. J Thorac Cardiovasc Surg. 1974;67(4):606–11.

92. Davidson AC, George RJ, Sheldon CD, Sinha G, Corrin B, Geddes DM. Thoracoscopy: assessment of a physician service and comparison of a flexible bronchoscope used as a thoracoscope with a rigid thoracoscope. Thorax. 1988;43(4):327–32.

93. Davidson AC, George RJ, Sheldon CD, Sinha G, Corrin B, Geddes DM. Thoracoscopy: assessment of a physician service and comparison of a flexible bronchoscope used as a thoracoscope with a rigid thoracoscope. Thorax. 1988;43(4):327–32.

94. Ishida A, Ishikawa F, Nakamura M, Miyazu YM, Mineshita M, Kurimoto N, Koike J, Nishisaka T, Miyazawa T, Astoul P. Narrow band imaging applied to pleuroscopy for the assessment of vascular patterns of the pleura. Respiration. 2009;78(4):432–9.

95. Chrysanthidis MG, Janssen JP. Autofluorescence videothoracoscopy in exudative pleural effusions: preliminary results. Eur Respir J. 2005;26(6):989–92.

96. de Campos JR, Cardoso P, Vargas FS, de Campos WE, Teixeira LR, Jatene FB, Light RW. Thoracoscopy talc poudrage: a 15-year experience. Chest. 2001;119(3):801–6.

97. Froudarakis ME. New challenges in medical thoracoscopy. Respiration. 2011;82(2):197–200.

98. Reddy C, Ernst A, Lamb C, Feller-Kopman D. Rapid pleurodesis for malignant pleural effusions: a pilot study. Chest. 2011;139(6):1419–23.

99. Chen J, Li Z, Xu N, Zhang X, Wang Y, Lin D. Efficacy of medical thoracoscopic talc pleurodesis in malignant pleural effusion caused by different types of tumors and different pathological classifications of lung cancer. Int J Clin Exp Med. 2015;8(10):18945.

100. Thethi I, Ramirez S, Shen W, Zhang D, Mohamad M, Kaphle U, Kheir F. Effect of chest tube size on pleurodesis efficacy in malignant pleural effusion: a meta-analysis of randomized controlled trials. J Thorac Dis. 2018;10(1):355.

101. Dresler CM, Olak J, Herndon JE, Richards WG, Scalzetti E, Fleishman SB, Kernstine KH, Demmy T, Jablons DM, Kohman L, Daniel TM. Phase III intergroup study of talc poudrage vs talc slurry sclerosis for malignant pleural effusion. Chest J. 2005;127(3):909–15.

102. Stefani A, Natali P, Casali C, Morandi U. Talc poudrage versus talc slurry in the treatment of malignant pleural effusion. A prospective comparative study. Eur J Cardiothorac Surg. 2006;30(6):827–32.

103. Mummadi S, Kumbam A, Hahn PY. Malignant pleural effusions and the role of talc poudrage and talc slurry: a systematic review and meta-analysis. F1000Res. 2014;3.
104. Bhatnagar R, Luengo-Fernandez R, Kahan BC, Rahman NM, Miller RF, Maskell NA. Thoracoscopy and talc poudrage compared with intercostal drainage and talc slurry infusion to manage malignant pleural effusion: the TAPPS RCT. Health Technol Assessment (Winchester, England). 2020;24(26):1.
105. Yim AP, Chan AT, Tak WL, Wan IY, Ho JK. Thoracoscopic talc insufflation versus talc slurry for symptomatic malignant pleural effusion. Ann Thorac Surg. 1996;62(6):1655–8.
106. Maier A, Anegg U, Renner H, Tomaselli F, Fell B, Lunzer R, Sankin O, Pinter H, Friehs GB, Smolle-Jüttner FM. Four-year experience with pleural abrasion using a rotating brush during video-assisted thoracoscopy. Surg Endosc. 2000;14(1):75–8.
107. Crnjac A, Sok M, Kamenik M. Impact of pleural effusion pH on the efficacy of thoracoscopic mechanical pleurodesis in patients with breast carcinoma. Eur J Cardio-Thoracic Surg. 2004;26(2):432–6.
108. Martini N, Bains MS, Beattie EJ. Indications for pleurectomy in malignant effusion. Cancer. 1975;35(3):734–8.
109. Fry WA, Khandekar JD. Parietal pleurectomy for malignant pleural effusion. Ann Surg Oncol. 1995;2(2):160–4.
110. Fry WA, Khandekar JD. Parietal pleurectomy for malignant pleural effusion. Ann Surg Oncol. 1995;2(2):160–4.
111. Bernard A, de Dompsure RB, Hagry O, Favre JP. Early and late mortality after pleurodesis for malignant pleural effusion. Ann Thorac Surg. 2002;74(1):213–7.
112. Wong PS, Goldstraw P. Pleuroperitoneal shunts. Br J Hosp Med. 1993;50(1):16.
113. Grossi F, Pennucci MC, Tixi L, Cafferata MA, Ardizzoni A. Management of malignant pleural effusions. Drugs. 1998;55(1):47–58.
114. Genc O, Petrou M, Ladas G, Goldstraw P. The long-term morbidity of pleuroperitoneal shunts in the management of recurrent malignant effusions. Eur J Cardiothorac Surg. 2000;18(2):143–6.
115. Sudharshan S, Ferraris VA, Mullett T, Ramaiah C. Effectiveness of tunneled pleural catheter placement in patients with malignant pleural effusions. Int J Angiol. 2011;20(01):039–42.
116. Doelken P. Management of pleural effusion in the cancer patient. In: Seminars in respiratory and critical care medicine. Vol. 31, no. 06. © Thieme Medical Publishers; 2010. p. 734–42.
117. Feller-Kopman DJ, Reddy CB, DeCamp MM, Diekemper RL, Gould MK, Henry T, Iyer NP, Lee YG, Lewis SZ, Maskell NA, Rahman NM. Management of malignant pleural effusions. An official ATS/STS/STR clinical practice guideline. Am J Respir Crit Care Med. 2018;198(7):839–49.
118. Roberts ME, Neville E, Berrisford RG, Antunes G, Ali NJ. Management of a malignant pleural effusion: British Thoracic Society pleural disease guideline 2010. Thorax. 2010;65(Suppl 2):ii32–40.
119. Walker S, Mercer R, Maskell N, Rahman NM. Malignant pleural effusion management: keeping the flood gates shut. Lancet Respir Med. 2019.
120. Lentz RJ, Lerner AD, Pannu JK, Merrick CM, Roller L, Walston C, Valenti S, Goddard T, Chen H, Huggins JT, Rickman OB. Routine monitoring with pleural manometry during therapeutic large-volume thoracentesis to prevent pleural-pressure-related complications: a multicentre, single-blind randomised controlled trial. Lancet Respir Med. 2019;7(5):447–55.
121. Tremblay A, Michaud G. Single-center experience with 250 tunnelled pleural catheter insertions for malignant pleural effusion. Chest J. 2006;129(2):362–8.
122. Tremblay A, Mason C, Michaud G. Use of tunnelled catheters for malignant pleural effusions in patients fit for pleurodesis. Eur Respir J. 2007;30(4):759.
123. Sivakumar P, West A, Hak CC, Noorzad F, Ahmed L. Late-Breaking Abstract: spontaneous pleurodesis rates in chemotherapy and non-chemotherapy patients undergoing indwelling pleural catheter insertion for malignant pleural effusion.

124. Fortin M, Tremblay A. Pleural controversies: indwelling pleural catheter vs. pleurodesis for malignant pleural effusions. J Thorac Dis. 2015;7(6):1052–7.
125. Chalhoub M, Harris K, Castellano M, Maroun R, Bourjeily G. The use of the PleurX catheter in the management of non-malignant pleural effusions. Chron Respir Dis. 2011;8(3):185–91.
126. Warren WH, Kim AW, Liptay MJ. Identification of clinical factors predicting Pleurx® catheter removal in patients treated for malignant pleural effusion. Eur J Cardiothorac Surg. 2008;33(1):89–94.
127. Wahidi MM, Reddy C, Yarmus L, Feller-Kopman D, Musani A, Shepherd RW, Lee H, Bechara R, Lamb C, Shofer S, Mahmood K. Randomized trial of pleural fluid drainage frequency in patients with malignant pleural effusions. The ASAP trial. Am J Respir Crit Care Med. 2017;195(8):1050–7.
128. Bertolaccini L, Viti A, Terzi A. Management of malignant pleural effusions in patients with trapped lung with indwelling pleural catheter: how to do it. J Visualiz Surg. 2016;2.
129. Efthymiou CA, Masudi T, Charles Thorpe JA, Papagiannopoulos K. Malignant pleural effusion in the presence of trapped lung. Five-year experience of PleurX tunnelled catheters. Interact Cardiovasc Thorac Surg. 2009;9(6):961–4.
130. Qureshi RA, Collinson SL, Powell RJ, Froeschle PO, Berrisford RG. Management of malignant pleural effusion associated with trapped lung syndrome. Asian Cardiovascular Thoracic Annals. 2008;16(2):120–3.
131. Miller CR, Chrissian AA, Lee YG, Rahman NM, Wahidi MM, Tremblay A, Hsia DW, Almeida FA, Shojaee S, Mudambi L, Belanger AR. AABIP evidence-informed guidelines and expert panel report for the management of indwelling pleural catheters. J Bronchol Intervent Pulmonol. 2020.
132. Ahmed L, Ip H, Rao D, Patel N, Noorzad F. Talc pleurodesis through indwelling pleural catheters for malignant pleural effusions: retrospective case series of a novel clinical pathway. Chest J. 2014;146(6):e190–4.
133. Reddy C, Ernst A, Lamb C, Feller-Kopman D. Rapid pleurodesis for malignant pleural effusions: a pilot study. Chest. 2011;139(6):1419–23.
134. Bhatnagar R, Maskell NA. Indwelling pleural catheters. Respiration. 2014;88(1):74–85.
135. Burgers JA, Kunst PW, Koolen MG, Willems LN, Burgers JS, van den Heuvel M. Pleural drainage and pleurodesis: implementation of guidelines in four hospitals. Eur Respir J. 2008;32(5):1321–7.
136. Lee P, Colt HG. State of the art: pleuroscopy. J Thorac Oncol. 2007;2(7):663–70.
137. Feller-Kopman DJ, Reddy CB, DeCamp MM, Diekemper RL, Gould MK, Henry T, Iyer NP, Lee YG, Lewis SZ, Maskell NA, Rahman NM. Management of malignant pleural effusions. An official ATS/STS/STR clinical practice guideline. Am J Respir Crit Care Med. 2018;198(7):839–49.
138. Lee P, Colt HG. State of the art: pleuroscopy. J Thorac Oncol. 2007;2(7):663–70.
139. Bhatnagar R, Zahan-Evans N, Kearney C, Edey AJ, Stadon LJ, Tremblay A, Maskell NA. A novel drug-eluting indwelling pleural catheter for the management of malignant effusions. Am J Respir Crit Care Med. 2018;197(1):136–8.
140. ClinicalTrials.gov. Identifier: NCT02649894.
141. Heffner JE, Nietert PJ, Barbieri C. Pleural fluid pH as a predictor of survival for patients with malignant pleural effusions. Chest. 2000;117(1):79–86.
142. Yildirim H, Metintas M, Ak G, Metintas S, Erginel S. Predictors of talc pleurodesis outcome in patients with malignant pleural effusions. Lung Cancer. 2008;62(1):139–44.
143. Hassan M, Gadallah M, Mercer RM, Harriss E, Rahman NM. Predictors of outcome of pleurodesis in patients with malignant pleural effusion: a systematic review and meta-analysis. Expert Rev Respir Med. 2020:1–0.
144. Leemans J, Dooms C, Ninane V, Yserbyt J. Success rate of medical thoracoscopy and talc pleurodesis in malignant pleurisy: a single-Centre experience. Respirology. 2018;23(6):613–7.

145. Corcoran JP, Hallifax RJ, Mercer RM, Yousuf A, Asciak R, Hassan M, Piotrowska HE, Psallidas I, Rahman NM. Thoracic ultrasound as an early predictor of pleurodesis success in malignant pleural effusion. Chest. 2018;154(5):1115–20.
146. Shafiq M, Feller-Kopman D. Management of Malignant Pleural Effusions. Clin Chest Med. 2020;41(2):259–67.
147. Frost N, Ruwwe-Glösenkamp C, Raspe M, Brünger M, Temmesfeld-Wollbrück B, Suttorp N, Witzenrath M. Indwelling pleural catheters for non-malignant pleural effusions: report on a single centre's 10 years of experience. BMJ Open Respir Res. 2020;1:7(1).
148. Majid A, Kheir F, Fashjian M, Chatterji S, Fernandez-Bussy S, Ochoa S, Cheng G, Folch E. Tunneled pleural catheter placement with and without talc poudrage for treatment of pleural effusions due to congestive heart failure. Ann Am Thorac Soc. 2016;13(2):212–6.
149. Shojaee S, Rahman N, Haas K, Kern R, Leise M, Alnijoumi M, Lamb C, Majid A, Akulian J, Maldonado F, Lee H. Indwelling tunneled pleural catheters for refractory hepatic hydrothorax in patients with cirrhosis: a multicenter study. Chest. 2019;155(3):546–53.
150. Patil M, Dhillon SS, Attwood K, Saoud M, Alraiyes AH, Harris K. Management of benign pleural effusions using indwelling pleural catheters: a systematic review and meta-analysis. Chest. 2017;151(3):626–35.
151. Hallifax RJ, Goldacre R, Landray MJ, Rahman NM, Goldacre MJ. Trends in the incidence and recurrence of inpatient-treated spontaneous pneumothorax, 1968-2016. JAMA. 2018;320(14):1471–80.
152. Hallifax RJ, Yousuf A, Jones HE, Corcoran JP, Psallidas I, Rahman NM. Effectiveness of chemical pleurodesis in spontaneous pneumothorax recurrence prevention: a systematic review. Thorax. 2017;72(12):1121–31.
153. Lippert HL, Lund O, Blegvad S, Larsen HV. Independent risk factors for cumulative recurrence rate after first spontaneous pneumothorax. Eur Respir J. 1991;4(3):324–31.
154. Videm V, Pillgram-Larsen J, Ellingsen O, Andersen G, Ovrum E. Spontaneous pneumothorax in chronic obstructive pulmonary disease: complications, treatment and recurrences. Eur J Respir Dis. 1987;71(5):365–71.
155. Gupta D, Hansell A, Nichols T, Duong T, Ayres JG, Strachan D. Epidemiology of pneumothorax in England. Thorax. 2000;55(8):666–71.
156. Vanderschueren RG. Pleural talcage in patients with spontaneous pneumothorax (author's transl). Poumon Coeur. 1981;37(4):273–6.
157. Casali C, Stefani A, Ligabue G, Natali P, Aramini B, Torricelli P, Morandi U. Role of blebs and bullae detected by high-resolution computed tomography and recurrent spontaneous pneumothorax. Ann Thorac Surg. 2013;95(1):249–55.
158. Baumann MH, Strange C, Heffner JE, Light R, Kirby TJ, Klein J, Luketich JD, Panacek EA, Sahn SA. Management of spontaneous pneumothorax: an American College of Chest Physicians Delphi consensus statement. Chest. 2001;119(2):590–602.
159. MacDuff A, Arnold A, Harvey J. BTS pleural disease guideline group. Management of spontaneous pneumothorax: British Thoracic Society pleural disease guideline 2010. Thorax. 2010;65(Suppl 2):ii18–31.
160. Almind ME, Lange PE, Viskum KA. Spontaneous pneumothorax: comparison of simple drainage, talc pleurodesis, and tetracycline pleurodesis. Thorax. 1989;44(8):627–30.
161. MacDuff A, Arnold A, Harvey J. Management of spontaneous pneumothorax: British Thoracic Society pleural disease guideline 2010. Thorax. 2010;65(Suppl 2):ii18–31.
162. MacDuff A, Arnold A, Harvey J. Management of spontaneous pneumothorax: British Thoracic Society pleural disease guideline 2010. Thorax. 2010;65(Suppl 2):ii18–31.
163. Baumann MH, Strange C, Heffner JE, Light R, Kirby TJ, Klein J, Luketich JD, Panacek EA, Sahn SA. Management of spontaneous pneumothorax: an American College of Chest Physicians Delphi consensus statement. Chest. 2001;119(2):590–602.
164. Waller DA, Forty J, Morritt GN. Video-assisted thoracoscopic surgery versus thoracotomy for spontaneous pneumothorax. Ann Thorac Surg. 1994;58(2):372–7.

165. Mierzejewski M, Korczynski P, Krenke R, Janssen JP. Chemical pleurodesis–a review of mechanisms involved in pleural space obliteration. Respir Res. 2019;20(1):1–6.
166. Lee P, Folch E. Thoracoscopy: advances and increasing role for interventional pulmonologists. In: Seminars in espiratory and critical care medicine (Vol. 39, no. 06). Thieme Medical Publishers; 2018. p. 693–703.
167. Lamb C, Li A, Thakkar D, Lee P. Pleurodesis. In: Seminars in respiratory and critical care medicine (Vol. 40, no. 03). Thieme Medical Publishers; 2019. p. 375–85.
168. Fysh ET, Wrightson JM, Lee YG, Rahman NM. Fractured indwelling pleural catheters. Chest. 2012;141(4):1090–4.
169. Chalhoub M, Saqib A, Castellano M. Indwelling pleural catheters: complications and management strategies. J Thorac Dis. 2018;10(7):4659.
170. Fysh ET, Wrightson JM, Lee YG, Rahman NM. Fractured indwelling pleural catheters. Chest. 2012;141(4):1090–4.
171. Thomas R, Budgeon CA, Kuok YJ, Read C, Fysh ET, Bydder S, Lee YG. Catheter tract metastasis associated with indwelling pleural catheters. Chest. 2014;146(3):557–62.
172. Michaud G, Berkowitz DM, Ernst A. Pleuroscopy for diagnosis and therapy for pleural effusions. Chest. 2010;138(5):1242–6.
173. Rodríguez-Panadero F. Medical thoracoscopy. Respiration. 2008;76(4):363–72.
174. Alihodzic-Pasalic A, Maric V, Hadzismailovic A, Pilav A, Grbic K. Comparison of efficiency of pleurodesis between video assisted thoracoscopic surgery (VATS) and standard thoracostomy. Acta Informatica Medica. 2018;26(3):185.
175. Puri V, Pyrdeck TL, Crabtree TD, Kreisel D, Krupnick AS, Colditz GA, Patterson GA, Meyers BF. Treatment of malignant pleural effusion: a cost-effectiveness analysis. Ann Thorac Surg. 2012;94(2):374–80.
176. Tschopp JM, Boutin C, Astoul P, Janssen JP, Grandin S, Bolliger CT, Delaunois L, Driesen P, Tassi G, Perruchoud AP. Talcage by medical thoracoscopy for primary spontaneous pneumothorax is more cost-effective than drainage: a randomised study. Eur Respir J. 2002;20(4):1003–9.
177. Torresini G, Vaccarili M, Divisi D, Crisci R. Is video-assisted thoracic surgery justified at first spontaneous pneumothorax? Eur J Cardiothorac Surg. 2001;20(1):42–5.
178. Tassi GF, Davies RJ, Noppen M. Advanced techniques in medical thoracoscopy. Eur Respir J. 2006;28(5):1051–9.
179. Bridevaux PO, Tschopp JM, Cardillo G, Marquette C, Noppen M, Astoul P, Driesen P, Diacon AH, Froudarakis ME, Janssen JP. Safety of large-particle talc pleurodesis after talc poudrage under thoracoscopy for primary spontaneous pneumothorax. A European multicentre prospective study. In: Swiss medical weekly (Vol. 139, no. 13–14). Farnsburgerstr 8, Ch-4132 Muttenz, Switzerland: EMH Swiss Medical Publishers LTD; 2009. p. 2S.
180. Lee P, Colt HG. Rigid and semirigid pleuroscopy: the future is bright. Respirology. 2005;10(4):418–25.
181. Chrysanthidis MG, Janssen JP. Autofluorescence videothoracoscopy in exudative pleural effusions: preliminary results. Eur Respir J. 2005;26(6):989–92.

Index